TRAUMA AND LIFE STORIES

Traumatic experiences and their consequences are often the core of life stories told by survivors of natural disasters, war or other kinds of violence. In this volume leading academics explore the relationship between the experiences of terror and helplessness that have caused trauma, the ways in which survivors remember, and the representation of these memories in the language and form of their life stories.

International case studies include accounts of:

- the migration journal of Ethiopian Jews to Israel
- the life stories of Guatemalan war widows
- violence in South Africa
- persecution of political prisoners in South Africa and the former Czechoslovakia
- war in the Malvinas
- lynching in the Mississippi Flats
- resistance in Zimbabwe's liberation war
- sexual abuse
- the Irish Troubles.

The volume reveals the complexity of remembering and forgetting traumatic experiences, and shows that survivors are likely to express themselves in stories containing elements which are imaginary, fragmented or disjointed, and loaded with symbolism.

Trauma and Life Stories is a ground-breaking work of relevance across the social sciences. This new perspective on trauma will be of particular importance to researchers in psychology, history, women's studies, anthropology, sociology and cultural studies.

Selma Leydesdorff is based at the Belle van Zuylen Instituut, University of Amsterdam, The Netherlands. **Kim Lacy Rogers** is Professor of History and American Studies at Dickinson College, Pennsylvania, USA. **Graham Dawson** is a Senior Lecturer in Cultural and Historical Studies at the University of Brighton, UK.

ROUTLEDGE STUDIES IN MEMORY AND NARRATIVE

Series editors: Mary Chamberlain, Paul Thompson, Timothy Ashplant, Richard Candida-Smith and Selma Leydesdorff

If you are interested in finding our more about the series, please see our website at:
http://www.livjm.ac.uk/mcctashp/memory

TRAUMA AND LIFE STORIES

International perspectives

Edited by
Kim Lacy Rogers,
Selma Leydesdorff
and Graham Dawson

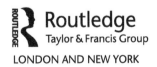

Routledge
Taylor & Francis Group

LONDON AND NEW YORK

First published 1999
by Routledge
2 Park Square, Milton Park, Abingdon, Oxfordshire OX14 4RN

Simultaneously published in the USA and Canada
by Routledge
711 Third Avenue, New York, NY 10017
First issued in paperback 2014

Routledge is an imprint of the Taylor & Francis Group, an informa business

Editorial material and selection © 1999
Kim Lacy Rogers, Selma Leydesdorff and Graham Dawson

Individual chapters © 1999 the contributors

Typeset in Garamond by Curran Publishing Services

British Library Cataloguing in Publication Data
A catalogue record for this book is available from the
British Library

Library of Congress Cataloguing in Publication Data
Trauma and life stories: international perspectives / edited by Kim
Lacy Rogers and Selma Leydesdorff with Graham Dawson.
272 pp. 15.6 x 23.4 cm
Includes bibliographical references and index.
ISBN 978-0-415-20688-4 (hbk)
ISBN 978-0-415-75775-1 (pbk)

1. Psychic trauma Cross-cultural studies. 2. Post-traumatic stress
disorder Cross-cultural studies. 3. Reminiscing - Therapeutic use
Cross-cultural studies. I. Rogers, Kim Lacy. II. Leydesdorff, Selma.
III. Dawson, Graham, 1956–
RC552.T7T736 1999   99–28901
616.85'21—dc21   CIP

CONTENTS

ILLUSTRATIONS

Figures

Tables

CONTRIBUTORS

Selma Leydesdorff is Chair of Women's Studies and Women's History at the Belle van Zuylen Instituut, Graduate Centre for Comparative and Multicultural Gender Studies at the University of Amsterdam. She has published extensively in women's history, oral history and Jewish history. Recent major books include *We Lived with Dignity: The Jewish Proletariat of Amsterdam 1900–1940* (1994). She is supervising a research project comparing the stories of three generations of migrant women from the Dutch Antilles and Surinam.

Kim Lacy Rogers is Professor of History and American Studies and Director of the Community Studies Center at Dickinson College in Carlisle, Pa. USA. She is the author of *Righteous Lives: Narratives of the New Orleans Civil Rights Movement* (1993) and co-editor with Eva M. McMahan of *Interactive Oral History Interviewing* (1994). She has also written several articles on African-American narrative traditions, literary subjects and interviewing. Between 1995 and 1998 she co-directed with Professor Jerry W. Ward Jr. the Delta Oral History Project, a collaborative effort of Tougaloo and Dickinson Colleges.

Gadi BenEzer is a clinical and organizational psychologist who has been working with Ethiopian Jews in Israel. He has written extensively on their absorption and adaptation after migration to Israel. He has acted as consultant to various Israeli and international agencies and teaches at Ben Gurion University in the Negev.

Judith Zur is a clinical psychologist and social anthropologist. Currently she is setting up a mental health service for refugees within the NWL Mental Health Trust and directing and running workshops in mental health and restitution in Guatemala. Her book about Guatemalan widows, *Violent Memories*, is forthcoming (San Francisco: Westview Press).

Sean Field is a research officer for the Western Cape Oral History Project in the Department of History, University of Cape Town, South Africa. He teaches oral history methodology and is also turning his doctoral thesis into a book. His research explores the social construction of memories and identities within the local communities of Cape Town.

Jan Coetzee is Professor of Sociology at Rhodes University, Grahamstown, South Africa. He is a member of the board of Research Committee 38: Biography and Society of the International Sociological Association. He is author of *Development is for the People* (Southern Book Publishers, 1989) and co-author of *Reconstruction, Development and People* (International Thomson Publishing 1996).

Otakar Hulec is a Senior Researcher in the Department of Africa and the Near East in the Oriental Institute Academy of Sciences of the Czech Republic, Prague. He is a member of the Scientific Council of the Oriental Institute and author of *A History of South Africa* (in Czech).

Federico Guillermo Lorenz is a history teacher and lives in Argentina. He researches the oral history of the Malvinas War and recently won a grant from the SSRC for researching the memory of repression in South America. He is also involved in a project for applying oral history techniques in primary and secondary schools, as a member of the Oral History Programme of the University of Buenos Aires.

JoAnn McGregor lectures in the Department of Geography, University of Reading. Her research has focused on Zimbabwe and Mozambique. She is joint author (with Jocelyn Alexander and Terence Ranger) of the forthcoming *Memory and Violence: One Hundred Years in the 'Dark Forests' of Matabeleland* (James Currey), and has published articles in the *Journal of South African Studies, Environment and History,* and *Past and Present.*

Susan Rose has a Ph.D. from Cornell University and is Professor and Chair of Sociology at Dickinson College, Carlisle, Pa. USA. She has written extensively on gender, sexuality, violence and religious fundamentalism, is the author of *Exporting the American Gospel: Global Christian Fundamentalism* (Routledge 1996) and *Keeping them Out of the Hands of Satan: Evangelical Schooling in America* (Routledge 1988) and has co-produced a video documentary, *Clothesline*, on childhood sexual abuse, which has been screened at many national and international forums including the Fourth World Conference on Women in Beijing.

Graham Dawson teaches Cultural and Historical Studies at the University of Brighton and is the author of *Soldier Heroes: British Adventure, Empire and the Imagining of Masculinities* (Routledge 1994). He is currently writing a book on cultural memory and the Irish Troubles.

CONTRIBUTORS

Reviewers

J. P. Roos, University of Helsinki.

Arthur Hansen, California State University, Fullerton.

Paul Thompson, University of Essex.

Susannah Radstone, University of East London.

Tina Papoulias, University of East London.

INTRODUCTION

Trauma and life stories

Selma Leydesdorff, Graham Dawson, Natasha Burchardt and T. G. Ashplant

> Deep
> in the time-crevasse,
> by the
> honey-comb ice, there waits, as breath crystal
> your unimpeachable
> testimony
> (Paul Celan 1971, quoted in Rosenfeld 1990: 227)

The life-long impact of traumatic experience is the subject of the essays in this volume, *Trauma and Life Stories*. Traumatic experiences and their consequences often constitute the core of the life stories told by those who have survived natural disasters or war, or other kinds of social, state, or interpersonal violence. In this volume, we explore the relationship between the experiences of terror and helplessness that have caused trauma, the ways in which survivors remember, and the representation of these memories in the language and form of their life stories. The impact of trauma makes the processes of remembering and forgetting more complex than in other situations, and survivors are therefore particularly likely to express themselves in stories containing elements which are imaginary, fragmented or disjointed, and loaded with symbolism. This in turn means that the understanding and analysis of these stories is inevitably complicated and challenging.

The notion of 'trauma' has no straightforward definition (see BenEzer, this volume). The term has been used in a variety of ways by researchers of different persuasions and disciplines, not to speak of its many popular uses (Sandler *et al.* 1991, Dawes 1992, Furst 1986). This breadth of definition is also reflected in this volume. In its original sense (derived from the Greek 'traumatizo', meaning to wound) trauma signified a blow or shock to the bodily tissues which led to injury or disturbance. Later this medical concept

1

was extended to encompass the structures of the mind, developing a broader psychological and social reference. The American sociologist Kai T. Erikson, in his work on the trauma of major disasters, points out that if 'trauma' in its customary medical usage refers first and foremost to the shock and the event causing it (rather than to the impact of the injury on the body and mind), in the psychological literature the term is redefined to refer to the state of mind resulting from the shock, which disconnects the person involved from their relationship to the world. Erikson writes: 'Something alien breaks in on you, smashing through whatever barriers your mind has set up as a line of defence. It invades you, possesses you, takes you over, becomes a dominating feature of your interior landscape, and in the process threatens to drain you and leave you empty' (Erikson 1994: 228). Erikson's own work rests on a further redefinition of the concept. Rather than conceiving trauma as caused solely by a discrete happening, he argues that it should be considered as the outcome of a constellation of life experiences; that, in fact, trauma may arise not only from an acute event but also from a persisting social condition.

Graham Dawson, writing in this volume on trauma in the context of the Irish Troubles, points to the importance of psychoanalysis in the historical redefinition of trauma as a psychic as well as a bodily phenomenon (see Chapter Nine). As Dawson says, from his earliest work on hysteria in the 1890s Freud identified and set about theorizing the possibility that certain intractable 'illnesses' might be more correctly described as states of psychic disturbance and disconnection, whose underlying causes could be traced back to traumatic experiences in the past. According to psychoanalysis, the traumatic effects of a shocking event or circumstance upon the psyche are manifested unconsciously in a range of bodily symptoms and disturbances, in neurotic behaviours, in nightmares and hallucinations, and in amnesia. These can all be read as symbolic expressions of an experience which is difficult or impossible to make sense of, assimilate, or integrate with the 'ordinary' sense of oneself. Dori Laub, a Jewish-American psychoanalyst and survivor of the Shoah, who has worked extensively with other survivors, argues that the horror of the Nazi labour and death camps 'was beyond the limits of human ability (and willingness) to grasp, to transmit, or to imagine':

> [T]he imperative to tell the story of the Holocaust is inhabited by the impossibility of telling, and therefore, silence about the truth commonly prevails . . . [S]urvivors who do not tell their story become victims of distorted memory . . . The events become more and more distorted in their silent retention and pervasively invade and contaminate the survivor's daily life. The longer the story remains untold, the more distorted it becomes in the survivor's conception of it, so much so that the survivor doubts the reality of the actual events.
>
> (Laub 1995: 68, 64)

2

Psychoanalysis, the 'talking cure' (Breuer and Freud 1895: 83), was founded on the necessity of articulating the traumatic experience to a listener or witness, 'so as to reassert the veracity of the past and to build anew its linkage to, and assimilation into, present-day life' (Laub 1995: 62).

If psychoanalysis provided a vocabulary and framework to name and understand the psychic effects of traumatic experience, it is certainly apparent from historical accounts that these phenomena were by no means new. Samuel Pepys, writing his diary in 1667, describes how, five months after the Great Fire of London, his sleep is still disturbed by recurrent memories and images: 'it is strange to think how to this very day I cannot sleep a night without great terrors of fire, and this very night could not sleep till almost 2 in the morning through thoughts of fire' (Pepys 1667). Nor was psychoanalysis the only tradition in psychology to investigate the phenomena of trauma. Throughout the latter part of the nineteenth and early twentieth centuries there developed an increasing medical awareness of possible psychological and neurological effects of physical injuries, such as 'railway spine' – a term coined to describe the experience of persistent severe back pain after train accidents, without any apparent injury to the back itself (Miller 1961). A fierce medical debate also raged at this time about 'compensation neurosis': whether a patient engaged in litigation inevitably has a prolongation of physical and psychological symptoms, or whether, as more recent research has suggested, this is irrelevant to the time taken for resolution of symptoms for a given individual. This remains a matter or intense controversy even in the present day (Cohen 1987: 485).

However, arguably the most important focus for the study of trauma from the mid-nineteenth to the mid-twentieth century, was the soldier. The Crimean War (1854–6) and the American Civil War (1861–5) brought to the attention of doctors various states of physical and mental exhaustion arising in soldiers exposed to combat. The term 'neurasthenia' gained wide currency, and was used to include those described as suffering from phobias, nightmares and nervousness, arguably a male equivalent of 'hysteria' (Showalter 1997: 65–7). During the First World War, medical controversies about this condition – popularly known as 'shell shock' – were fought out in Britain. On one side of the debate were psychologists who acknowledged that anxiety, sleeplessness and repetitive battle dreams were symptoms of 'mental origin' afflicting the 'genuinely ill'; for 'hard-line' neurologists, in contrast, these were symptoms of organic illness affecting the nerves and brain (Bourke 1996: 118, 120). As Joanna Bourke has shown, these debates were 'related to fears about malingering' and cowardice (especially concerning working-class rank-and-file soldiers) on the part of military authorities, who became increasingly prepared to side with the psychologists as the war progressed (ibid.: 109, see also 107–22).

If the study of wartime trauma affecting soldiers was, as Bourke argues, 'instrumental in the growth of psychiatry as a discipline' (ibid.: 120), the shell shock debates also make plain the powerful institutional imperative for trauma research that derives from the military: namely to promote effective combat behaviour through the 'scientific' management of soldiers. According to Nikolas Rose, the very emergence of mainstream psychology as a science in the period from 1875 to the Second World War came about as a means to classify and measure 'dysfunctional' behaviour within new regimes of social regulation, spanning schools, prisons and factories as well as the army (Rose 1985). The continuing stimulus to research on trauma by military institutions (especially in the USA) is evident throughout the twentieth century, from studies of 'combat fatigue' in the Second World War to 'post-traumatic stress disorder' (PTSD) in the aftermath of Vietnam (Ellis 1980, Bartemeier *et al.* 1946).

A further major focus for the study of trauma has been the experiences of survivors of concentration camps in Europe and Japan. The long-term effects on brain and mind of conditions of pervasive fear, continuous threat to life of self and others, prolonged extreme assaults and physical hardship, starvation and epidemic illness are still insufficiently understood, but it has sometimes been suggested that survivors of such conditions may well have a higher risk than others of developing organic brain disorders such as dementia in later life. Certainly, the enduring high risk of suicide in concentration camp victims is well-known with Primo Levi, Bruno Bettelheim and Jean Améry among the most famous instances. Psychologists and physicians have long recognized that trauma may fundamentally affect the processes of memory and indeed they have maintained that traumatic experiences may affect neu-rological functions, changing the way that survivors *think*. These changed thinking processes tend to produce memories of trauma which are at the same time unusually vivid and unusually fragmented. Primo Levi draws on this psychological literature to distinguish those survivors 'who repress their past *en bloc*' from those (like himself) for whom 'memory of the offense per-sists, as though carved in stone . . . as if at that time my mind had gone through a period of exalted receptivity, during which not a detail was lost' (Levi 1986).

Recent advances in the endeavour to integrate psychological and neuro-logical understandings of trauma and memory have been made by Bessel van der Kolk and his colleagues (van der Kolk and Fisler 1996: 352–61). They have pointed to important differences between memories of stressful events (such as the memories of witnesses to a murder) and memories of trauma. The former may be especially vivid and detailed, with almost no change over time, while the latter can lead to 'extremes of retention and forgetting', including amnesia which may last for 'hours, weeks or years' (ibid.: 353–5). They contrast the often very specific memory of a stressful event, which can stand up even in a court of law as reliable, with so-called 'flashbulb' memo-ries of public events, such as the assassination of President Kennedy, for which people believe they have accurate recall, but for which research has shown there is likely to be considerable distortion and disintegration over time. To explain these differences they draw upon advances in brain imaging which are beginning to clarify how stressful, traumatic and ordinary memory can each be associated with specific areas of the brain (Broca's area, for example, which has long been known to have specific importance for various speech and language functions). Different kinds of dissociation, characteristic of the remembering and forgetting of trauma, are seen to involve distinctive neurological processes of storage and retrieval (ibid.: 353, 355, 357).

Alongside these scientific debates, trauma as a term has also entered popular discourse in many different ways. Images of collective trauma are now brought to us on screen into the intimacy of the living room, from all over the world. Trauma, has, in the latter half of this century, and especially in the last decade or so, become part of a public and media-dictated discourse in a way that never previously existed. As a consequence, mass audiences may empathize or be moved by the trauma of others, for example by the plight of starving children, by those who are victims of war and atrocities, by genocides (Bosnia, Rwanda); or by trauma affecting individuals. Some collective traumas have attracted widespread media coverage – the Heysel and the Hillsborough football stadium disasters, for example, or the plane crashes at Amsterdam and Lockerbie. Similarly, the dramatic deaths of high profile public figures, such as Ayrton Senna, the Formula 1 racing driver seen crashing to a premature death on track in controversial circumstances, or the death of Diana, Princess of Wales, have been seen to cause profound and unforeseen emotional responses in some onlookers.

The increasing public familiarity with the language of trauma used in the news media to describe such events has led to a gradual acceptance of the idea that both survivors and witnesses can suffer forms of delayed and continuing psychic disturbance. The term most commonly used now in medical, journalistic and other contexts, is post-traumatic stress disorder or PTSD, a term which first entered the American psychiatric literature in the 1980s in the aftermath of the war in Vietnam, referring to the disturbances experienced by US military veterans of that conflict on their return home. It has gone through successive revisions in the psychiatric manuals since then, in an attempt to define it more closely, to exclude related conditions, and to provide a basis for more reliable research. The core syndrome of PTSD, as defined in the American Psychiatric Association's *Diagnostic and Statistical Manual* (1987), involves exposure to a psychologically distressing event 'outside the range of human experience' (quoted in Brown 1995: 100). This leads to a characteristic collection of symptoms which involve mental reliving of the trauma, the numbing of general responsiveness to the external world, and paradoxically, a state of 'high arousal' or hyper-alertness to certain stimuli, particularly those which evoke reminders of a the original trauma. It is perhaps an irony that while psychiatrists have continued to pursue the seemingly elusive goal of defining PTSD ever more specifically, the popular usage of the new term has tended to expand to include the long term consequences of a wide variety of stressful experiences, whether communally or individually experienced.

Significantly, this wider public acceptance and understanding of PTSD has been deeply influenced by the campaigns of survivors themselves – whether these be Vietnam veterans, victims of domestic violence or incest, or the relatives of those who died in the Lockerbie air crash – to speak out and secure recognition of the damaging reality of their condition. As Susan Rose argues in her essay about sexual abuse in this volume, 'recovering from trauma is not just an individual act but a collective process', in which the struggle of survivors towards 'naming and claiming the experience of abuse and survival as their own story' requires a reciprocal willingness on the part of the others to listen, bear witness and (as Judith Herman has put it) to 'share the burden of pain' (Herman 1992: 7). To speak out about the trauma is to 'break through the silence' that surrounds it: a silence that is socially as well as psychologically determined, by defence mechanisms and survival strategies deployed by survivors, witnesses, and abusers themselves to minimize or deny the pain of abuse and the violence that caused it (Rose, this volume: 163–4). Thus, argues Rose, 'Speaking out is a political as well as a therapeutic act, and as such, is a claim to power . . . Trauma narratives . . . point to the unjustified violence done to people, and hold abusers rather than victims accountable'. Inevitably, then, they meet with a great scepticism and resistance, especially from those responsible and now called to account (ibid.: 163, 174).

The psychological debates about trauma need to be understood within this wider social and political context, because different theoretical paradigms have implications for – and are actively made to serve – competing interests and ideologies. This is clearly evident in the current attack on the veracity of so-called 'recovered memory', a term used to refer to apparent memories of trauma that have been therapeutically 'rediscovered' (or brought to light for the first time) after a lengthy period of amnesia, particularly in the case of adults recovering memories of sexual abuse in childhood.

This attack has stimulated heated debate in psychoanalytic and psychiatric circles in the United States from the late 1980s onwards (Brandon 1998), and much more recently has been taken up by the psychiatric establishment in Britain, Sweden, New Zealand and elsewhere (Conway 1997). In Britain, for example, a reductionist view has been taken by the Royal College of Psychiatrists in an official report making recommendations for good practice, which essentially denies the possibility of ever recovering genuine memories of trauma from the unconscious (Brandon *et al.* 1998: 296–7). At the core of the debate is the Freudian concept of 'repression', in which the unconscious is conceived as a kind of pit with a false bottom from which memories can be dredged up into consciousness by hard-working subjects (patients) in combination with committed therapists. This debate is self-evidently of crucial importance to historians concerned with life-history trauma, and in this volume J. P. Roos spells out the complexities with both irony and wit (this volume: 207–19).

At one level, these arguments about 'false memory' are part of a broader intellectual critique of Freudian psychoanalysis as a flawed science lacking conclusive empirical evidence for its propositions about unconscious memory (e.g. Crews *et al.* 1997). Studies grounded upon alternative psychological theories have fuelled this critique. For example, in a lucid and temperate discussion two psychologists, Ira Hyman and Elizabeth Loftus, demonstrate precisely how it has been shown that a proportion of people – typically around a quarter – can be quite easily convinced, through a mixture of true and false suggestions from people whom they trust, that they remember important experiences which never actually happened (Hyman and Loftus 1997). From a different perspective, van der Kolk and Fisler have also intervened in the recovered memory debate. They argue that, in the case of people suffering from traumatic amnesia:

> The combination of lack of an autobiographical memory, of continued dissociation, and of meaning schemes that include victimization, helplessness and betrayal, is likely to make those individuals vulnerable to suggestion and to the construction of explanations for their trauma-related affects that may bear little relationship to the actual realities of their lives.
>
> (van der Kolk and Fisler 1996: 355)

On the other hand, Judith Herman (1992) has assembled a number of studies indicating that traumatic memories from childhood have been retrieved after a period of dense amnesia and later confirmed beyond a reasonable doubt; and Lenore Terr (1990: 1–5) has demonstrated that, when abuse has taken place in early childhood, the lack of later childhood or adult access to the memory may have especially devastating consequences. Moreover, to problematize the specific tenets of Freudianism is not necessarily to deny that the psychological impact of trauma too painful to contemplate and thus not remembered may have far-reaching effects on people's lives; nor indeed that many who have suffered such trauma will benefit from therapeutic intervention. As Sidney Brandon concludes in discussing the creation of false memory by over-zealous therapists, 'there seems no room to doubt that false memories can occur or be created, but it does not follow that all recovered memories are therefore false' (Brandon 1998: 279). That the debate about 'false memory' is structured in such terms is due less to psychologists as such, and more to what Susan Rose describes as 'formal resistance to memory recovery' (this volume: 173) instituted by organizations such as the False Memory Syndrome Foundation, formed in the USA to discredit the claims of abuse survivors, if necessary in the courts.

Trauma and life histories

For life historians, the nature of traumatic memory has become a salient issue neither because it may be the key to healing the mentally suffering, nor because of a wish to understand the memory processes of the brain, but because of the effects of trauma upon storytelling about the self. In common with other social scientists and cultural analysts interested in exploring personal memory narratives in relation to forms of collective memory and amnesia, life historians interested in trauma have inevitably been attracted to those traditions in psychology, like Freudian psychoanalysis, which emphasize storytelling as a construction of meaning – an attempt to come to terms with or master intensely disturbing experiences. Ever since Breuer and Freud's notion of the 'talking cure', of course, such an understanding of the patient's need to talk and tell stories has been basic to modern psychotherapeutic approaches. Thus Jeremy Holmes and Glenn Roberts, co-authors of a recent volume on *Narrative Approaches in Psychiatry and Psychotherapy,* call their discussion on working with trauma 'stories in search of a voice'. They write of the torment of the solitude in not talking, of the 'curse' of a 'toxic story'; and of the therapist's role in helping the suffering to rework the meaning of their narratives, but above all, to draw out the story. 'It is in naming that silence that the beginning, and only the beginning, of a healing journey becomes possible' (Holmes and Roberts 1999).

A key figure in the historical development of such approaches – and one who has been relatively neglected until Pat Barker portrayed him as a central character in her award-winning *Regeneration* trilogy of novels – was the psychiatrist W. H. R. Rivers, who sheltered Siegfried Sassoon from humiliation and disgrace during the First World War. In the early debates on mental illness Rivers was an exceptional figure, for he was not only a psychiatrist but also a highly esteemed anthropologist, who had worked particularly in Melanesia, and brought his two interests together in various studies of medical anthropology. Interestingly, in his subsequent work in treating shell-shocked officers in the First World War, Rivers was a pioneer in introducing a more social dimension to his interpretations, for he linked their recurring nightmares to an earlier boarding school socialization in which they had been taught to suppress their feelings, and to meet frightening situations without any sign of fear. His tactic for treating them was therefore to encourage them to share with him the otherwise repressed feelings which haunted them through their dreams. Day after day, 'he looked at twitching mouths that had once been clenched. Go on, he said, though rarely in so many words, cry. It's all right to grieve' (Barker 1995: 96; see also Rivers 1920: 209).

In general both oral historians and life-story sociologists initially tried to avoid rather than seek out those who might have traumatized memories, for the double reason that they were looking for memories whose significance was clear, and they had no wish to cause further pain to those who had suffered traumatic life experiences. The relatively recent interest of life historians in this topic has emerged from wider social, cultural and political developments since 1945, especially from the radical protest and liberation movements in Western Europe, the USA, the former colonized world, and the Soviet Union. In various ways these movements demonstrated that trauma has social roots in structural oppression, persecution, devaluation, and official indifference to the sufferings of socially subordinated and powerless groups. Furthermore, these movements – whether for women's liberation or anti-colonial national liberation, whether protesting against American bombing of Vietnam or against the Gulag – created a context in which the voices and stories of the victims (or, in that crucial redefinition, 'the survivors') could speak and be heard.

Thus especially since the mid-1970s, an explosion of publications of testimony has taken place, as an integral element of 'history from below' and other forms of radical social analysis. Notably, researchers in America and Britain have become increasingly interested in uncovering the ongoing effects of interpersonal, face-to-face violence enacted within intimate and familial relationships (Pynoos *et al.* 1996). Rape, incest, domestic violence, and criminal assault have been studied by psychologists, social scientists and other researchers, many using life histories in their methodology; and this work has been instrumental in demonstrating how violence to individuals may lead to lasting damage over the whole life course. Violence and sexual abuse within families was first recognized as a long-endured feature of the domestic lives of many women, and later as suffered also by children. Much of this interest originated in the women's movement, which since the 1970s has argued that 'the personal is political', and has insisted on the opening up of 'private' life to collective social scrutiny within the public domain.

More recently, critical investigation has shifted to other institutional contexts of abuse. Among such accounts have been startling exposures of religious abusers, of which a striking recent instance is a television documentary on the Magdalen institutions run by Catholic nuns in Ireland. Until as late as the 1960s many Irish women were locked away in these homes and made to earn their living through enforced laundry work. They included women who had had an illegitimate child, but also others who were stigmatized simply because they had protested against sexual abuse by a parent or a local priest or teacher. Although many potential witnesses had been located by the filmmakers in Ireland, all of them were still too fearful to speak in public, and the film was eventually based on four Irish women who had since come to live in England. Broadcast in March 1998 on British television as *Sex in a Cold Climate*, with a Channel Four 'helpline' telephone number as back-up support, the film produced an unprecedented response, with hundreds of calls from women in the Irish Republic who now wanted for the first time to tell in public the story of their own traumatic experience of abuse.

As so often in the history of trauma, a recurring theme of such investigations has been not only the reluctance of the afflicted to speak, but also the reluctance of society for them to be heard – and, if heard, to be believed. The process of witnessing requires space within the symbolic order of a culture, a 'listening space' that is not granted automatically, but very often has to be won through struggle. Telling a story of trauma, then, frequently depends upon a politics of memory to force the issue into the public domain. In this respect, groups within the women's movement have been crucial in organizing rape crisis centres, refuges for battered women and their children, and survivors' groups.

A similar process is evident in relation to other collective struggles within the public political arena. In the years following the Vietnam War, American veterans of that conflict formed support groups to explore their own traumatic experiences and pressurize the US Veterans' Administration to treat thousands of them for PTSD. As Kim Lacy Rogers shows in this volume (Chapter Six), the black civil rights movement in the USA transformed the lynching stories of the southern states into signs of white racist oppression, capable of inspiring and mobilizing political resistance to the underlying causes of trauma. Massive oppression by the Western imperial powers against resistance and liberation movements throughout the colonized world has also given rise to political recognition of trauma and of the importance of giving expression to silenced memories. Frantz Fanon, one of the leading figures of the Algerian Revolution, argued in *Les Damnés de la Terre* that:

> In the period of colonization when it is not contested by armed resistance. . . [t]here is . . . a regular and important mental pathology which is the direct product of oppression. Today the war of national liberation which has been carried on by the Algerian people for the last seven years has become a favourable breeding-group for mental disorders, because so far as the Algerians are concerned it is a total war.
>
> (Fanon 1961: 201)

In a section of the book entitled 'Colonial War and Mental Disorders', Fanon analysed the psychic effects of the conflict upon 'a whole generation of Algerians, steeped in wanton, generalized homicide with all the psychoaffective consequences that this entails' (ibid.: 202; see 200–50). Moreover, the success of anti-colonial movements in the fifties and sixties provoked a situation in which western cultures had to acknowledge that imperialist aggression had inflicted trauma on a vast scale. In France, for example, the fight for openness about mass slaughter and torture during the Algerian war created the cultural space to talk about the effects of trauma, which appealed especially to those who doubted the moral supremacy of the West. Jean-Paul Sartre, in his famous preface to Fanon's *Les Damnés*, wrote that: 'Our victims know us by their scars and by their chains . . . you, who are so liberal and so humane . . . pretend to forget that you own colonies and that in them men are massacred in your name' (Sartre 1961: 12).

10

Over the past decade, psychologists, historians, literary scholars, and sociologists have also focused on the personal as well as social consequences of political terror, systematic oppression, and genocide in former totalitarian and authoritarian regimes. In inquiring into the long-term effects of mortal terror, torture, and the witnessing of torture, they have been stimulated by the literary, visual, and verbal narratives of the survivors of the Shoah and the Gulag. This new focus of interest is well symbolized in the extraordinarily powerful national Holocaust Memorial Museum in Washington, which almost seeks to impose a form of witness on the visitor, who is given an individual concentration camp number on entry, taken up in a prison-like elevator, and overwhelmed by the cumulative witness of photographs, documents, films, and audio and video interviews with survivors. Where there is silence, when there are no witnesses, it may seem as if an event has not occurred. Still now, over fifty years after the Second World War there are many survivors of the Shoah who need to be heard – and many who feel they will never be understood. Yet as Bruno Bettelheim (1952) has reminded us, only when such personal histories are acknowledged can mourning hope to begin. The wish to bear witness is the key to the extraordinary growth of the Spielberg project, in which hundreds of survivors are participating because they fear that unless they do so their history will be forgotten.[1]

In Europe too, major changes resulting from the fall of the former communist regimes in the late 1980s and early 1990s have resulted in an intense focus on the subjects of trauma and social rupture. One of the largest movements in the former Soviet Union has been aptly named *Memorial,* based, significantly, on the wish to give the memories of victims a proper place. Coming to terms with the communist past involves confronting a trauma that is both collective and, for individuals who suffered directly, deeply personal. Many of them had not previously been publicly recognized as victims. Speaking out – telling one's own story about the traumatic past – is both a personal necessity, and inescapably social in its significance.

What is occurring in all these societies is an attempt to come to terms with a traumatic past that is collective in its impact and scale, the result of major historical forces and conflicts that have produced ruptures between the society's past and its present. Often, this process of coming-to-terms has to confront institutional amnesia and official denial by the state itself, as forms of social and ideological control. In this volume Graham Dawson and Judith Zur write about such conflicts in Northern Ireland and Guatemala respectively (Chapters Nine and Two). Much more rarely, in other circumstances, such as post-apartheid South Africa, the need to tell has been recognized at a formal political level. The extraordinary Truth and Reconciliation Commission which began sitting in 1996 under the chairmanship of Archbishop Tutu is partly a consequence of the amnesty which the Afrikaner police and military extracted as their price for allowing a peaceful transition to majority rule in South Africa. But it is also the outcome of a much wider reflection on the process of transition which included comparisons with the Nuremberg trials which followed the end of Nazi rule in Europe, or the ambiguous silences following the transition from settler rule in Zimbabwe, and from military dictatorships in Brazil and Chile, or the transition in Argentina with its much more limited commission on the disappeared.

In the event the wish of Nelson Mandela's government to put the needs of the future above those of the past, and so to emphasize reconciliation rather than legal justice and retribution, led to a combination of amnesty with 'truth-telling', by both victims and perpetrators, in a single process. Perpetrators who convinced the hearing that they were telling the truth and that they acted from a genuine political motive on either side of the apartheid struggle are given their amnesty, but at the price of public shaming that confession usually implied for them, while victims were promised some undefined, but probably largely symbolic, compensation. The draft constitution draws on the African communalist concept of *ubuntu*, with its implications of 'compassion', 'restorative justice', and 'recognizing the humanity of the other'. And undoubtedly some of the most powerful moments in the Commission's hearings were when a murderer or torturer had to look in the eyes of a victim who had survived, or a bereaved spouse, or an orphaned child.

There have certainly been many serious criticisms of the Truth and Reconciliation Commission. It was not easy to work out suitable procedures for such a novel process. Many of the poorer victims had clearly hoped for a material and substantial compensation for their losses, and the absence of this makes it much less easy to accept that perpetrators do not have to accept punishment for their offences. There are doubts about the religious basis of Archbishop Tutu's philosophy of forgiveness, of healing, of redemption through bearing witness. There are ethical difficulties too about the exposing of intimate sorrows in hearings which have a mass audience on television, and whose final report, like that of *Nunca Mas* on the Argentinian disappeared, is likely to become a best-seller.

There can be no doubt, however, that the Commission has proved profoundly influential in the South African situation, and that all over the country people have picked up its language. It was based on the recognition that people have a moral and political urge to speak out about their suffering. The telling itself gives a meaning to the trauma: suffering may not have been in vain. One widow looks forward to a little compensatory money: 'some day I would like once again to own the vegetable stall'. But even without that, she says that 'the Truth Commission has done a lot for me: I know what happened to my husband. And it is better that way. I don't want any more blood spilled in South Africa, what these people did was enough (Garton Ash 1997, O'Hagan 1998, Boraine *et al.* 1997).

Issues in constructing life histories of trauma

Life stories are particularly useful in understanding the significance of trauma in people's lives. The life story approach allows room for contradiction, a holistic richness, and complexity. It gives the opportunity to explore the relation between personal and collective experience, by focusing on remembering and forgetting as cultural processes. It also offers a means of making sense and interpreting the experience of marginalized peoples and forgotten histories. It allows us to explore the relation between individual memories and testimonies, and the wider public contexts, cultural practices, and forms of representation that shape the possibilities of their telling and their witnessing. But while life history approaches bring rich resources to the study of trauma, the study also poses particular difficulties and problems for those approaches. These centre on the relation of social histories to the psychic dimensions of trauma, and the effects of trauma upon life-history narration. This is why historians need to be familiar with some of the psychological debates on the effects of trauma discussed above. This is not simply a matter of grafting a social dimension onto an existing psychology, nor of 'psychologizing' a historical analysis. The study of trauma challenges and invites a fundamental rethinking of these received categories across disciplinary boundaries (Antze and Lambek 1996).

Whose voices should be listened to and how? We need to distinguish more clearly between different kinds of trauma, since experiences may have widely different impacts according to the specifics of personal experience and context. Among the subjects of life-history narration may be those who have been directly affected by a traumatic event or process in which some have died and others survived; others may have witnessed a traumatic event or series of events, and consider themselves, in a sense, survivors. Some may have been bereaved, suffering trauma through the loss of others, in addition to the direct trauma they themselves have suffered. Others may be witnesses or listeners to stories of trauma told by any of the above. In each case we need to be aware of the different effects which such experiences and stories may have upon their subjects' consciousness and their memories.

Survivors who have lived through concentration camps or bomb attacks or have suffered other violations or disasters may silence their own fears. It therefore takes a particular form of courage, and a painful effort, to call to mind those phases of life in which excessive stress, sadness and violence have been experienced. Robert Lifton has written about the long-term diminution of the capacity to speak and feel following trauma. The phenomenon which he describes as 'numbness' is a psychic defence which contributes to a loss of contact with the surroundings, and a lack of awareness of a problem's existence. As a result of such psychic defences, speaking about trauma may, in some cases, prove altogether impossible. In this volume, a graphic example of the mechanism of psychic defence is found in Judith Zur's account of the Guatemalan war widow who had forgotten her own husband's name (Caruth 1995: 130–1, Zur, Chapter Two).

Another metaphor for 'numbness' is 'frozen memory'. The theme of frozen memory appears in many testimonies of people's experiences during the

Second World War. Thus Lawrence Langer paraphrases Kafka when he compares the testimonies he heard to icebergs – 'to freeze the warm coursing blood within us' – and this constitutes a threat as well as a challenge (Langer 1991: 36). Hence in addition to the inherent difficulty in coming to terms with a traumatic event, a 'frozen' moment may exist that isolates it from the surrounding recovery. This frozen quality complicates verbalization. Such inability is an important literary theme (Rosenfeld 1980). The world has become so dark that visualizing cruelty is impossible. This same idea underlies Claude Lanzmann's film *Shoah*. Silence signifies acknowledgement of the painful difficulty of metaphoric representation.

Victim populations and groups also frequently remain reticent out of shame, for fear of not being heard, or because of self-imposed censorship. Indeed, some psychological researchers suggest that the process of articulating and verbalizing trauma can re-traumatize and can awaken terrors and depressions that were long blocked from the mind (van der Kolk 1996). Such intellectual and emotional consequences of trauma significantly affect the narrative in survivors' life stories which are frequently fragmented and distorted by blocks and gaps in memory. Indeed, personal and social trauma may cause the self to be split apart into disconnected fragments. The life stories of survivors relate what is conscious and can be narrated, and provide insight into that which is subconscious and often remains unverbalized and unintegrated with other experience.

Such narratives therefore require particularly sensitive kinds of readings. They concern an experience that is likely to be re-enacted in the subconscious through illusions, nightmares, and physical and psychological symptoms. In Chapter One of this volume Gadi BenEzer describes how the black Ethiopian Jews whom he interviewed gave their accounts of the traumas which they had suffered during their migration, not only through particular oral forms, including repetitions or long silences, and changes in voice tone, but also through their body language, including trembling, and foetal postures. As the American literary scholar Cathy Caruth puts it, 'trauma seems to be much more than a pathology or a simple illness of a wounded psyche: it is always the story of a wound that cries out, that addresses us in an attempt to tell us of a reality or truth that is not otherwise available' (Caruth 1996).[2] This is fundamentally why such memories are so difficult to read, to hear, and to witness.

In some cases the personal and cultural codes that survivors develop to convey the unspeakable, and to name that which defies verbal and emotional expression, can be analysed linguistically and as narrative forms, to reveal the impact of trauma within a life story. Variations and discontinuities in narrative structure may sometimes enable researchers to trace the terror's shattering and life-changing impact. This task is far from simple. Trauma codes and narratives are very likely to be as culturally specific as other life story forms. Moreover, experiences considered traumatic in some cultures may not be interpreted as such in others. One factor which helps to shape such narratives is the quality of language and the symbolism available to the narrator. Because of their apparent spontaneity, life histories may seem to operate outside a theoretical or narrative framework, with every narrator creating an individual matrix. But no matter how spontaneous and personal this may appear, it is an illusion: a closer look reveals that this matrix is influenced by narrative styles and genres. These forms are aids for verbalizing the silences and for overcoming the block to expression created by the trauma. The patterns which unite the stories told by different individuals are fascinating.

Perhaps best known is the coding in descriptions of the Shoah. The first eyewitness accounts of the Shoah were conventional testimonies. Survivors wrote their stories to inform the world and to disseminate a moral message, Primo Levi's works being an outstandingly influential example. This warning and moralizing framework was the only way in which many survivors could verbalize the hell they had experienced. Levi's own approach was in fact particularly original, for he was able, partly because he was a professional scientist, to develop an exceptionally plain and straightforward style, which contrasts strikingly with the flowery elaboration much more typical of contemporary Italian literary fashion. For others, conveying the images before their eyes proved impossible, except perhaps in poetry, as in the work of Paul Celan. Yet other survivors attempted to solve the problem by using well known forms from earlier literature that led both author and reader through the terra incognita of the narration. The acknowledgement of suffering in such works brought about recognition for their own suffering. Motifs from Dostoeyevsky's novels and Dante's *Inferno* (1998) permeate early stories about the Nazi camps, and reappear in Solzhenitsyn's *The Gulag Archipelago* (1974). Episodes from *The Bible* provide an organizing framework for many narrations of trauma.

Stories and life histories of traumatized individuals rarely reflect continuity: typically they are structured in terms of a 'before' and an 'after', hinging on one or several ruptures that have permanently affected these lives. In this respect a trauma is not an isolated event in a life story but may in itself often play a decisive role in a person's perception of life afterwards, interpretations of subsequent events, and consequently, memories of preceding experiences. Thus, the study of trauma in life stories – whether based on oral or literary texts – entails investigating discontinuities and fragmentation. Life stories may attempt to place trauma in the context of a whole life, to integrate it with other life experiences; but they can also show us how connections with others may have been distorted and what dissociations may have resulted.

Lenore Terr (1990), who pioneered the study of trauma in childhood, has demonstrated how it can colour every subsequent experience. Even though the children she studied seemed at first sight to have recovered from the shock of a group kidnapping, she found that many of them continued to have serious emotional and behavioural disorders, and severe difficulties in living their lives. Patterns of fear that had emerged during the trauma, continued to have a profound influence on their life experience. In addition she has shown how the symbolism and imagery of an originating trauma – albeit only partially remembered – can colour and inflect the perception of memories of other life events. Thus trauma may become the prism that refracts self-understanding and perception of the surrounding environment. It seems that even dimly-remembered trauma, and even trauma that has never surfaced in conscious awareness, can define the shape of a life and a life narrative by conditioning all other intellectual, emotional, and sensory processes.

A crucial part of the contribution which the life-history approach can make to the study of trauma lies in its interest in – and its ability to analyse – how different cultural contexts affect the production and reception of trauma narratives. Any particular culture may make available, or may lack, suitable narrative codes or other forms of representation, as well as publics prepared to believe and witness – or not. These variable cultural conditions are themselves part of the experience of trauma, and may contribute either to the perpetuation of traumatic silence, or to the viable expression and representation of traumatic experience.

Change in the collective context of telling can sometimes radically reshape the story. Lutz Niethammer (1992) has analyzed the importance of changing contexts of domination in the lives of his East German interviewees, who as a result had to adapt their life histories repeatedly over time. Their categories of good and evil changed with their successive adaptations to the chronology of fascism, communism, and democracy. Such fairly rapid changes are also visible both in post-communist societies and elsewhere in Europe, especially where entire peoples – as in the Baltic states – produce new and varied historiographies. These new versions of history are often based on trauma inflicted on the population by, for example, Soviet military occupation: the trauma and the heroic struggle thus become constituents of a new mythology and form the core of a new type of nationalism.

In Russia itself a whole society became wrapped in silence for almost three generations, from the 1920s to the late 1980s. For six decades millions of Russian families suffered traumatic deprivation and loss through wars, economic chaos and famine (at moments so severe that neighbours became cannibals) or, much more often, through the death or disappearance of family members, especially men, either through war or through political repression. Informing became so widespread that Soviet Russia was a society in which even intimate family members concealed basic experiences from each other: that a grandfather had fought in the White Russian army, that the family had been *kulaks*, that a close member had spent years in the Gulag. Sometimes even a husband or wife did not know that their spouse had formerly been named as an 'enemy of the people'. Family stories had mysterious gaps; in family photograph albums pages were torn out, or a single face, or even just a tell-tale medal, scissored from a group scene. From the late 1980s, with the advent of *glasnost*, suddenly memories came pouring out: even to the point that some people wanted to claim, apparently fictitiously, that they themselves not only knew about a prison whose very existence they had denied two or three years earlier, but that they themselves had been warders or prisoners there (Sherbakova 1992, Khubova *et al.* 1992, Pahl and Thompson 1994).

As long as the telling of stories of trauma continues to meet with resistance and denial, the psychic effects of the past remain to poison the present. However, creating more receptive social, political and cultural conditions does not necessarily mean that all resistances to recognizing the existence of trauma can be overcome, or that a 'full' version of the past can be recovered from amnesia and dissociation, and restored. It may not be possible for trauma ever to be fully overcome. Moreover recent research suggests that trauma is contagious, transmissible from survivors to their listeners and witnesses; and, both within families and by means of wider, collective processes, to subsequent generations (Burchardt 1993). Studies of the children of Shoah survivors, for example, have demonstrated how distortions in the mental life and life styles of the parents may have profound and confusing effects on some of their offspring, especially when a particular child appears to carry the burden of representing the aspirations of murdered ancestors (Wardl 1992, Hass 1991).

We need to end on a last note of caution. Life history interviewing about trauma may, as we have seen, unwittingly stir up memories which victims have fought hard to keep out of consciousness in order to get on with their lives. Lutz Niethammer (1985) has shown some of the dilemmas involved. Historians need to be aware of these inherent risks, while remaining clear that (for the most part) their role and responsibilities differ from those of psychologists and therapists (though, as the work of Dori Laub (1995) demonstrates, for example, these are not necessarily incompatible). On the positive side, however, it is the experience of many life-story historians that interviewees may benefit from the opportunity to unburden themselves, sometimes speaking for the first time of matters so profoundly troubling that they have never previously found expression (see also Thompson 1988: Chapter Five).

Narratives of trauma

Each of the studies presented in this volume focuses on particular instances which exemplify the potential of life histories to reveal, represent, and unravel trauma – and also the various limitations upon this process. The studies focus on a wide variety of social and political contexts, in Africa, Europe, and the Americas; and draw on the work of anthropologists, sociologists, psychologists and oral historians.

The black Ethiopian Jews, of whom Gadi BenEzer writes, suffered multiple traumas in their passage to Israel. Between 1977 and 1985, pushed by fear of persecution and drawn by hope of the promised land, whole families migrated in large numbers. They walked the mountains and desert at night, and then were held up in refugee camps in Sudan where they struggled for food, a fifth perishing on the journey; they lost parents, brothers and sisters; and when the survivors reached Israel, they not only had to adapt from a traditional rural culture to a modern one but, perhaps worst of all, their very Jewishness was challenged. BenEzer worked with them as a psychologist (both clinician and researcher) in Israel, and has also carried out life-story interviews, especially with the younger migrants. In an especially innovative insight, he describes their 'linguistic-narrative behaviour'; their particular gestures and ways of speaking about their memories of trauma, in special detail. He also suggests how an interviewer might proceed when such trauma signals, verbal or non-verbal, are detected.

Judith Zur lived as an anthropologist in a remote Indian village in the mountains of Central America. She writes of the traumatic memories of widows in a mountain Indian village whose husbands were murdered by the army during Guatemala's civil war, 'La Violencia', an assault by the military on the indigenous rural population which lasted from 1978 until 1985. Even today, although the war itself is over, the government has not accepted its responsibility for the massacres, and defends its reputation by an official prohibition on remembering. In Guatemala the Indians had been traditionally used by the '*ladinos*' as cheap seasonal agricultural labour, and were viewed with a mixture of contempt and fear. This was intensified when a section of the Indians were converted to a radical Catholicism which was linked with rural development by the communities. Partly because market agriculture was leading to an increasing land shortage, conflict escalated to the point when progressive but peaceful communities like that subsequently studied by Zur in the late 1980s were labelled as 'subversive' and 'Marxist', and regarded by the army as indistinguishable from the guerrillas with whom they were almost forced to join. The cumulation of the civil war was the deliberate engendering of terror by the army, which forced the women of the village to witness the public massacre of their own men, and even after that encouraged marauding 'civil patrols' who indulged in rapes of many surviving widows.

Despite being forced to witness the murders of their husbands, the widows are forbidden to speak about what they saw. This is a deliberate part of the government's propaganda strategy: 'historical amnesia is a means of social control'. To provide a basis for the official ideology, which explains the war in terms of a defence against Marxist subversives, the dead are constantly vilified and criminalized. Through such 'symbolic domination', as Bourdieu (1991: 72) has termed it, not only is evidence suppressed, but the personal identity of surviving victims is weakened, and hence their capacity to counter-organize. Nevertheless these Indian widows showed exceptional bravery in their refusal to keep absolute silence. They speak about their memories in small groups of women, mostly at home, but also in the fields, at religious shrines, and in the hills. Zur describes the kind of memories they share: how even among them some things, such as their shame at being prevented from helping their men at the massacre, remain unspeakable; and the constant reshaping and restructuring of memories which takes place within the group.

Sean Field writes of a more persistent violence, that of Cape Town neighbourhoods under apartheid and through to the present. He describes the process of carrying out an oral history study with former residents of the once vibrant, racially mixed and part-squatter township of Windermere, which was torn apart under the apartheid laws in 1958–63, when the township was zoned as 'coloured'. The majority of the black population was therefore forcibly removed to the new township of Guguletu, which has become notorious for its violence, both from crime and from its struggles with the police and the army. Interviewing at all in Guguletu was clearly very hazardous, for as Field demonstrates, neither his political credentials nor the company of a black assistant could give more than 'minimal protection' and on one particular day in 1993 it is likely that only a sixth sense of danger saved him from being murdered himself.

Both the relationship with the interviewees and the quality of the memories are affected by this context. Field discusses how the intensity of emotion heightens the potential for a process of transference and counter-transference in the interviews: 'there are often unexpected times when the interviewer has to be a safe container for the interviewee's emotions'. He found that men were more likely to cry with him than women, and attributes this to 'our common gender'. In the memories themselves he notes both silences and idealizations. On the one hand, in many interviews there were 'frightened silences produced by the violence of apartheid, poverty and social upheavals': often shown through a 'fearful passivity and at times a stubborn protectiveness', which he interprets as reflecting 'a numbing fear of who to trust or distrust', persisting even with the dismantling of apartheid. On the other hand, above all for blacks who had been forced out, the pre-apartheid past of Windermere was often idealized as 'a place of peace and togetherness' in contrast to today's violence and loss of community help and trust. Only a minority of those whom he interviewed could also recall the burnings of wooden houses, the killings of blacks by blacks, that made Windermere itself, even if less violent than today's townships, also violent in the past.

Jan Coetzee and Otakar Hulek also write partly about apartheid South Africa, but this time of imprisonment under apartheid, in comparison with the experience of dissenters imprisoned under communism in Czechoslovakia. While life in prison under both regimes could certainly bring traumatic experiences through lack of food, hard labour in quarries and elsewhere, and beatings, the contrast they bring out is rather of how such experiences can be mitigated by solidarity. South African political prisoners were gaoled as recognized participants in a mass struggle and resistance against the apartheid regime. They were successful in maintaining their organization even in the prison itself, always discussing, sending delegations, studying, debating and teaching each other, and all this gave a meaning to their experience which helped them to survive it. Dissenters against communism, by contrast, were a small minority whose political motivation was never recognized, so that they were herded together with the ordinary criminal population. They faced a material struggle above all for food, in which they could trust nobody, and necessarily confronted their traumatic deprivation and ideological non-recognition alone.

Lack of social recognition is also at the heart of the traumatic memories which the Argentinian veterans of the Malvinas War continue to suffer. In the account given by contemporary historian Federico Lorenz, we hear echoes of the better-documented experiences of Vietnam veterans in the United States. On their return home after the national humiliation of defeat, so far from their sufferings being acknowledged or the local population giving support, they found themselves at best ignored, at worst spurned or ostracized. The physical and psychological scars of the combat which they had endured brought them no sympathy. They were greeted with an indifference or hostility which greatly added to their difficulties in readjusting to civilian life.

In view of the small number of life stories which he collected, Lorenz is tentative in his conclusions. Nevertheless he is conscious of how the oral historian, through studying social myths, can influence their social construction – in the case of the social myth of the Malvinas, as he puts it, effecting 'a transition from a jingoistic nationalism to an infinitely more human and less blindfolded position': a position from which the healing of such traumatic memories might begin.

Kim Lacy Rogers explores as an oral historian the lynching stories from the Mississippi Delta, told to her by African-Americans who were often active in civil rights struggles in the 1950s and 1960s. She situates them both in a family context (as memorials and warnings handed down to the next generation), and in a political generational context (as indicative of a racist system which was no longer bearable and had to be overthrown). Her analysis stresses the two-sided nature of these narratives. On the one hand, they performed a range of positive functions. They were a remembrance of members and others who had been victims of atrocity. They were a testament of the survival, resilience and agency both of older generations who had survived this regime, and of a younger generation who had successfully struggled for educational and political rights. That affirmation of initiative countered the earlier attempt to crush black agency which lynching often represented. And they acted politically to warn blacks of what they had to fear, to name the perpetrators and their system, and thereby discredit white supremacist claims to civilized values, and to indicate the necessity for federal intervention to establish justice and the rule of law. On the other hand, they necessarily encoded a massive sense of communal trauma among blacks, and both enacted and encouraged a profound protectiveness towards family members against arbitrary and unchecked white violence. On the political level, they revealed a continuing sense of the fragility of the political gains made over the last thirty years, and an unease that this represents any deep shift in white attitudes.

Despite its concern with traumatic events – the deaths of guerrillas through poisoning in the Dandanda area of Zimbabwe during the liberation war, and the resultant killings of suspected witches – the focus of JoAnn McGregor's contribution, which draws together both oral history and documentary sources, is as much on the (partially-successful) struggle to contain trauma. The success of the Rhodesian government special forces in supplying guerrilla groups with poisoned clothing and food led to unexplained deaths – deaths especially traumatic because of their mysterious origin. Pre-existing cultural beliefs left the way open for the practice of witchcraft to be blamed; and accusations against individuals soon followed. The cycle of trauma then intensified when one of those subsequently killed, a suspected witch who was burned to death, appeared to have laid a posthumous curse on the guerrillas, since they continued to die mysteriously. Various traditional methods deployed to allay her spirit failed to stop these deaths, and more witch hunts and civilian killings followed.

McGregor tracks the efforts made, in the tense wartime atmosphere, to halt the cycle of killings, by both local communities and the guerrillas. The former involved traditional mediums and Zionist prophets in an attempt to forestall random or grudge-motivated identification of witches. The guerrilla forces and their political organization demanded evidence rather than denunciation, and insisted that the killing of witches was not consonant with their constitution and vision of the future. She concludes with an examination of efforts made by various parties since the war to understand what happened. McGregor's study not only reveals the crucial importance of strongly-articulated political and cultural structures in partially containing the spiral of trauma which threatened to get out of control; it also shows the extent to which the Rhodesian tactic, though it ultimately failed to affect the outcome of the war, nevertheless to a degree 'poisoned the future'.

Two further papers address themselves to the issue of public acknowledgement of trauma. Susan Rose, writing as a sociologist, is concerned with the traumatic effects of sexual abuse, and with the struggle waged by female survivors to name the experience and thus to claim a part of themselves hitherto split off and lost. The life-enhancing importance of this effort to articulate the meaning of traumatic experience is demonstrated with reference to the Clothesline Project developed in the USA during the mid-1990s. Women were invited to design and make tee-shirts expressing the personal significance of the violence they had suffered through abuse, its subsequent impact on their lives and sense of self, and the healing process (of which the Clothesline Project was itself a part) in which they were not engaged. A number of women were then interviewed about the way they had symbolized the damaging and the recovery of the self, expressing their current feelings and understandings about what had happened to them.

Rose addresses both the tee-shirt representations and the life stories told in interview. Drawing on psychological theory of trauma, she explores the central importance of narration to remembering and recovery. In her account, psychic defence mechanisms mobilized in self-protection whilst abuse is taking place – mechanisms of dissociation and denial – split off the experience of abuse and separate it out from ordinary experience. As a result the self becomes divided, so that the trauma becomes the experience of someone else; as in the case of one who symbolically leaves her body and watches the action of abuse from another place (from the ceiling or through a window). Recovering the memory of abuse, argues Rose, involves the re-integration of these divided part-selves, or at least the establishment of a dialogue between them. This process depends on telling the story of the abuse; that is, on naming it as such, and claiming it as a part one's own full experience, integrated into a life story with a before and an after. To do so, the survivor must necessarily challenge the abuser's story of events, with its power to deny any acknowledgement that abuse has indeed been perpetrated, or any recognition of the suffering entailed. In these circumstances, Rose suggests, to remember trauma is to fashion a new form of narrative that calls in question the received knowledges of a culture. The existence of a listener who is prepared to hear and recognize the truth of the survivor's story is fundamental to her empowerment. The politics of trauma, for Rose, lies in this relationship between telling and listening.

Graham Dawson's contribution is concerned with a key theme in contemporary politics: the immense difficulty of coming to terms with the legacy of violent civil conflict within a society. He offers a very precise analysis of the concept of trauma, arguing its applicability to the impact of the Northern Ireland conflict of the past thirty years. He carefully delineates the ways in which the Unionist/Loyalist and Nationalist/Republican communities commemorate their own losses, situating them within a much longer historical narrative stretching back to 1916 (Easter Rising/Battle of the Somme) and before. This serves to commemorate the dead, as well as the suffering of the bereaved; and to locate these losses within a continuing political struggle which gives them meaning. Successive British governments, however, have been able largely to disavow both their share in this traumatic history, and its reciprocal impact on British policy and people.

The commemoration of death and suffering strengthens the political identity of the separate traditions. The impact of trauma within selective narratives of political memorializing or amnesia, makes it extremely difficult for either Northern Irish tradition to recognize the trauma of the other, or for the British government to acknowledge its own role. Dawson shows this in tracing Republican, Loyalist and government stances towards the Bloody Sunday killings in Derry in 1972. This relatively enduring, if mutually

22

hostile, tradition of public commemoration of loss during the Troubles, has in recent years come into conflict with the demand orchestrated by the British and Irish governments to 'overcome the legacy of history', to leave behind the bitterness of the past and move on. This approach, Dawson argues, risks abandoning those individuals and communities who have suffered trauma, with no public recognition of, or accounting for, the causes and impact of their loss. Against this he counterposes recent efforts in Northern Ireland during the paramilitary ceasefire to embark upon efforts of reparative remembering, to create spaces in which all deaths and maimings can be recognized, and their traumatic effects acknowledged. In a postscript he notes the impact of this agenda on the terms of the April 1998 Agreement.

All these contributions, whatever part of the world they focus on and whatever methods and perspectives they employ, are concerned with very painful aspects of the past which live on in the present, whether as private nightmares or as public conflicts. Researching trauma – even editing a volume on the theme – can be a difficult experience on all sides, both ethically and emotionally. We believe that it is a crucial theme to address, not only intellectually but also because the legacy of trauma raises such immediate personal and political issues and dilemmas. And as we read these stories it is important for us to remember that all the words printed here can have little significant impact on the ultimate loneliness of those who suffer such deep psychic wounds from social dislocation and violence.

> To stand in the shadow
> of the scar up in the air
> To stand-for-no-one-and-nothing
> Unrecognized,
> for you alone.
> With all there is room for in that,
> even without,
> language.
> (Paul Celan 1971, quoted in Rosenfeld 1980: 105)

Notes

1 The Survivors of the Holocaust Visual History Foundation is an international project for the video-recording Second World War Holocaust survivors, initiated by filmmaker Steven Spielberg in 1994.
2 Caruth refers to the French film *Hiroshima mon Amour*, screenplay by Alain Resnais and Marguerite Duras, transl. Richard Seaver (New York, 1961).

References

Antze, P. and Lambek M. (eds) (1996) *Tense Past: Cultural Essays in Trauma and Memory*, London.

Barker, P. (1995) *The Ghost Road* in *The Regeneration Trilogy*, London.

Bartemeier, L. H. *et al.* (1946) 'Combat exhaustion', *Journal of Nervous and Mental Diseases* vol. 104.

Bettelheim, B. (1952) *Surviving and Other Essays*, New York.

Boraine, A., Levy J. and Scheffer, R. (1997) *Dealing with the Past: Truth and Reconciliation in South Africa*, Cape Town.

Bourdieu, P. (1991) *Language and Symbolic Power*, London.

Bourke, J. (1996) *Dismembering the Male: Men's Bodies, Britain and the Great War*, London.

Brandon, S. (1998) 'Recovered memory: the nature of the controversy', *Psychiatric Bulletin* vol. 22.

Brandon, S., Boakes, J., Glaser D. (1998) 'Recovered memories of childhood sexual abuse: implications for clinical practice', *British Journal of Psychiatry*: 172.

Breur, J and Freud, S (1895) *Studies on Hysteria,* London.

Brown, L. S. (1995) 'Not outside the range: one feminist perspective on psychic trauma' in C. Caruth (ed.), *Trauma: Explorations in Memory*, Baltimore.

Burchardt, N. (1993) 'Transgenerational transmission in the families of Holocaust survivors in England', in D. Bertaux and P. Thompson (eds), *Between Generations: Family Models, Myths and Memories* (International Yearbook of Oral History and Life Stories, vol. 2), Oxford: pp. 121–37.

Caruth, C. (1995) 'An interview with Robert J. Lifton', in C. Caruth (ed.), *Trauma: Explorations in Memory*, Baltimore.

Caruth, C. (1996) *Unclaimed Experience: Trauma, Narrative and History*, Baltimore.

Celan, P. (1971) *Speech-Grille and Selected Poems*, trans. J. Neugroschel (New York, 1971), quoted in A. H. Rosenfeld, *A Double Dying: Reflections on Holocaust Literature*, (1980) Indiana.

Cohen, R. L. (1987) 'Post–traumatic stress disorder: does it clear up when the litigation is settled?' *British Journal of Hospital Medicine* vol. 37.

Conway, M. (ed.) (1997) *Recovered Memories and False Memories*, Oxford.

Crews, F. C. *et al.* (1997) *The Memory Wars: Freud's Legacy in Dispute,* London.

Dante Alighieri (1998) *The Divine Comedy, 1: Inferno*, Oxford.

Dawes, A. (1992) 'Psychological discourse about political violence and its effects on children', International Seminar on the Mental Health of Refugee Children Exposed to Violent Environments, Refugee Studies Programme, Oxford University.

Ellis, J. (1980) *The Sharp End of War: The Fighting Man in World War Two*, Newton Abbot.

Erikson, K. T. (1994) *A New Species of Trouble: The Human Experience of Modern Disasters*, New York.

Fanon, F. (1961) *Les Damnés de la Terre*, translated as *The Wretched of the Earth* (1967) London.

Furst, S. (ed.) (1986) *Psychic Trauma*, New York.

Garton Ash, T. (1997) 'True confessions', *New York Review of Books,* 17 July.

Hass, A. (1991) *In the Shadow of the Holocaust*, London.

Herman, J. L. (1992) *Trauma and Recovery: From Domestic Abuse to Political Terror*, New York.

Holmes, J. and Roberts, G. (eds.) (1999 forthcoming) *Narrative Approaches in Psychiatry and Psychotherapy*, Oxford.

Hyman, I. E. (Jnr) and Loftus, E. (1997) 'Some people recover memories of childhood trauma that never really happened', in P. S. Appelbaum, L. A. Uyehara and M. R. Elin (eds), *Trauma and Memory*, Oxford, pp. 3–24.

Khubova, D., Ivankiev, A. and Sharova, T. (1992) 'After glasnost: oral history in the Soviet Union', in L. Passerini (ed.), *Memory and Totalitarianism*, (International Yearbook of Oral History and Life Stories, vol. 1), Oxford, pp. 89–102.

Langer, L. L. (1991) *Holocaust Testimonies: The Ruins of Memory*, New Haven.

Laub, D. (1995) 'Truth and testimony', in C. Caruth (ed.), *Trauma: Explorations in Memory*, Baltimore.

Levi, P. (1986) *Moments of Reprieve*, New York, cited in S. Friedlander (1993) *Memory, History and the Extermination of the Jews of Europe*, Bloomington.

Miller, H. (1961) 'Accident Neurosis', *British Medical Journal*, vol. 1., pp. 919–25.

Niethammer, L. (1985) 'Fragen antworten fragen', in L. Niethammer and A. von Plato (eds), *Wir Kriegen Jetzt andere Zeiten: Auf der Suche nach der Erfahrung des Volkes in Nachfaschistische Länder. Lebensgeschichte und Sozialkultur im Ruhrgebiet 1930–1960,* Berlin, pp. 392–448.

Niethammer, L. (1992) 'Where were *you* on 17 June? A niche in memory', in L. Passerini (ed.), *Memory and Totalitarianism* (International Yearbook of Oral History and Life Stories, vol. 1), Oxford, pp. 45–71.

O'Hagan, A. (1998) 'To forgive – and not forget', *Guardian Weekly*, 4 January.

Pahl, R. and Thompson, P. (1994) 'Meanings, myths and mystifications: the social construction of life stories in Russia', in C. M. Hann (ed.), *When History Accelerates: Essays on Rapid Change, Complexity and Creativity*, London, pp. 143–77.

Pepys, S. (1667) quoted in R. J. Daly (1983), 'Samuel Pepys and post–traumatic stress disorder', *British Journal of Psychology*, no. 143, pp. 64–8.

Pynoos, R. S., Steinberg A. M. and Goenjian, A. (1996) 'Traumatic stress in childhood and adolescence: recent developments and current controversies', in B. A. van der Kolk, A. McFarlane and L. Weisaeth (eds), *Traumatic Stress: The Effects of Overwhelming Experience on Mind, Body and Society,* New York, pp. 331–59.

Rivers, W. H. R. (1920) *Conflict and Dreams*, London.

Rose, N. (1985) *The Psychological Complex: Psychology, Politics and Society 1869–1939*, London.

Rosenfeld, A. H. (1980) *A Double Dying: Reflections on Holocaust Literature*, Indiana.

Sandler, J. *et al.* (1991) 'An approach to conceptual research in psychoanalysis illustrated by a consideration of psychic trauma', *International Review of Psychoanalysis*, vol. 18 pp. 113–41.

Sartre, J.-P. (1961) Preface to Fanon, *Les Damnés de la Terre* (1961), translated as *The Wretched of the Earth* (1967) London.

Sex in a Cold Climate, dir. S. Humphries, broadcast in the UK Channel 4 series *Witness* (16 March 1998).

Sherbakova, I. (1992) 'The Gulag in memory', in L. Passerini (ed.), *Memory and Totalitarianism*, (International Yearbook of Oral History and Life Stories, vol. 1), Oxford, pp. 103–16.

Showalter, E. (1997) *Hystories: Hysterical Epidemics and Modern Culture,* London.

Solzhenitsyn, A. (1974) *The Gulag Archipelago, 1918–1956: An Experiment in Literary Investigation*, London.

Terr, L. (1990) *Too Scared to Cry: How Trauma Affects Children and Ultimately Us All*, New York.

Thompson, P. (1988) *The Voice of the Past,* 2nd edn, Oxford.

van der Kolk, B. A. (1996) 'Trauma and memory', in B. A. van der Kolk, A. McFarlane and L. Weisaeth (eds), *Traumatic Stress: the Effects of Overwhelming Experience on Mind, Body and Society*, New York, pp. 279–303.

van der Kolk, B. A. and Fisler, R. (1996) 'Dissociation and the fragmentary nature of traumatic memories: overview', *British Journal of Psychotherapy*, vol. 12, no. 3.

Wardl, D. (1992) *Memorial Candles: Children of the Holocaust,* London.

Part 1

CASE STUDIES

1

TRAUMA SIGNALS IN LIFE STORIES

Gadi BenEzer

The concept of trauma does not have a straightforward definition. It is used by psychologists, psychoanalysts and researchers in a variety of meanings (Sandler *et al.* 1991; Dawes 1992; Furst 1967). I shall not attempt here to add theoretically to the concept or even to discuss in full its lack of clarity. For the purpose of this article suffice it to say that psychoanalysts and psychologists use the term to denote two main meanings: first, an event which happened in the external world, *together* with the way it was subjectively experienced. The external and internal reality are put together through the common reference to a 'traumatic state' or 'situation' which is their nexus. The second main meaning refers to some pathological consequences which are interpreted – through extrapolation backwards in time – as having been initiated by the trauma. These dimensions of meaning (Sandler and Sandler 1983; Sandler *et al.* 1991) can also be found in the literature on refugee trauma as, for example, in Millica's Harvard Trauma Questionnaire, HTQ (Mollica *et al.* 1992) and in many others. In this paper I shall mainly use the term trauma referring to the first meaning mentioned above.

Life stories seem to be particularly suitable for gaining an understanding of the significance of trauma in people's lives. Traumatic events create a multifaceted complex of reactions, which may even be contradictory at times. The life story method enables these contradictions and complexities to be legitimately included within the various parts of the story (while questionnaires and even question and answer modes force the person to 'choose' and to 'decide' between optional reactions).

Trauma is a very intimate experience; its meaning very personal. A life story technique with its non-interfering focus (in narrative interviews in particular (Rosenthal 1991)), enables the person to share his/her most intimate experiences which involve, in many cases, feelings of shame, guilt, and the like, which are not otherwise easy to express.[1] It also enables the person to reconstruct the meaning of the traumatic experiences to him or herself, as well as to the interviewer. In many cases, traumatic events change their meaning during the course of a person's life. Life stories, as Gelia Frank has suggested (Frank and Vanderburgh 1986), are not only a list of events but include evaluations of the experience. Thus, life stories can reveal these changes in the meaning of trauma at various stages of a person's life.

It is apparent, too, that traumatic events never happen in a social vacuum. They are connected to the social context in which they take place. In many if not most cases, they are related to the norms of society and to what is spoken about and what is kept silent in public. Life stories include an exposition of the relation between the private and the collective context. They can thus give a better understanding of both the personal trauma, as it is viewed within a social context, and of the social milieu, as reflected in the individual's life.

Only a few researchers have studied trauma using life story (or narrative) interviews (Heizner 1994). Labov analysed difficult experiences within stories of black youth in New York as part of his evaluation theory. Dan Bar-On (1994) and Dwork (1991) have researched the life stories of Holocaust survivors. Rosenthal (1991) and Bar-On (1989) have studied the psychological legacy of the Holocaust for the German people of various generations through their life stories. Lomsky-Feder (1995) has looked at the effects of war on the life stories of young Israeli men; Leiblich (1994) has studied the life stories of those who went through the traumatic experience of captivity, and Agger (1994) has studied narratives of refugee women who were subjected to sexual and other torture.

These different studies centred on the context and thematic organization of the text rather than on the linguistic-narrative behaviour of the interviewees.

Some researchers have studied the rhetoric of trauma. Osgood (1960), for example, researched written texts. He studied suicide letters and looked at the general influence of mental stress on linguistic abilities; and more recently, Heizner (1994) looked at the rhetoric of trauma in both oral and written texts, in personal narratives as well as in the literary reconstructions of traumatic experiences.

This paper tries to add to this developing scientific literature by charting possible verbal and non-verbal trauma signals within the life story. It considers the various ways in which trauma is expressed within the form of personal narrative, both verbally and in non-verbal communications. I suggest that traumatic experiences, even if the person has come to terms with them, are narrated in a unique way within narratives, and that these ways could be 'charted' and detected within the stories. This paper is based on narratives of the journey of young Ethiopian Jews migrating on foot to Israel. It is part of a larger study on the subject (BenEzer 1992, 1995), which I shall describe briefly below.

The study of the journey stories

During the period 1977–85, some 20,000 Ethiopian Jews left their homes in Ethiopia and – motivated by an ancient dream of returning to the land of their ancestors, to 'Yerussalem' – embarked on a secret and highly traumatic exodus to Israel. Due to various political circumstances, they had to leave their homes in haste, and go a long way on foot through unknown country towards the Sudan. They stayed for a period of one to two years in refugee camps there until they were brought to Israel. Conditions on the journey were extremely difficult, including incarcerations, attacks by bandits, walking at night over mountains, illness and death. A fifth of this group of migrant-refugees, 4,000 people, did not survive the journey. Each and every family suffered some loss of life. They also faced problems connected with their Jewish identity and the fact that they were heading for Israel. The trauma was thus perceived as collective as well as personal.

The study I conducted focused on the experience of this journey, its meaning for the people who made it and its relation to the initial encounter with Israeli society. It aimed to fill a gap in the existing literature in relation to migration journeys and refugee studies. It argued that powerful processes occur on such journeys which affect the individual and the community in life-changing ways, including the initial encounter with, and adaptation to, the new society.

Forty five young people were interviewed in the tradition of the narrative interview and their personal stories of the journey were then analysed. Three main themes expressed the major dimensions of meaning through which Ethiopian Jews constructed their experiences along the journey: the theme of Jewish identity, the theme of suffering and that of bravery and inner strength. The kinds of experience relating to these themes were presented and discussed in full in the study. The psycho-social impact of the journey on the individual and on the community was also analysed, focusing mainly on the relationship between coping and meaning, on trauma and on personal development and growth.

The three major themes derived from the journey, which also constitute dimensions of self-concept, correspond to the three main aspects and myths prevalent in Israeli society during the 1980s. However, Israeli society failed to acknowledge Ethiopian Jews' self-perception, thus causing considerable difficulties in their adaptation. The study concludes by showing how Ethiopian Jews use the story of their journey in order to assert their own self-concept and identity and to find their place within Israeli society. It is also suggested that the story of the journey is in the process of itself turning into a myth.

Trauma and trauma signals

This paper takes up a subsidiary issue of the study: the ways in which traumatic experiences are expressed in the narratives.

Ethiopian Jewish adolescents experienced on their journey one or more painful experiences that constituted traumatic events for them.[2] For some adolescents, the whole experience of the journey was coloured by their traumatization and was accordingly perceived mainly as a traumatic experience.

Trauma was brought about by a range of situations. These included situations in which their lives were in danger; when they suffered the loss of a parent, relative or close friend; went through separation or disintegration of the family; experienced a total inability to walk any further; were subjected to hunger, thirst, or what seemed to be fatal disease; suffered persecution and torture and were subjected to violation of body boundaries; underwent painful events connected to their Jewish identity; or witnessed any or all of these in others, whether as a single incident or repeatedly.

I should add here that many of the events of this particular migration journey would have traumatized anyone who had experienced them. Traumatization, however, is related to, and imbued with, the *meaning* of the event for the individual (Klein 1976, Garbarino 1992). The meaning given to any of a series of events is related, among other factors, to one's life history and personal biases, priorities and sensitivities.

Let me emphasize, however, two aspects of the journey that had an impact on the whole community. They were both sources of trauma and also raised the overall level (baseline) of pain, thus lowering the threshold for traumatization. I refer, first, to the separation from parents and, second, to the shock following the realization that they would have to stay in the Sudan for a long period. I shall elaborate below.

Many Ethiopian adolescents set out on their journey without their parents. Some had been sent by their parents in order to ensure that at least the adolescents' migration might be secured, if at all possible; others were sent ahead of the family in order to check whether there was really a passage to Israel via the Sudan; and many ran away with their peers, without their parents' consent.

Separation affected the adolescents because, first of all, it forced them to experience the journey without the particular and almost irreplaceable support that the proximity of parents normally gives to children.[2] As well as protecting them against real dangers, parents supply children and adolescents with a feeling of safety which affects the way that they deal with events and whether they experience them as traumatizing. Moreover, by their verbal and non-verbal responses parents also interpret the environment for their children, supplying children with the meaning of occurrences, and thus of their traumatic or non-traumatic significance.[3]

In the Ethiopian context, where decision making is maintained by familial authority, parents and family serve as an even stronger protective and supportive layer for the individual child. Adolescents had thus been less accustomed to handling their multi-generational social world and to making important decisions by themselves. Moreover they were also accustomed to being more 'emotionally refuelled' within the intensive relations of the Ethiopian family so that an individual would often feel incomplete when separated from his or her parents for a long time.[4] Separation, therefore, left these adolescents particularly vulnerable, and made them more prone to traumatization.

The shock of arriving in the Sudan, and discovering that it was not Jerusalem, was a second factor that affected their vulnerability to trauma. The wayfarers had been convinced that once they arrived in the Sudan they would immediately be transferred to Israel. Their 'part' was to arrive in the Sudan; the Israeli government's 'part' was to get them to Israel straight away. The thought of that, the inner conviction that their mission was only to complete the tough walking section of the journey, helped them to cope with the difficult and demanding trail. In their stories they report that although they had known that the Sudan was not Israel, they kept concentrating their minds on arriving in the Sudan, feeling and thinking that it was actually the end of their journey, the arrival in the promised land. Some even tell of people throwing away extra clothes at the border because they felt they had arrived in Israel, or were just about to do so. One youngster recounts how, upon arriving in the Sudan, he had sent a letter back to his parents in Ethiopia telling them that he had indeed arrived in Jerusalem.

Thus, realizing that they would have to stay for a very long time in the Sudan came as a complete shock to them. It turned the immediate gratification of getting to Israel, which they had anticipated during their journey, into a deep and painful disappointment. It demoralized them. Instead of finally being able to settle down peacefully, they had to call once again on their inner resources in order to deal with conditions in the Sudan. In order to cope with the harsh refugee existence, they had to reorientate themselves and to review their ideas of their immediate future. They were also faced with self-doubt and questions about the wisdom of their initial decision to set out. The shock of crossing into the Sudan and realizing that it was not the end of their journey put the sacrifices they had already made into a new light and resulted in many personal crises.

The impact of separation from parents and the shock of arriving and staying in the Sudan thus lowered the overall resistance of the adolescents to those potentially traumatizing events which had occurred on the journey and in the Sudan.

Before discussing the specific trauma signals, it is important to note one additional methodological aspect of this study: I refer to the adaptations in interviewing techniques which took into account the cross-cultural context. These adaptations were partly developed through many years of work as a clinical psychologist/psychotherapist with Ethiopian Jews, as well as specifically for this research. They were intended to overcome the problem of trust in the inter-cultural situation, and the misunderstandings that could arise from the different cultural communication codes of interviewee and interviewer (BenEzer 1987, 1995). In particular, techniques were invented to circumvent the Ethiopian cultural dictum of reserve and containment concerning painful experiences, suffering and trauma, so they could be included in the stories. These adaptations, however, are not elaborated here.

Trauma signals

How then are traumatic experiences detected in the life stories? Are there specific signals of trauma within narratives?

I would like to suggest that when an interviewee is recounting a traumatic experience – even if it is an experience with which he/she has come to terms – it will still produce particular forms of expression within the narrative. In other words, traumata are related differently from the rest of the story. These signals of traumata within the narration are listed below. They are not proposed as diagnostic criteria of trauma in the clinical sense but as a way of detecting traumatic experiences within narratives. It is worth adding that in many of the cases two or more of these narration signals of trauma are found within the account. Thirteen of these narrative signals of trauma were identified within the present study:

1 *Self-report*: the individual reports that a certain event was traumatic (carries a traumatic significance through its related emotions, meaning, or consequences). Examples include telling of an event's special painfulness, emphasizing it as being extremely distressing or wounding, or referring to its particularly negative (and/or long term) unsettling effect on the individual. This may also take the form of reporting an 'image of ultimate horror'; an event or a scene which serves as a symbol of a series of traumata experienced or witnessed. These traumata are thereby represented by one which is related as being the most horrifying of them all, due to its particular meaning for the individual.[5]

2 A *'hidden' event*: an event which was not narrated in the main story comes up during the probing phase, accompanied by distressing emotions such as mourning, grief, shame or guilt which were not previously expressed during the telling of the story.

3 *Long silence*: a long silence occurs before or after the narration of a certain event (or a particular part of it), which seems to have a particularly painful or tormenting quality for the individual.

4 *Loss of emotional control*: sudden loss of control over emotions relating to an event which is being narrated is expressed in sobbing, rage, or other responses which are uncharacteristic of this person's recounting.

5 *Emotional detachment or numbness*: individuals report events which seem to have had a horrifying quality or horrifying consequences for them but show no emotions during the narration. It is as if there is a forced detachment, due to the event's traumatic quality, isolating it from the

emotional life of the individual. The individual seems to be staying rigorously within the verbal mode of reporting (frequently with an unvarying tone of voice and 'frozen' facial expression and body gestures) not engaging his or her feelings at all in this act, as if suffering from what has been described as 'psychic numbness'.

6   *Repetitive reporting:* a distressing experience is re-told in its entirety or with an extraordinary reiteration of its minute details, time and time again, as if the narrator is unable to move on, which is in contrast to his or her style of narration in the rest of the account.

7   *Losing oneself in the traumatic event:* speakers seem to disappear from the reality of the interview while narrating a traumatic event. They appear to sink into themselves, submerged and overwhelmed by the event in the middle of recounting it. They may be unable to emerge without the help of the interviewer; or without some shaking of themselves (sometimes physically as well as emotionally) as if trying to lift themselves up from a hole, maybe a mental hole they fell into via the trauma. This often expresses itself in an extraordinarily extended period of silence but, unlike the long silence described above, this one seems to be unending, and there are clear signs that the person is not there, is not experiencing the *current* situation. Rather he or she is completely submerged in the traumatic event.

8   *Intrusive images:* scenes or images of a traumatic event, or a particular fraction of it, come up involuntarily throughout the narration as quick 'flashes', which clearly distract the persons' train of thought and interrupt the intended flow of the narrative. The person sometimes apologizes, or verbally expresses uneasiness, while admitting the recurrence of an image.

9   *Forceful argumentation of conduct within an event:* narrators stress the reasons for their behaviour within a situation instead of relating the facts, as if the traumatic quality of the event is connected to their conduct in that situation which they feel they should justify. The argumentation seems to reflect a wish to prevent an independent conclusion by the interviewer about what happened.[6]

10 *Cognitive-emotional disorientation:* this is characterized by a disappearance of the boundaries between the event which is being recounted and the situation of the interview. This may be expressed in relating to the interviewer as a figure within the story (without the 'as if' quality that is sometimes used in recounting). For example, the narrator may shout at the interviewer in answer to an interrogative figure within the narrative. Speakers may lose their sense of exactly where they are, within the story as well as in reality, yet continue to recount the event or utter unintelligible words in trying to express themselves, until they break down in tears, or come back to themselves, or until they are comforted and relaxed by the interviewer.[7]

11 *Inability to tell a story at all:* the speaker may wish to tell the story but is

35

unable to speak of it, getting stuck, typically, at the starting point of the narration. If repeated attempts at narration fail, the interviewer is obliged to resort to a question and answer mode of interview, which will circumvent the particular contents of the trauma (unknown to the interviewer at the start).

12 *Changes in voice:* the narration of trauma is often accompanied by changes in voice. The tone of the voice, its pitch or its 'colouring' will change while narrating a traumatic event. It may turn quiet, or hoarse, or the opposite of these, but in any event, it is different from the person's usual voice.

13 *Changes in body language:* facial expressions and body posture may also change during the recounting of a traumatic event. People may 'retreat into' themselves by adopting a 'foetal' posture in the chair, signifying pain (which is a universal genetically-based posture of humans when experiencing pain) (Morris 1977). They may attempt to cover trembling lips with hands, trying to control emotional expression but then giving way to crying. Some may clutch their legs strongly together, or wrap one around the other, during the whole time that they are recounting the trauma, and then release them again. Particular gesticulations with the hands also sometimes appear during narration of traumatic experiences, and end when the narration is completed. All these serve as additional, non-verbal signals for detection of a traumatic event during narration.

Let me now exemplify various signals of trauma by presenting some excerpts from life stories. Each includes more than one signal of trauma. As mentioned above, when a traumatic experience is recounted in the life story, more than one signal of trauma is commonly expressed during the narration.

One girl in our study, for example, was unable to narrate her journey experience at all. She froze immediately after starting her account. After a few unsuccessful attempts to continue, she paused for a long time and then said: 'I cannot do it.' She wept. It turned out that her traumatic separation from her parents, who had been left in Ethiopia, came between her and the act of narration. This separation had not yet been processed in a way which would allow her to tell her story. She had not made a story out of it, not even for herself. It was unnarrateable then. And since it was supposed to be the beginning of her story, that is where she got stuck.

The process underlying this inability to tell a story could be understood as follows: when a trauma remains alive, active, not processed, people will have difficulty in connecting it to their life histories. In such cases this will also affect the life story as a whole. People will find it difficult to construct a story for themselves which will include trauma in a 'manageable' way (so that they can successfully' sail through it'). The trauma will still be too emotionally (psychically) charged for that to happen, and will interfere with any recounting of the event to others. Roy Schafer (1981) argues that when we tell our life story to others we are always telling it to ourselves as well. An inability to tell it to ourselves thus prevents us from narrating it to others. What he means is that the boundaries between the experiencing self (the self of the event) and the constructing self (that of the present, in fact a re-constructing self) cannot be maintained; they will keep dissolving. In such cases, therefore, the life story cannot be narrated.

A thirteen-year-old boy named Yoav, who came from the village of Keftah, Wolkite, went through the traumatizing experience of death within the family.[8] He lost his nephew during their stay in the Sudan. He did not recount it at first. Apparently it was too painful. The story only came up in the probing phase of the interview. When asked about deaths on the way he became silent and then recounted:

> My sister's son – he was three years younger than me [pauses]. I was there [in the Sudan] when he died. I do not know the cause of his death. It is hard. [silence]. Hard. A child, you grow up with him, are fond of him, and suddenly – [silence]; especially for the family, they do not have [another] son, only girls. . .

Yoav stops his story, there is a very long silence, his eyes become wet, and he begins to sob. After a cry, he rolls into himself and keeps silent. At times, he still rubs his eyes as if trying to block another wave of tears. A very long silence ensues. I try to help him by gently asking a question but he is still very much immersed within himself and does not hear it. He just raises his head asking 'Eh?' [pardon?]. I repeat my question but he still seems far away, and answers a different question. After another long silence he seems ready to continue. He remembers: 'We needed to bury him. There was a problem, one had to look for a place and so on. I do not know – I do not think . . .' Yoav stops. He cannot continue his story.

It is not surprising, it seems to me, that this event was not recounted in the first phase of the interview. Yoav had grown up with the boy and loved him. Most distressingly, as he perceived it, the boy was his sister's only son and she had not had another child since. He empathized with her pain at the loss of her only son among seven children.

The various signals of trauma appear in the telling of this experience. It is a 'hidden event' which is not told in the first flow of the narration of the story; there are long silences; there is a loss of emotional control which did not happen in the rest of the interview/story; and he loses himself in the traumatic event, to the point of actual blocking or not receiving auditory stimuli; and at the end, there is an inability to continue the narration of the traumatic experience. All these signals, as we have noted, signify the traumatic nature of the experience.

A trauma related to humiliation was experienced by Daniel, a seventeen-year-old boy from the Gonder region in Ethiopia. During their stay in the Sudan, he tried to escape with a group of friends from the refugee camp of Um-Rakuba to the town of Gedaref. Unfortunately they were captured by the Sudanese and imprisoned. Daniel was shouted at, beaten, and accused of being head of a *shifta* gang (outlaws in Ethiopia). He continues his account of the event:

> Then, on the second day there the prison commander came, called me, and when I approached him he took out a big pair of scissors and told his people to shave my hair. I was frightened but even more I was *angry*. Because . . . the commander said all kinds of things to me [insults related to his Jewishness]. And so they started, two of his men, one started here [points to one side of his head] and the other [silence] they took off all my hair! On that day I was . . . on that day . . . [finds it difficult to go on] I went inside myself [quiet]. [I realized that] if I said anything, if I let out one word, then they could do as they wished. So eh – I shut down my mind. They cursed me with all kinds of curses [talks in a very quiet tone] and so on – and later, [long pause] the sun was, what shall I tell you, the sun was *strong* and I was thinking of the sun, [being] without hair [whispers] . . . I shall never forget that day [keeps quiet for some time] . This is the worst, I suffered worst, I suffered very much. They made me bold, they did – [unclear]. So I became enraged. On that day I thought of my parents. Why had I come? How had I come to be separated from them? What did I have in the Sudan? And so on. I had a day [which was] very sad [extremely long silence] . . . they were laughing at me while they were cutting my hair, they were making fun of my hair . . . [stops].

Some of the trauma signals in this example are different from those in the previous one. First of all, there is 'self-report'; he himself says that it was the most painful and traumatic event of his journey. He reports that 'I went inside myself' and that he 'suffered worst' from this experience. He reports, also, the painful questions that he asked himself during and immediately after this event, which relate to the original motivation and bravery in going on a journey where such events could happen to him. Then there are other signals of trauma within the narration of the incident. There are long silences, changes in tone of voice which are not typical in the rest of his narrative, some loss of emotional control, connected to his rage within the traumatic situation, which lead him to end his account.

In my view, the subject of humiliation as a distinct source of trauma has not been sufficiently studied within the literature on children in war, refugees and migrants. In this study it comes out as a common source of trauma, perhaps because the sufferers were refugees, people without status and protection, and also culturally different. But even more so, they were

Jews, members of a despised professional caste in Ethiopia and the Sudan, belonging to an enemy country (Israel) and to a rival ethno-religious group.

The experience of deliberate humiliation by another human being constitutes for many individuals a 'narcissistic hurt' of an enormity which traumatizes them. Their self-image and self-esteem are affected and they find this hurt difficult to absorb and to recover from. As the [freely translated] Ethiopian proverb claims in relation to verbal abuse: 'Curses [insults] are of such a nature that, once uttered, they keep being [hurtfully] spoken in your mind.' Of course, it is not curses alone that we are concerned with here, but with other humiliating measures as well.

Rivka was twenty-four when she started her journey. She was married but had no children of her own. When she set out her eldest sister asked her to take her thirteen-year-old daughter (Rivka's niece) with her to Israel. The sister was very attached to this daughter, who was very beautiful and she found it difficult to part with her. Nevertheless, she wanted her to have a chance of reaching Israel and was not sure when she would be able to set out herself because her husband's parents were old and sick.

As it was a request from her eldest sister, whom she respected almost like a parent, Rivka agreed to do it. She knew how special this girl was for her sister and she also loved the girl as if she was her own younger sister. It was a grave responsibility and Rivka was determined to look after the girl and to make sure that she came to no harm on the journey.

When they arrived in the Sudan, there was a chaotic situation: refugees everywhere, famine and diseases. At night the camps turned into 'a different place', and she witnessed people being knifed and killed daily. Prostitutes were all around, and even during daylight the situation was dangerous, especially for the Jews who were the least organized group there. She tried to manage as best she could, attempting to confine herself and her sister's daughter to the tent or its immediate surroundings. The heat was unbearable and they had to go to look for water, of which there was never enough and which was always filthy.

One day, on coming back from her search for water, Rivka found that the girl had vanished. Rivka asked people round about what had happened, and they told her that they had seen the girl being led away by some fierce looking young men. It was later assumed that these young men were from the Tigrean community in the camp, but this knowledge did not help bring the girl back. What could Rivka do? She could not complain to the Sudanese police because she feared that that would mean revealing her Jewish identity. She had no one to turn to.

She kept looking for the girl, relentlessly, among the thousands of refugees. She searched the camp from end to end. Eventually, she discovered the girl but could not get her back. The Tigreans would not let her go. She was too beautiful, and they had sexually abused her. Rivka waited in hope. Her turn to go to Israel finally arrived but she would not go. People were dying around her in great numbers and she herself became sick as well. Her turn came for the third time, and, fearing that she too would soon die, she decided to go. The girl was left behind.

Rivka exemplifies what seems to be a condition of psychic numbness following an extremely traumatic event. She told her story with no emotion at all – without emotional expression on her face or in the sound of her voice, merely the repetition of the verbal utterance: 'Difficult. Difficult.' And this repeated word expressed it all. She would not allow herself to dwell on any moment of her journey. Restraining her emotions in relation to the trauma was her central inner task, and she kept to it like a dedicated guard to his post. At the end of her narration when the tape recorder was no longer running, she mentioned, as if in passing, that her brother-in-law had never written to her since then, because he was so angry with her for leaving his daughter in the Sudan.

Concluding remarks

This article shows the possible contribution of clinical psychology/psychotherapy to the analysis and understanding of life stories of trauma. We have seen how one can detect various communication signals, verbal and non-verbal, in order to get a better understanding of the emotional influence of various events on the interviewee's life. Specifically, we suggested thirteen signals of trauma within the form of the narrative.

I believe that sensitivity to these signals might enable researchers in various disciplines to detect traumatic events in interviews. Their understanding and interpretation of life stories would thus be enriched and become more accurate.

Understanding these signals might also have major practical implications. One example is for the analysis of the testimony of refugees seeking political asylum in other countries. In such cases accurate description and evaluation of the experiences the person has undergone, including their emotional impact, is crucial for decision-makers in deciding the fate of the application for asylum.

I will conclude this paper by giving some thought to the role of the interviewer faced with such sensitive and emotionally laden material. Most frequently, the researcher/interviewer is not a psychotherapist trained to deal with such matters. How then may the lay interviewer react to the recounting of a traumatic event? Two points seem relevant to this issue.

The first relates to the attentiveness of the interviewer. During any interview it is quite common for the interviewer's attention to fluctuate. Sometimes he or she is orientated towards the interviewee, trying to understand the content of the story, and noticing the ways in which the story is being told, or what the person felt about the situation, etc. At other times, the interviewer is orientated towards him or herself (i.e. thinking of the relevant issues beyond the content presently being recounted; or of questions to be asked in order to expand on the subject; or dealing with personal associations; or being partially absorbed with emotions aroused by the interview, etc.). The interviewer also has responsibility for aspects of the management of the interview, such as keeping time limits and avoiding unexpected external interruptions of the interview.

It is important to stress that once trauma signals are detected, interviewers should make a special effort to minimize these normal fluctuations of attention, and try to orient themselves entirely towards the interviewee. This is suggested because one aspect of trauma is that people feel 'enwrapped' in the traumatic experience, which segregates them from other people and makes them different in a range of ways. As a result they feel very much alone and isolated from others. They find it difficult to believe that people who have not gone through such an experience could indeed understand or empathize with them (Herman 1992: 214). Interviewers in these circumstances should try to become especially attentive to what the interviewee is going through. They should be more empathic and considerate than usual, listen with all senses and by doing so help the interviewee to feel that now he or she is not alone.

The second point relates to the issue of space within the interview. In many instances, traumata are related to experiences of violation of personal boundaries. These may be either body boundaries or boundaries of the psychic self. It is thus important to be particularly sensitive to the question of boundaries during the interview. Interviewers should give enough space to the interviewee and refrain from interventions which might be considered intrusive. They should respect what the person wants to give and not press too hard for further information. They should let the person narrate the traumatic event at his or her own pace, avoid asking too many questions and allow for longer silences in which the person can relive the experience if he or she needs to do so.

Notes

1 On 'cumulative trauma' see Khan 1963; on 'sequential trauma' see Keilson 1979.

2 See Bowlby (1951); (1960); (1980); Mahler (1979); Roberton and Robertson (1971); Anna Freud (1965); Burlingham and Freud (1943); Ainsworth (1969); Pine and Furer (1963); and Spitz (1950).

3 Reuven Feurstein *et al.* (1979) wrote of this process as 'mediation' and developed hypotheses in relation to the nature of such mediation and the degree to which it is needed by the child during different phases of development. Feurstein also developed a revolutionary diagnostic approach based on mediated learning.

4 Margaret Mahler used the concept of refuelling in respect of the infant or toddler in relation to its mother or 'mothering' figure (Mahler *et al.* 1975; Mahler 1979).

5 Robert Lifton (1979: 172) has suggested that people's vulnerability to intrusive

images is a defining feature of the 'traumatic syndrome'. These are images that 'can neither be enacted or cast aside'. In particular he focuses on the 'image of ultimate horror' which 'condenses the totality of the destruction and trauma and evokes particularly intense feelings of pity and self-condemnation in the survivor' (ibid.). Although Lifton's work did not specifically concern itself with how this was expressed in detail in narrative interviews, he did give some examples from interviews.

6 See also Gabriele Rosenthal (1989; 1991) on 'argumentation' as distinct from what she calls 'narration' within the narratives of different generations of German people in relation to their Second World War experiences.

7 A particularly dramatic example is reported by Abramowitch (1986) who interviewed a Greek Holocaust survivor in Israel. This interview took place in the interviewee's car, while parked outside his workplace. This was the only place where he would agree to meet the interviewer, due to a long 'forced silence' in which he had not told his traumatic experience to his family or work colleagues (or anyone else). Sitting in the car with the windows shut, the interviewee told his story of horror which included, at its centre, a partial castration by the Nazis: one of his testicles was removed in the immoral experiments on human beings in the concentration camp. Then, in the midst of telling his story, reaching a point where he spoke about the infamous 'selections' in the camp, he suddenly burst out: 'You mean Mengele? What do you mean?'. The interviewee was, as the interviewer emphatically describes, obviously disorientated. Abramowitch goes on to say that it seems as if the boundaries between the person's current speaking self and his Holocaust self had abruptly dissolved. For a moment he did not know if he was the person suffering in the camp or the one speaking about it. For this person, it seems to me that the 'image of ultimate horror' was also the 'melting point' of the two selves.

8 All names are pseudonyms.

References

Abramovitch, H. (1986) *There Are No Words: Two Greek-Jewish Survivors of Auschwitz,* unpublished manuscript.

Agger, I. (1994) *The Blue Room: Trauma and Testimony among Refugee Women: A Psycho-Social Exploration,* London and New Jersey: Zed Books.

Ainsworth, M. D. S. (1969) 'Object Relations, Dependency and Attachment: A Theoretical Review of the Infant-Mother Relationship', *Child Development,* vol. 40, pp. 969–1025.

Bar-On, D. (1989) *The Legacy of Silence: Encounters with Children of the Third Reich,* Cambridge, Mass.: Harvard University Press.

—— (1994) *Fear and Hope,* Tel-Aviv: Ghetto Fighter's House.

BenEzer, G. (1987) 'Cross-cultural misunderstandings: The case of Ethiopian immigrant Jews in Israeli society', in M. Ashkenazi and A. Weingrod (eds) *Ethiopian Jews and Israel,* New Brunswick and Oxford: Transaction Books.

—— (1990) 'Anorexia Nervosa or an Ethiopian Coping Style?', *Mind and Human Interaction,* vol. 2, no. 2, pp. 36–9.

—— (1992) *As Light Within A Clay Pot: Immigration and Absorption of Ethiopian Jews,* Jerusalem: Rubin Mass.

—— (1995) *Narratives of a Migration Journey: Ethiopian Jews on their Way to Israel (1977–85),* unpublished Ph.D. dissertation, University of Essex.

Bowlby, J. (1995) *Maternal Care and Mental Health,* Geneva: WHO, London: HMSO.

—— (1960) 'Separation and Anxiety', *International Journal of Psychoanalysis,* vol. 41, pp. 89–113.

—— (1980) *Loss: Sadness and Depression (Attachment and Loss vol. 3),* London: Hogarth Press and the Institute of Psychoanalysis.

Dawes, A. (1992) 'Psychological discourse about political violence and its effects on children', International Seminar on the Mental Health of Refugee Children Exposed to Violent Environments, Refugee Studies Programme, University of Oxford.

Dwork, D. (1991) *Children With A Star: Jewish Youth In Nazi Europe,* New Haven and London: Yale University Press.

Erikson, E. (1969) *Gandhi's Truth: On the Origins of Militant Non-Violence,* New York: Norton.

Feurstein, R., Rand, Y. and Hoffman, M. (1979) *The Dynamic Assessment of Retarded Performance: The Learning Potential Assessment Device. Theory. Instruments and Techniques,* Glenview, Ill.: Scott, Foresman and Co.

Frank, G. and Vanderburgh, R. M. (1986) 'Cross-cultural use of life history methods in gerontology', in C. L. Fry and J. Keith (eds) *New Methods for Old Age Research,* Massachusetts: Bergan and Garey.

Freud, A. (1965) *Normality and Pathology in Childhood:Assessments of Development,* New York: International University Press.

Furst, S. (ed.) (1986) *Psychic Trauma,* New York: Basic Books.

Garbarino, J. (1992) 'Developmental consequences of living in dangerous and unstable environments: the situation of refugee children', in M. McCallin (ed.), *The Psychological Well Being of Refugee Children: Research, Practice and Policy Issues,* Geneva: International Catholic Child Bureau.

Heizner, Z. (1994) *The Rhetoric of Trauma,* unpublished Ph.D. dissertation, Hebrew University of Jerusalem, in Hebrew.

Herman, J. L. (1992) *Trauma and Recovery: From Domestic Abuse to Political Terror,* New York, Basic Books.

Keilson, H. (1979) *Sequential Traumatisation Among Jewish Orphans,* Stuttgart: Ferdinand Enke Verlag.

Khan, M. M. R. (1963) 'The concept of cumulative trauma', *The Psychoanalytic Study of the Child, vol. 18,* pp. 286–306.

Klein, G. S. (1976) *Psychoanalytic Theory: An Explanation of Essentials,* New York: International University Press.

Labov, W. (1972) *Language of the Inner City: Studies In The Black English Vernacular,* Philadelphia: University of Pennsylvania Press.

Lieblich, A. (1994) *Seasons of Captivity,* New York: New York University Press.

Lifton, R. J. (1979) 'Survivor experience and traumatic syndrome', in *The Broken Connection: On Death and the Continuity of Life,* New York: Schuster.

Lomsky-Feder, E. (1995) 'The meaning of war through veterans' eyes: A psychological analysis of life stories', *International Sociology,* vol. 10, pp. 463–82.

Mahler, M. S. (1979) *The Selected Papers of Margaret S. Mahler, vols 1 and 2,* New York: Jason-Aronson.

Mahler, M. S., Pine, F. and Bergman, A. (1975) *The Psychological Birth of the Human Infant,* New York: Basic Books.

Morris, D. (1977) *Manwatching,* London: Jonathan Cape.

Osgood, C. H. (1960) 'Some effects of motivation on style of encoding', in T. A. Sebeok (ed.), *Style in Language,* Cambridge, Mass.: MIT Press.

Pine, F. and Furer, M. (1963) 'Studies of the separation-individuation phase: A methodical overview', *The Psychoanalytic Study of the Child, vol. 18,* pp. 325–42.

Robertson, James and Robertson, Joyce (1971) 'Young children in brief separation: a fresh look', *The Psychoanalytic Study of the Child, vol. 26,* pp. 264–315.

Robinson, V. (1992) 'Introduction', in V. Robinson, (ed.), *The International Refugee Crisis: British and Canadian Responses,* Basingstoke: Macmillan.

Rosenthal, G. (1945) 'The biographical meaning of a historical event', *International Journal of Oral History,* vol. 10, no. 3, pp. 183-93.

—— (1991) 'German war memories: Narrability and biographical and social functions of remembering', *Oral History,* vol. 19, pp. 34–42.

RPN (1992) *Refugee Participation Network: Issue on Refugee Children,* no. 12.

Sandler, J., Dreher, A. U., and Drews, S. (1991) 'An approach to conceptual research in psychoanalysis illustrated by a consideration of psychic trauma', *International Review of Psychoanalysis,* vol. 18, pp. 113–41.

Schafer, R. (1981) 'Narration in the psychoanalytic dialogue', in W. J. T. Mitchel (ed.), *On Narrative,* Chicago: Chicago University Press.

Spitz, R. A. (1950) 'Anxiety in infancy: A study of its manifestations in the first year of life', *International Journal of Psychoanalysis,* vol. 31, pp. 138–43.

2

REMEMBERING AND FORGETTING

Guatemalan war-widows' forbidden memories

Judith Zur

Re-membering and forgetting are two sides of the same phenomenon: the past in the present.[1] Both are employed, whether consciously or not, for a variety of social and political purposes. The Guatemalan government uses public, official memories for rhetorical and political purposes; widows, through reworking unofficial, secret memories, turn personal tragedies into narratives, thereby repositioning themselves in the past, constructing a sense of continuity and restoring a semblance of dignity.

The past which is in dispute is *La Violencia* (1978–85), the military dictatorship's assault on the country's rural population. In order to promote their version of the past, remembering the atrocities which comprised *La Violencia* is forbidden by the authorities.

La Violencia resulted from a collision between conflicting elements in Guatemala's socio-economic structure. Guatemala's export-led, labour-intensive plantation economy depends on subsistence farmers for its cheap, seasonal labour. This system allows Indians to retain their culture whilst simultaneously marginalizing them from the wider national society. Contact between *Ladinos* and Indians is generally distant, causing stereotypes of the other to fester.[2] *Ladinos* disparage Indians for their insistence on their traditional way of life but fear their 'natural' ('magical') powers. This mixture of fear and contempt probably accounts for the ferocity of the assault on indigenous communities.

The cultural, economic and social distance between *Ladinos* and Indians was emphasized when some indigenous communities converted to Catholicism in the 1950s, took liberation theology to heart and began self-help development projects: building their own schools, health clinics and so on. Aided by Catholic Action, agriculturalists also formed co-operatives and peasant unions, which brought down the wrath of the *Ladino* State which viewed these projects as a challenge to the status quo. Villages with 'progressive' institutions were said to be 'organized [against the State]' and labelled 'subversive'.

Despite the dictatorship's efforts to maintain the status quo, advances in agri-business technology since the I 960s undercut its social base by enabling the land-hungry plantation economy to expand into areas previously only tilled by Indians. Sometimes expropriation was partial, increasing pressure for land within a community and fracturing the fragile facade of village harmony; sometimes it was total. Resistance to eviction was labelled 'subversive'. The military was involved in village clearances and sometimes massacred recalcitrant Indians. Such events drove many Indians to join the guerrilla cause.

Nominally, *La Violencia* was a battle against guerrilla forces who had begun to regroup by the mid-1970s. Guatemala's military regime, headed by General Lucas Garcia from 1978 to1982, declared war on 'Marxist communism', which it viewed as an armed and dangerous menace within (McClintock 1985); dissidents and dissidence were to be eliminated once and for all. The concept of dissidence or, more accurately, 'otherness', soon led Guatemala's military machine – which has been called the most proficient, albeit brutal and corrupt, in Central America (Painter 1993) – to target the indigenous population. Millions of civilians were thus subsumed under the 'subversive' label.

By 1988, at least 130,000 political killings (GGIS 1992) and 38,000 'disappearances' had been committed by army, police and paramilitary government forces (Simon 1987). Most of the victims were indigenous. By 1985, when the first democratic elections were held for thirty years, at least 120,000 women (mostly of Mayan descent) had been widowed as a result of The Violence. The vast majority of these widows also lost other relatives as *La Violencia* cut a swathe through some families and communities.

Over 90 per cent of the population of the remote, highland province of El Quiché (where I worked between 1988 and 1990) is indigenous.[3] They refer to themselves as *naturales* and are part of the largest of Guatemala's twenty-two Indian sub-groups, the K'iche'. They speak a K'iche' dialect; most men but few women also speak rudimentary Spanish; very few have achieved basic literacy in Spanish.

Most K'iche' live in dispersed settlements grouped into villages. The mountainous terrain means that hamlets comprising a village can be an hour's walk from each other. The village of Emol is typical: it consists of five hamlets collectively known by the name of the largest.[4]

In the late 1970s, nearly 3,000 Emoltecos lived in over 500 households. Two-thirds of the villagers had converted to Catholicism in the 1950s. It was a relatively poor village, although some hamlets were poorer than others; one hamlet, Kotoh, organized several successful development projects. As Kotoh progressed and the more conservative Emol became comparatively poorer, the traditional rivalry between them developed into oven hostility. These local enmities were not perceived as relating to the wider, national unrest and villagers were shocked when, in late 1981, the army surrounded Kotoh and virtually destroyed it. Survivors claim that 1,000 villagers were killed in the following six months. The large number of decimated families and the burnt-out houses littering the landscape gives credence to these claims.

Exacerbating existing tensions within and between villages, setting one hamlet against another, was a standard army tactic. The resultant fragmentation of indigenous communities allowed the military to impose control with greater ease and also to obscure their involvement. Thus, after they had brutally suppressed guerrilla activity in the province, the army's public massacres and other atrocities in occupied villages were often viewed in terms of local relationships. Pacification also included the establishment of ostensibly voluntary civil patrols, which committed further atrocities within their communities not only on the army's behalf but, as the military had anticipated, to settle personal scores.[5]

Most Emoltecos promptly convened to evangelical Protestantism, the religion associated with the military. People who remained faithful to the traditional Mayan religion, known as *Costumbrismo,* found themselves lumped together with Catholics; both were accused of being 'subversive'. Today, all three religions co-exist within Emol, even in the same family. The widows presented here are Catholics or *Costumbristas* from Kotoh who cling tenaciously and publicly to their faiths which, in the culture of terror in which they live (Taussig 1984), shows considerable courage. But these women are not representative of all women, nor of all widows: their bravery and tenacity are exceptional.

The widows have experienced repeated acts of violence against themselves and their families. Their kin have been abducted, either singly or *en masse,* some privately from their homes at night and others publicly in daylight; they themselves or their younger female kin had been raped and sometimes gang-raped. Virtually all of El Quiché's estimated 11,000 war-widows can tell similar stories.

The most shocking and painful event of *La Violencia* for Emolteco widows was their enforced 'participation' in the public massacre of village men by other village men to whom both victims and witnesses were related. The victims' families and neighbours provided the necessary audience to this gruesome act of political theatre which destroyed not only the traditional way of doing things (*costumbre*) but also the emerging local alternatives (Catholic-based self-help). It imposed army-dictated power relationships mediated by violence in their stead. Speaking about the massacre and its victims was strictly prohibited.

Keeping silent in front of outsiders is a long-established indigenous coping stratagem. Keeping silent on the orders of village men, albeit men whose authority rests on external support, is totally new. The accompanying threats are equally new inside indigenous communities. The boundaries between inside and outside, private and public were completely re-drawn during *La Violencia*: in most households, the public sphere entered the private realm though the men's enforced patrol duty. The system provides a conduit for the State to promulgate its version of recent history to the country's indigenous citizens; it also provides the means to enforce this official 'truth'.

Both military and paramilitary leaders, on national and local levels respectively, are active in historical construction and historical amnesia, that is the suppression and neglect of alternative and oppositional voices (Williams 1977) such as those of human rights groups and relatives of the dead and disappeared.[6] Historical amnesia is a means of social control because it 'furnishes a base for undisputed triumph of official ideology, and because by weakening the sense of personal identity (by negating people's own history) it deprives them of a sense of efficacy and thus the capacity to organize and initiate actions' (Pateman 1980: 35).

Villagers also face insidious intimidation resulting from 'symbolic domination' (Bourdieu 1991: 72) for example, the same images of the dead are constantly vilified in the context of the political theatre of national security. They are criminalized as enemies of the State, portrayed as communists, as rebels excised from the national body in a cleansing of 'impure elements'; their surviving kin are accused of subversion by association. War-widows are labelled 'wives of the guerrilla', an army-endorsed license for mistreatment. Thus local patrol commanders and military commissioners, the perpetrators of much of the violence in the early 1980s, remain as village authorities to the present.[7] They continue to threaten, control, persecute and occasionally rape and kill widows with impunity.[8] Yet these men fear the power of women's speech.

The deliberate violence to people's memories is less tangible but just as profound as physical violence. Both kinds of violence continue today, because the terror machinery created during *La Violencia* remains intact. Political repression in Guatemala (and elsewhere) aims to ensure that citizens will psychologically repress or 'not see' the atrocious aspects of the government. And, if they do see, it is better that they do not remember. The entire history of *La Violencia* can be read as a war against memory, an Orwellian falsification of memory, a falsification and negation of reality.[9] The army attempts to deny people access to truth, thus contaminating their morality and their memory.

The terrorization which exists in El Quiche creates a divided reality which refuses to credit any particular explanation of a violent act as definitive. Memories of what actually happened are 'popular memories' (cf. Foucault 1975) which make a different truth-claim from official history. These unofficial memories can be studied as the politics of forgetting or as forms of counter-memory (cf. Nora). They are the residual or resistant strains which withstand official versions of historical continuity (Foucault 1977). Remembering in Emol, where leftist sympathies had been strong, therefore contradicts the official 'truth' which is that subversives and potential sympathizers need to be eradicated to protect the nation from being overwhelmed by armed rebels. This 'truth', enacted through an ideology of anti-communism, has become an official ideology of the Guatemalan Nation State in the post-war era.[10]

Women's refusal to accept the official version, which effectively silences them, immediately confronts the military government's agenda and turns private thoughts into unobtrusive political acts. Whatever the person's intentions, these actions reinterpret the political domain and challenge the 'natural order of things' proposed by State discourse in which the official historical past is a coherent, unified and self-explanatory narrative which blames the dead for *La Violencia*.[11]

War-widows re-member against and in spite of the military forces' direct and indirect instructions to forget. They talk about their experiences with women perceived to be '*de la misma cabeza*' (literally, 'of the same head'). The smaller and more intimate the group of close confidantes, whether friends, family or new acquaintances from other settlements who, prior to *La Violencia*, would not have spoken to each other, the safer the women feel to express themselves. In this new situation, the familiar concept of deference to elders is comforting, even though it denies equal rights of expression to all members of the group: for example, daughters-in-law have to defer to their mothers-in-law, who therefore seem to have greater powers of memory articulation.

From the extreme margins of society, K'iche' women create a secret oral discourse which is condemned to remain unofficial, as a 'public secret' (cf. Bourdieu 1977). The social sites for discussing such dangerous topics are narrowly restricted. The safest locations for speaking of forbidden subjects are in the least patrolled and most autonomous social sites: in other words, in exclusively female spheres such as their sweat baths in which up to four women can bathe together. Equally unpatrolled, though not beyond suspicion, are women's visits to sacred hills to perform *costumbre* with a female shaman. The danger here is that both *Costumbrismo* and the hills themselves have become associated with the guerrillas.

More guarded conversations take place in widows' houses, when out grazing their sheep, or tending their gardens. Such sites are less secure and women are constantly vigilant for informers. In insecure sites women employ linguistic codes and gestures which are not understood by members of the dominant regime.

I heard women speak in all these places. At first they were very wary of me, even though I had been introduced to them as an associate of the non-governmental organization which had been working with them for five years. My obvious interest in *La Violencia* frightened them. As trust developed between us, I began to be regarded as someone who gave them permission to speak; I believe that my presence became a reassuring one. Sometimes, once engaged in vigorous conversation, the women forgot my otherness.

I can only assume that what women called up from memory in my presence was edited according to their changing perceptions of me. Their memories and their general conversation are certainly influenced by contemporary events and their frame of mind at any particular moment.

In response to my questions, some women spoke for the first time about aspects of their experiences, revealing memories which, although shaped by their cultural and personal history, were more idiosyncratic and 'raw'.[12] Sometimes a single question triggered a flow of memory from one woman to another; revelations and reflections ricocheted from woman to woman. The spontaneous expression of memories, though unusual, is occasionally prompted by the arrival of a time when their missing menfolk would have performed some agricultural task, the sudden recognition of a site where an atrocity had occurred, or, more dramatically, the unanticipated occurrence of violence in the present. Only then, or when inebriated, do women's narratives seem to be impulsive. But I doubt that memories are released with entire abandon even then, because hyper-vigilance seems to be second nature to K'iche' women.

All villagers are active in the process of forgetting and adopt a variety of stratagems to cope with the State's demands to forget. Forgetting is something people are forced to do, do unwittingly, or consciously choose to do. Consciously employed tactics include silence, mutism, negation, forging, and confusion.

A less conscious device for forgetting is repression (Favret-Saada 1991); a similar, unconscious device is denial. Women seem to deny aspects which are especially painful and disturbing to them; men's accounts of the same event contain more painful details.[13] Denial and repression protect one from psychic dangers, that is, the pain of the memories of atrocity which people experience within themselves.

People also defend themselves from painful memories by impeding their entry. The memory is logged at some level but people do their best to avoid attending to it; however, they cannot resist its subliminal entry. Sometimes the memory is taken in and transformed and, in that state, remains in mind but not as the original experience.[14]

Some women found that although they had not forgotten what had happened, neither could they access their memories properly. They had been unable to cope with the experience when it happened and/or were unable to integrate it into cultural categories or codes of significance. Memories which cannot be remembered properly cannot be laid to rest.

While employing various strategies to forget, women also rework the material which is left which, paradoxically, includes the 'forgotten'. Silence and forgetting are not lackings; rather, they are present absences or negative spaces which shape what is remembered. This has a communal aspect, in that there is tacit agreement about what is to be remembered or forgotten. The 'forgotten' is, therefore, as much shared as what is remembered.

Which memories are forgotten and which retained is defined by the women's needs in the present. The widows are less concerned with the historicity of their experiences or the chronology of events (which I tried, unsuccessfully, to establish), than with how this past relates to their present lives. For example, the women chose, consciously and unconsciously, not to remember or speak of their unbearable guilt and shame. Their guilt is more than 'survivor guilt'; it stems from the paralysis which prevented parents who witnessed the murder of their children from acting to protect them. K'iche' women's guilt and shame is exacerbated by the fact that they cannot fulfil their obligations to the dead; funerary and commemorative rituals were banned during *La Violencia*: there was often no body to bury anyway. Perhaps the only way to deal with intolerable emotions is by forgetting.

The constant review of traumatic incidents and the construction of various alternative outcomes has been identified as the classic syndrome of obsessional review (Lifton 1967); among Guatemalan widows, however, the activity is creative and has a healing quality. Uncovering memories and turning them into narratives is a way of re-living, re-working, making sense of, coming to terms with, and integrating violent events which dramatically altered their lives. In telling each other stories, women place order on traumatic events and normalize their reactions to them; they also create a boundary to their suffering. Through re-membering incidents and relating them to the group, women reconstruct and reshape events for themselves and each other. Together they produce altered drafts of the past, discarding one in favour of the other. There is never a final version. Their memories change as they change; they alter as the state of oppression fluctuates. The women and their memories, which are sites of disguised repression, reflect and re-present a specific moment in the process of history.

There seems to be an implicit understanding among the women of the problems of memory in situations of unprecedented trauma. It is always possible, in any oral account of a shared experience, to incorporate other people's memories into one's own, but here the process is encouraged in order to create narratives which make sense to the group. Oral memories have an advantage over written history because the narrator retains control over its dissemination – the audience, site, the particular version. A memory can be withheld or retold; it can be summarized or magnified; altered or uttered in disparate forms corresponding to the interests, intents and fears of the speaker.[15]

Every retelling provides an opportunity for including new material or changing detail as the women attempt to understand what happened and why. In recounting their memories and interpretations of violent events, they correct each other's views on what actually happened. For example:

Eugenia: The men were tied up. They had thrown them on the ground like pigs who are about to be slaughtered.

Candelaria: They were on the ground with their faces bloodied. Some shouted, 'Please forgive us, forgive us', out of devotion and because they were suffering so much.

Flora: They asked the patrols to forgive them. Many of the murderers were evangelicals. After the killings, they told people that those assassinated had begged to 'ask our pardon and our help to convert to our religion'.

Eugenia: But I know everything that happened and they [the dead men] didn't say anything like that . . . In fact, many didn't even utter a word. They couldn't even if they wanted to, because they were hurt so badly that they couldn't talk at all.

Candelaria: Perhaps a few of them said a few things but nothing about that.

Eugenia: Only my child said something when they first captured him. He said, 'Mother, ask the patrol commander to get help to free me. Tell him I have not done anything wrong.' So I went to Mr. Justice [one of the commanders] and I asked him, 'What did he do to make you take him? Why not let him go?' But he didn't respond; he just ignored me. I then followed him until we reached the centre of the village. He didn't stop there, he just continued on a path which led to the ravine where they were digging the pits where the men would be buried. This is what happened. And, I tell you, I heard nothing about what you said, about conversion. That's all a big lie . . . Indeed, what they [the commanders] shouted was that the men they had rounded up were to be slaughtered because they had left the village and become 'organized'. They accused them of being guerrillas.

Discrepancies between the official truth and the women's private truth, between different women's versions of the same events, and distortion arising from psychic distress or other causes, all give rise to concern about the lack of correspondence between what actually happened and received narratives of the past. The process of 'adjusting the fit is an ongoing one' (Knapp 1989). Candelaria continues her narrative:

Candelaria: We were all there sitting in the school waiting . . . And when they had buried them, they all returned to the school to threaten all of us. They warned us, 'None of you had better utter a word about what you have just seen. And if we should learn that one of you has, then what you have just seen will also happen to you and you'll go with them!' . . . Because of this I realized that the commanders themselves decided to kill the men.

Candelaria implies that the massacre was not ordered by the army, which causes Eugenia to rethink her position. Both women are right but ultimately, the army is responsible because it deliberately created the conditions which encouraged the perpetrators to act upon local animosities. This is generally unrecognized by survivors, who remain burdened with their role in *La Violencia*.

Retelling narratives can alter the memory which is being related. Memory is constantly in flux, continuously transformed by social experience, membership of the group and the narratives they produce. In turn memory transforms the narratives, the social experience and, for some, even behaviour itself. Such memories can be characterized as provisional rather than fragmented (Halbwachs 1950).

Incorporating other people's memories has its drawbacks. Images can be based on 'false recognition, in accordance with others' testimonies and stories' (ibid.: 71). Memory not only invents the past out of the fluctuating imagery of the mind but also clings to its fabrications in the face of changing realities. Memory is a social phenomenon. Memories become whole only in social contexts; they are shaped by the cultural past and the conceptual structures and processes of the group in the present, be it family, church, communal association (ibid.: 22–49) or, following *La Violencia*, new groups such as widows.

The widows found themselves relating narratives in a moral vacuum. The social structure they knew had been smashed, their families shattered. They spoke about the disconcerting sensation of a disjuncture in their lives and in themselves as people. Women's self-observations in this respect relate not only to the different types of action, roles and responsibilities that they claimed to, and sometimes did, assume during *La Violencia*, but to the moral space in which they now live. Thus, when Ana confessed that she could neither think nor feel during *La Violencia*, she described the mental and emotional numbness which accompanies shock and grief, the confusion resulting from the abrupt alteration in her identity, and her inability to function in a totally alien atmosphere which was antipathetic to K'iche' concepts of 'the right thing to do'.

The women's recollections of the 'amoral' behaviour forced upon them during *La Violencia* are very painful, despite their awareness that it was impossible to act according to customary definitions of morality during 'that time' without putting their own lives, and those of surviving kin, at risk. They did not, for example, search for their lost kin, including their children; values such as parental care lose their reference in situations which preclude their expression. Although their behaviour was determined by the situation, not their values, women are unable forgive themselves for what they retrospectively judge as their own failings. Thus, although the circumstances of *La Violencia* did not permit the luxury of doing the 'Christian' thing, this does not prevent women from condemning others as a way of lifting themselves or, in more candid moments, from condemning themselves directly for not operating according to the morality of better times. When Flora remarked that a 'good Christian' would have denounced the killings and abductions, which she herself did not do, this harsh self-judgement led to a diminished self-perception with which her memory and her continuing 'self' has to contend.

La Violencia demanded novel and unconventional definitions of the 'self' in order for people to function at all. Widows feel divided by the past and are therefore unable to forge an integrated vision of themselves. Part of the diminished 'self' stems from the effect of this discontinuity of the integrity of the 'self'. This disunity alienated the widows from their own conception of personhood.[16] This conception develops as one moves through life and, for various culturally specific reasons, not everyone becomes 'fully a person'; for those who do, 'personhood may be partly or fully rescinded later' (Harris 1989).

The feeling that their personhood has been diminished is a genuine problem for widows, who sometimes remark that they 'do not feel like a person'; some even gave me the impression that their sense of themselves was no longer of someone real but as somehow 'other'. This stems partly from the inauthenticating effect of living behind a lie (the official truth) for several years and partly from their constructions to protect the 'self' at a time of disruption, loss and failure. The issues are a magnification of those facing people in less drastic situations when it is easier to maintain their 'ordinary masks' (cf. Giddens 1979), when the discrepancy in the way one perceives oneself to act and the 'reality' is not so large. In dire situations, there is an even greater need to protect the 'self' by minimizing the need for radical shifts in 'self-concept'.

Women's references to their broken personhood tend to be expressed allegorically. Their talk of their inability to keep their animals alive is a reference to themselves as inadequate carers; it expresses their self-perceptions of negligence towards their families. Unable to save their children, they view themselves as failing to fulfil the quintessentially female function of protection. This unavoidable failure is also reflected in the women's preoccupations with the violent removal of their traditional skirts which are a metonym for Indian women in shamanic prayers.[17] The implied exposure also reflects the fact that this appalling indignity, the loss of ownership of the status of motherhood, occurred in public. That Emol is a face-to-face community in which reputation is important increases the women's humiliation. Their sense of failure continues into the present.

Sharing re-membered memories is an important part of the women's ongoing attempts to make sense of their ruptured past. In the process, women also create a shared identity. Identity depends on the memory state, in other words, a 'self' that remembers its earlier states. Having identity, or knowing who one is, is 'to be oriented in moral space . . . where questions arise about what is good or bad, what is worth doing and what not, what has meaning and importance for you and what is trivial and secondary' (Taylor 1989: 28). These are precisely the issues which women address through their narratives.

Creating narratives also allows women to present themselves to themselves in a new light and to re-position themselves within memory and history. The starting point is the need to protect the psyche by rejecting intolerable truths and constructing different ones. The widow attempts to protect herself with 'cover-memories' (Freud 1899) not only from the events themselves but from her own retrospective self-criticism about not acting according to pre-existing values. In devastating situations, the process of re-elaboration of the past overshadows the actual event considerably more than in more mundane situations. An event's extreme resonance within, and emotional impact on, an individual or group can result in the fragmentation of memory, the omission of detail or the exaggeration of minutiae, and the insertion of fiction if not complete fabrication.

Widows create and re-create stories of how they survived *La Violencia* and its aftermath. They claimed the heroic quality usually attributed to men for themselves. Stories of heroism were told by the heroines themselves or by women who marvelled at their bravery.

The village massacre was the most common subject for this kind of revision. Eugenia presented herself as taking a leading role against this atrocity. Her story provoked horror because it 'broke the rules' which govern the behaviour of women and Indians.[18] Women are usually silent before unrelated men, so Eugenia's attempt to bribe patrollers into releasing her son was truly shocking. Patrollers clubbed her with their rifle butts, shouting 'XO!', which is how one normally scolds an unruly animal. This kind of oral testimony draws a veil over more tragic elements − the beaten men who were buried alive or 'chopped into pieces like a pumpkin' − and brings out the symbolic and, to some extent, actual overturning of order.

Eugenia's 'cover-memory' marked the beginning of the positive reconstruction of an identity for herself and her listeners. This was made possible by radical changes in the women's perceptions of their 'selves' and their surroundings following *La Violencia*. This change in the perception of personal identity, in turn, created new experiences and interpretations of the past. For example, the widows reject the symbolic devaluation implied by the label 'wives of the guerrilla', together with its implicit threat, as harmful to their sense of 'self'. There seems to be some realization that names do more than reflect and classify: they also create experiences. The labelling issue is important because, being social, new metaphorical language creates not just new references, but new 'forms of life' or 'events' (Parkin 1982: xxxiii). Here, the new language relates to the woman's 'self'-definition and the new form of life is her own.

The destruction of traditional relationships allowed women to assume novel positions in relation to others. That widows do not seem bound by the traditional structure of their society is reflected in their reformulations of the world and their narratives of this version of the 'self'. This seems to be where widows draw most strength. To some extent, they revel in their self-portrayals as 'disorderly', women who overturn gender roles; they cultivate the very disorderliness with which the patrol commanders taunt them. Yet the widows also stake a claim on cultural continuity: they see themselves as maintaining the K'iche' value system which is oriented towards the good. Even Eugenia insists that she conforms to K'iche' values within her family, thereby maintaining a sense of continuity within the chaos surrounding her own identity. The need to maintain a perception of order is also suggested by her revelation that her rebellious streak is consistent with the non-conformist tendencies of her family. Thus, while the disruption of relationships and the taking on of reconstructed identities is acknowledged, continuity is restored.

But the re-establishment of continuity is only partial; widows had to find other anchors in the past. Widows' groups foster the positive reconstruction of identity through linking contemporary widows with characters from both Mayan history and myth and the bible. One of the founders of CONAVIGUA, a young catechist named Petronila, repeatedly tells the women that they are 'like the heroines in the Bible, Ruth, Ester and Judith from the Old Testament, and saints such as the Virgin Mary from the New Testament'.[19] Petronila addresses the women in the name of the Virgin, whom she presents as a girl from the corn fields.

Petronila told me that it was not men who sacrificed their lives: 'The women were those who made the sacrifices – they sacrificed the lives of their men'. The women identify with this allusion and as they listen to Petronila, they become heroines, celibates and virgins who have sacrificed their sons. In contrast to most widows' tendency to idealize their dead kin as martyrs, some women now portray themselves and their murdered menfolk as heroes; this counteracts the psychological effects of the authorities' attempts to equate 'guerrillas' with 'sinners' and the devil. Women derive comfort from seeing themselves as worthy and from thinking that their kin do not suffer in the after-life.

Relating shared memories and discourses to biblical and historical characters diminishes the women's pain; collectivisation and then universalization through reference to historical figures puts their experiences in context, decreasing their alienation. But ancient battles are not merely the initial stages of a historical sequence which leads to feminism (although there are certainly the beginnings of a feminist proclivity to this group): the critical element is the creation of a sense of continuity through characteristics and events shared by both ancient and modern heroines which link past, present and future via historical sequence and analogy (Knapp 1989: 130). Women draw on analogies within their cultural repertoire which have not been usurped by the State; they construct sense and continuity via alternative routes, by-passing the unacceptable or unavailable aspects of their own history and provide a frame for the future. Some CONAVIGUA members see their future as a mission: as survivors, their ambition is to secure justice for the dead.

Biblical contexts applicable to the contemporary struggle also assist in the positive renewal of identity: they furnish the 'roots and beginning' of the 'continuous history' of 'women as the ekklesia (church or holy place) of God' (Fiorenza 1983: 344). The women's 'self'-constructions and reconfigurations of themselves work against the diminishing of identities caused during *La Violencia*.

The reconstructed identities can be considered fictional (exceeding the ordinary falsehoods upon which any of our identities are based) in so far as they are based on remembered past actions and future identity claims rather than on present pursuits. The women are unable to locate themselves in unmitigated reality (the lived present) and can only locate themselves in managed, re-presented reality, that is, fiction.

There is some concern that over the years 'silence can reshape memory, history, even the notions of right and wrong to the point that might makes right' (Stoll 1993: 302). However, this process has a limit which can be found in the private, women's sphere where the silence is broken. The public and private realms permeate one another, mutually and dynamically, each shaping and reshaping the other. Each domain is important when trying to understand the effects of repression on the shaping of memory and history. Violence and terror dismantle established categories which are reassembled in new ways, causing confusion and hindering people's attempts to integrate the 'self' of the past with the 'self' of the present. Memories connected with dissociated aspects of the 'self', frozen in the chaos of 'that time', become inaccessible or unspeakable. And, in the end, they can neither be re-membered nor truly forgotten.

Notes

1 The added hyphen in 're-membering' emphasizes the women's constant review of memory fragments in an attempt to construct something whole.

2 Known as *mestizos* in other Central American countries, *Ladinos* claim mixed Spanish and Indigenous descent. In Guatemala this is more of a social classification as half of the population is estimated to be of entirely indigenous ancestry (Smith 1985).

3 El Quiché's few *Ladinos* live in town and tend to be landowners or their agents. They were the first to flee when *La Violencia* reached the province.

4 All local place and personal names are pseudonyms.

5 All village men between the ages of fifteen and fifty-five were induced to volunteer in the *Patrullas de Autodefensa Civil* (Civil Defence Patrols). In 1988, when villages were allowed to vote on whether or not to keep the system, the name was changed to *Comités Voluntarios de Autodefensa Civil* (Voluntary Committees for Civil Defense).

6 The State also promulgates its version of the 'truth' through the army's civic action or psychological warfare branch.

7 Military-commissioned civil authority. These are village men who have completed two years' military service.

8 For example, in May 1990, a widows' leader in Parraxtut, Sacapulas, was shot dead in her home by a local military commissioner.

9 A Swedish representative to the United Nations remarked that the rhetoric of General Rios Montt's government (1982-83) reminded him of George Orwell's novel *1984*: 'When they mean war they speak of peace,' he said, 'and when they mean repression, they speak of freedom . . . Guatemala is the same' (Simon 1987: 114).

10 By 'truth', I mean the Foucaultian concept, thoroughly historicized as discourse, which is constructed by 'the will to truth' (Foucault 1972).

11 Cf. the authoritarian Argentine state's articulation of a uni-dimensional theory of reality which describes all dissent in metaphors of illness. Official discourse uses the first person plural in an attempt to eliminate opposition, the sense of otherness and ambiguity of thought (Masiello 1987: 12–13).

12 I have borrowed this concept and that of 'cooked' from Lévi-Strauss (1969). 'Cooked' memories are more uniform and stereotyped, having been shared and worked on many times before.

13 Gender has a decisive impact on the way violence is experienced and the world reformulated. Men and women censor or select against different memories, owing to the differential resonance between genders.

14 I heard a story about a soldier who was haunted by a memory of a woman wringing a chicken's neck, a mundane activity in rural Guatemala. Later, in analysis, he was able to remember witnessing a woman being forced to strangle her baby; his disturbing memory then subsided.

15 I do not agree with the distinction between oral and written history, which has been described as a science built on durable evidence, because 'the historian, like the mnemonist, builds interpretative paradigms, and historical understanding relies heavily on retrospective reconstruction of the past from a present-minded point of view' (Hutton 1988: 317).

16 Personhood has been described as 'those attributes, capacities, and signs of "proper" social persons which mark a moral career' (Poole 1982).

17 Oral narratives, like written texts, have an unconscious intertext which can be decoded through the repressed meanings of metaphor and metonym.

18 Within limits, the situation allowed Eugenia to extend her 'habitus', i.e. the propensity of a particular social group to select responses from a particular cultural repertoire according to the demands of a particular situation or field (Bourdieu 1977).

19 CONAVIGUA, The National Organisation of Guatemalan Widows (*Coordinadora Nacional de Viudas Guaremalitecos*), was established in 1988.

References

Bourdieu, P. (1977) *Outline of a Theory of Practice*, trans. Richard Nice, Cambridge.

—— (1991) *Language and Symbolic Power*, ed. J. B. Thompson, trans. G. Raymond and M. Adamson, London.

Favret-Saada, J. (1991) 'Sale Histoire', *Gradhaven* 10.

Fiorenza, E. S. (1983) *In Memory of Her: A Feminist Theological Reconstruction of Christian Origins*, London.

Foucault, M. (1972) *Histoire de la Folie à l'Age Classique*, Paris.

—— (1975) *Surveiller et Punir: Naissance de la Prison*, Paris.

—— (1977) *Language, Counter-Memory. Practice: Selected Essays and Interviews*, Oxford.

Freud, S. (1899) *Uber Deckerinnerungen. Gesammelte Schriften*, I, Band 1, S 465–88, Leipzig.

Giddens, A (1979) *Central Problems in Social Theory*, London.

GGIS (1992) Guatemalan Geo-Violence Information System database, Washington.

Halbwachs, M. (1950) *The Collective Memory*, reprinted 1980, New York.

Harris, G. G. (1989) 'Concepts of individual self and person in description and analysis', *American Anthropologist*, 91, pp. 599–611.

Hutton, P. H. (1988) 'Collective memory and collective mentalities: the Halbwachs-Aries connection', *Historical Reflections/Reflexions historiques*, vol. 15, no. 2, pp. 311–22.

Knapp, S., (1989) 'Collective memory and actual past', *Representations*, vol. 26, pp. 123–49.

Lévi-Strauss, C. (1969) *The Raw and the Cooked*, New York.

McClintock, M. (1985) *The American Connection: State Terror and Popular Resistance in Guatemala*, Bath.

Massiello, Francine (1987) in René Jara and Hernán Vidal (eds), *Ficción v Politica: La Narrativa Argentina Durante el Proceso Militar*, Minneapolis.

Painter, J. (1993) *Guatemala: Transmission from Terror?* London.

Parkin, D. (1982) (ed.) *Sacred Void: Spatial Images of Work and Ritual among the Giriama of Kenya*, New York.

Pateman, T. (1980) *Language, Truth and Politics*, Lewes.

Nora, P. 'Between memory and history: les lieux de mémoire', *Representations*, 26 (special issue), pp. 7–25.

Poole, F. J. P. (1982) 'The ritual forging of identity: aspects of person and self in Bimin-Kuskusmin male initiations', in G. H. Herdt (ed.), *Rituals of Manhood*, Berkeley, pp. 99–154.

Simon, J. M. (1987) *Eternal Spring, Eternal Tyranny*, U.K.

Smith, C. (1985) 'Culture and community: the language of class in Guatemala', in M. Sprinkler (ed.) *The Year Left*, London.

Stoll, D. (1993) *Between Two Armies in the Ixil Towns of Guatemala*, New York.

Taylor, C. (1989) *Sources of Self: the Making of Modern Identity*, Cambridge.

Taussig, M. T. 1984) ' Culture of terror – space of death: Roger Casement's Putumayo report and the explanation of torture', *Comparative Studies of Society and History*, vol. 26, pp. 467–97.

Williams, R. (1977) *Marxism, Literature and Politics*, Oxford.

Zur, J. (1998) *Violent Memories, Mayan War Widows in Guatemala*, Colorado.

3

INTERVIEWING IN A CULTURE OF VIOLENCE

Moving memories from Windermere to the Cape Flats

Sean Field

I don't know really. I don't think it's going to be a nice future. You just wait for anything these days. You know sometimes, especially here near KTC [a township area]. You not sleeping yet you hear these 'Rrrrrr'. You hear the shooting. The next morning in the paper you hear people being shot, they don't know who. And you hear people coming, as they can open the door here and do those funny things. Shooting people for nothing. So the future is not, you can't say there will be a nice future. There's no future. I don't see no future.

(Mrs J. M.)

Acts of violence and the awareness of potential violence are constantly present within the black townships of contemporary South Africa.[1] The socially constructed boundaries between common law and political forms of violence blur, as the legacies of the apartheid past and the uncertain transitionary present exacerbate each other.[2] This paper will analyse neither the history nor the socio-political causes of the 'culture of violence' in South Africa.[3] Rather, it explores two interwoven questions: first, how does the culture of violence affect the fieldwork process of doing oral history interviews? And second, what implications does the violence of the present have on the ways in which former residents of the Windermere community remember the past?

This paper draws on fifty-four oral history interviews conducted for a study of the history of the Windermere community.[4] Windermere was an ethnically mixed, part squatter community, on the urban periphery of Cape Town. Culturally, it thrived from the 1930s to the 1950s, but was torn apart by apartheid laws during the 1958–63 period. The bulk of Windermere's African residents were removed to Guguletu. While some coloured residents were also forcibly removed, the majority were located in the Factreton township which now partly covers the area on which Windermere once stood.[5] Most of the stories documented in this paper are drawn from experiences in both Factreton and Guguletu. These townships are part of the 'Cape Flats': a cultural patchwork of suburbs on the flat outskirts of Cape Town.

I will argue that interviewing in a culture of violence requires a flexible set of research strategies that are appropriate to the specific political, cultural and community circumstances encountered. The interviewer also needs to be acutely sensitive to the emotional, transferential and power dynamics of the interviewer/interviewee relationship. It is also important to be attuned to the complex ways in which interviewees construct memories and myths in order to cope with their emotional experiences of the past and present.

Simply put, oral histories are always emotional histories. In the context of a culture of violence, the expressed and unexpressed feelings of interviewees (and interviewer) are persistently 'present' in different, sometimes disruptive, manifestations. The use of nostalgia, exaggerations and metaphors in remembering the past constitute emotionally sustaining myths that support a sense of self and identity in the present. On the one hand, the former residents of Windermere feel the emotional loss of an ethnically mixed community destroyed by apartheid. On the other hand, the mythical wholeness of the Windermere past reconstructed in memory provides important comfort and a means to face the uncertain present and future. In a sense, I explore what Scott (1990: 27) calls the 'hidden transcripts' that are created through the 'practice of domination'. The emotional legacy located within these 'transcripts' constantly shapes the recalling (and denial) of memories, and the telling (and silences) of stories. Nevertheless, this study is neither an 'emotional history' nor a 'psycho-history', but a social history which documents emotions as vital forms of historical evidence.

The Windermere/Kensington community originated on farmlands on the urban periphery of Cape Town in the first decades of this century. The area at this time consisted of a few scattered brick buildings and many more iron shanties. People squatted in the Windermere area beyond 6th Avenue in order to avoid municipal laws and taxes (Swart 1983). During this period most of these squatters were coloured, with several whites and Africans. Most of them came from rural areas in search of work. However, according to oral accounts, it is clear that the major African influx from the rural areas of Transkei and Ciskei only began in the 1930s and accelerated in the 1940s.

At its peak in the 1950s the Windermere/Kensington area was estimated to contain more than 30,000 residents. During the 1950s the African majority made up approximately 55–60 per cent, coloured people 40–45 per cent and whites 2–4 per cent of the Windermere/Kensington population.[6] The Windermere/Kensington area was notorious for its over-crowding, unscrupulous landowners, poor sanitary conditions and high incidence of diseases, especially tuberculosis (ibid.) Despite these poverty-stricken and squalid conditions there was a vibrant cultural milieu of shebeens, dance halls, gangs, brothels and even a sand horse race-track where people gambled on Sunday afternoons.[7]

Windermere was incorporated under the jurisdiction of the Cape Town City Council (CCC) in 1943. In the period 1943 to 1953 the CCC and the Native Administration Department (NAD) used sections under the 1934 Slums Act and Pass Laws to begin clearing Africans out of the area. These initial measures seemed to have little effect on the stream of African new-comers to Windermere. During the 1950s approximately 12,000 African men (so-called 'bachelors') were forcibly removed to single-sex hostels in Langa (Swaart 1983). It was when the area was racially zoned a coloured area in 1953 that dramatic changes occurred. Between 1960 and 1963 approximately 2,500 African families were removed to Nyanga West, which was later to become Guguletu. During this period approximately 1,000 white people were removed to areas zoned for whites in Maitland, Brooklyn and Ruyterwacht. Because Windermere/Kensington was zoned as a coloured area, most coloured residents of Windermere were re-housed into a section for economic and sub-economic housing, renamed Factreton.

The majority of Windermere's former residents are now living on the 'Cape Flats'.[8] In the popular imagination of Capetonians the term 'Cape Flats' is often associated with apartheid social engineering and, in particular, the Group Areas Act of 1950. The experience of removals, dispersal and dumping of people into apartheid-designated ethnic ghettos left an indelible, and usually violent, mark on the social fabric of Cape Town.

The African residents who were removed to Guguletu were promised their own houses. For people living in corrugated iron shanties in areas highly prone to floods, fires, poor sanitary conditions and violence, a new house in a new community seemed appealing. However, this was not to be. When they arrived in their new homes, they found, as an interviewee put it, 'a concrete shell'. No ceiling. No inside doors. No proper floor. No electricity. No hot water. No inside toilets. A powerful sense of disappointment and in many cases anger were felt by every interviewee. Justifiably they felt that they had been tricked.

Since 1976 Guguletu has experienced school boycotts, stayaways, and repeated periods of violent struggles between residents, police and army. From the 1980s anti-apartheid civic and youth organisations became prominent. The levels of violence have steadily increased in Guguletu with ongoing political conflicts, taxi wars and rising unemployment. Since the abolition of influx control in 1986 there has been considerable growth of new squatter camps in vacant lots on the perimeter of, and inside, Guguletu.

By 1993, when the fieldwork for this study was being conducted, several comparisons could be drawn between Guguletu and Factreton. Guguletu was going through violent upheavals, while the Factreton area was politically quiet. African National Congress (ANC) structures in Guguletu were comparatively well developed, whereas the ANC branch in Factreton had limited support and weak organisational structures. In short, Factreton had become a relatively settled coloured township. However, it too experienced (and continues to experience) gang wars and related violence. Nevertheless, the apartheid state's intention of creating a politically conservative coloured village had to all intents and purposes been realised. This was not the case in Guguletu where residents were continuously waging struggles around sociopolitical issues. For example, in the mid-1980s the Factreton tenants of council houses were permitted to buy the houses they had been renting, while in 1993, their former Windermere neighbours in Guguletu were still fighting for the right to own the houses for which they had been paying rent for over thirty years.

The destruction of Windermere was not simply a 'slum clearance' but a racist plan to separate coloured and African residents of Windermere from each other. There is also little doubt that the differential access to jobs, owing to the application of the Coloured Labour Preference Policy (CLPP) in the Western Cape region, also accentuated the sense of cultural difference between African and coloured people. This policy, together with other apartheid laws such as the Group Areas Act, and the years of differential treatment meted out by the apartheid state, fostered painful fissures between the coloured and African residents of the Cape Flats. It is from this sociopolitical context that the culture of violence has emerged within the townships of the Cape Flats.

Interviewing in a culture of violence requires careful attention to developing appropriate research and access strategies. In most research settings gaining access is not simply a question of gaining acceptance from one or two gatekeepers. Doing fieldwork and interviewing is a lengthy process of *repeatedly* gaining access. The research process is structured by negotiations between the researcher and various individuals, institutions and discourses. From the initial browsing through literature through to the interpretation of oral transcripts, and even the act of writing, the researcher is struggling to gain wider and/or deeper access to meanings.

As a young white male middle-class university researcher whose first language is English, I was (and still am) in a relatively more powerful position than my black working-class interviewees. This is not to say that I was omnipotent and the interviewees were powerless victims. On the contrary, my 'power' did not derive from an abstracted social position but depended on two factors: first, what the interviewee thought and felt I was, or in short what I represented for that individual; and second, the set of research and interpersonal skills that I brought into the dialogue. The power relations of the interview dialogue are also fundamentally embedded in language. For example, an ability to frame effective (and affective) questions is crucial to negotiating an interviewer/interviewee power relationship. The aim is not to try to overcome these power relations in the interview, as it is a fantasy to suppose that a power-free interviewing space can be reached. These power relations cannot be willed away, but need to be skilfully negotiated in different ways from one interview situation to the next.

For potential interviewees in all cultural communities a respectful, humble but confident manner is important. In the coloured community I generally had to be careful about disclosing my political identity. The majority of the coloured interviewees were politically conservative and openly presenting my ANC affiliations would either have blocked access to an interview or severely distorted the information collected. On the whole, with coloured interviewees I presented personal information about where I grew up (in the neighbouring suburb of Maitland) and where I studied, although I felt uneasy about withholding aspects of my political identity from interviewees. Nevertheless, I believe that the more honest approach usually allows for a better interviewing rapport to develop. In general terms then, by shifting away from positivist notions of the neutral and objective interviewer, I offered a strategic selection of differing aspects of my life to different interviewees. This selective self-disclosure had to be appropriate to the specific circumstances encountered.

My access strategy towards African areas and individuals was different in crucial respects. I was about to begin negotiating entry to Guguletu when Chris Hani, the chairperson of the South African Communist Party (SACP), was murdered. This triggered weeks of popular unrest throughout townships in South Africa, including Guguletu. From April to June 1993 army patrols had checkpoints at every entrance to the township and my fieldwork ground to a halt. Fortunately, during a relatively calm period in July and August I conducted most of the African interviews with the help of a black research assistant. As we moved around Guguletu we saw the angry glares of youths on street corners and the fresh scars of street battles.

In Guguletu I had to vouch carefully for my political credentials and past. Not to do so would simply have meant no access at all. However, overtly political credentials alone were not enough. Each day as I did the interviews, we also set up interviews for later in the week. Time was of the essence, as I knew that this lull in violent activities could end on any day. After a few days of this process in Guguletu, I realised that many of the interviewees at that point seemed to have prior knowledge of aspects of my identity. I questioned my assistant about it and he told me that one of the earlier interviewees had put out the story that I could be trusted. Gossip, channelled through overlapping political and social networks, had eased open access to several people.[9]

Given the volatile circumstances, it was essential from the first interaction with a potential interviewee to find ways to convey research fieldwork as an intelligible, safe and affirming process. Seeing the link between his or her interview and other interviews also provided the interviewee with reference points and a sense of being part of a broader process. Oral history interviewing makes sense to most informants because it feeds into and from the day-to-day conversations and gossip that go on in all communities. This affirming and open process was also a way of protecting myself. As a white individual entering a war-torn black township, I was the one under observation. Given the unpredictable circumstances, the presence of a black research assistant offered little protection.

Just before 5 p.m. on 25 August I conducted my last interview in Langa and was on my way (alone) to conduct a final interview in Guguletu. Inexplicably, I did not feel like doing another interview that day and went home. Perhaps it was the end-of-fieldwork tiredness. Perhaps it was the sight of the smoldering ashes of tyres in the streets of Langa. So, instead of driving down the main road (called NY 1) of Guguletu at 5 p.m., I went home. At 5 p.m. on that day a white American student named Amy Biehl was brutally murdered on NY 1, Guguletu. For a few days the township witnessed a series of street battles. Guguletu was once again a war zone. All the residents I interviewed bore the emotional, and at times physical, scars of these township wars. Most of them have experienced the trauma of having had either friends, relatives or children imprisoned, shot, whipped, or in some cases killed.

Despite this context, my prime aim was to create a safe and secure interviewing space for the interview dialogue to take place. Partly this meant resolving the issues of confidentiality, the physical location of the interview and how the information conveyed would be used. To establish the basis for a fruitful interview dialogue at least three basic essentials of the oral historian's trade must be employed: sensitive questioning, attentive listening and empathy to human experience and emotion. Perhaps most critical of all is not just being a good listener, but ensuring that the interviewee senses that you are listening attentively and that you are taking their stories seriously.

This is not psychotherapy (Figlio 1995, Samuel and Thompson 1990). Psychotherapy is not the job of an oral history interviewer, and neither should it be. Without the appropriate skills the interviewer can do more harm than good. Also, it could be unethical if the oral historian dismantled any of the interviewee's conscious or unconscious defensive mechanisms. While the interviewer does not have the therapeutic aims of the psychotherapist, both are attempting to create a safe space for people to talk about themselves and their past experiences. The focus is on the interviewee, as a social *and* emotional being who has lived, and lives, within a matrix of power relations. For many people living within the culture of violence, a limited space to talk about personal experiences without fear of repercussions is especially important.

A relatively safe space to speak, however, does not neutralize or equalize the power relations between the interviewer/interviewee. Power, to paraphrase Foucault, is not an object, but always a situational relationship (Foucault 1976). In my interviewing experiences for this study, my 'race' and gender and other identities are an unavoidable reality which I bring into the situation, and these must be negotiated. While interviewer/interviewee power relations were unequally slanted in my favour, two general points must be stressed. First, these power relationships were not fixed and in fact shifted between, and within, interviews. Second, unequal power relations are not inherently negative for conducting a productive and affirming oral history interview. Through the subtle complexities of these unequal power relations there is potential to negotiate an engaging rapport that is mutually beneficial.

All interviews were conducted in either English or Afrikaans. For white and coloured interviewees (whose home language is either English or Afrikaans) the interview was conducted in the language of their choice. In contrast, with African interviewees whose home language in most cases is Xhosa, either English or Afrikaans was used because I cannot speak Xhosa. With African interviewees I did not use a translator but preferred to speak directly. In terms of power relations this obviously put African interviewees at a relative disadvantage. However, there were several instances where benefits were negotiated out of this dynamic. While a non-mother tongue can hamper story-telling, the process of working through language and cultural barriers often produces a more intimate relationship. In fact, very often non-mother-tongue speakers tell shorter and more vivid stories. Furthermore, using a translator invariably results in loss of detail and hampers the development of an interviewer/interviewee rapport.

In some cases interviewees' positions and skills acquired through political work minimized the unequal power relationship in the interview. It is also important that the interviewer should not underestimate the knowledge of working-class informants, especially the extent to which they are able to see beyond the stereotypes which the interviewer represents. The worldly survival skills of many of these older interviewees meant that they were quite capable of negotiating the interview relationship. Also, the basic premise of the interview situation, that the interviewee has information the interviewer does not have, ultimately means that the interviewee has relative power to withhold and to regulate which fragments of his or her life are revealed.

Concerning questions of 'race' and ethnicity, some interviewees distinguished between me as an individual and the broader cultural community from which I came. Coloured and African interviewees alike tended not to view me in stereotypical terms. For example, they were able to express their hurt and anger towards white people directly and indirectly. However, this was not always the case. Some African interviewees never seemed sufficiently comfortable to make the above distinction, even with my openly presented political identity and the presence of a black research assistant.

There was a fearful passivity and at times a stubborn protectiveness hindering the process of telling a life story. This I attribute partly to my 'race'/ethnicity (and in some cases gender) and partly to non-mother-tongue difficulties. But I would argue that the more persuasive reasons were the forms of silence that were created within the culture of violence.[10] These external silences were internalized as silences of the individual self, and were brought into the interview dialogue. At times they seemed to be rooted in a numbing fear of not knowing who to trust or distrust, a set of frightened silences produced by the violence of apartheid, poverty and social upheavals. But in many instances these silences were created by my inability to 'hear' what interviewees were 'saying'. Ultimately I suspect most interviewees had made strategic decisions not to disclose certain kinds of information as a way of maintaining a sense of personal security and control.[11]

In contrast, some coloured interviewees displayed an unsettling combination of crude racism towards Africans and an admiration of whites. This group of coloured interviewees were virtually 'too nice' and accommodating towards me. Here again, but with different consequences, I was being viewed in stereotypical terms. However, many coloured interviewees did tend to make the distinction between stereotype and person. They presented mixtures of anger, hurt and respect towards white people, and were not racist towards Africans.

Gendered power relations also intersect with 'race', and with ethnic, class, educational and generational relationships and images which are brought into the interview dialogue. Many female interviewees, I suspect, did not tell particular stories because I am male. The pattern of patriarchal discourses within African and coloured working-class communities also probably created a set of gendered silences, although many African and coloured women occupy relatively powerful positions in their families and even in the broader community. Many of the female interviewees were domestic workers for white families and they tended to show an ambiguous mixture of submissiveness and strong maternalism towards me.

As for male interviewees, I had good interviews with most coloured men who tended to speak freely. African men varied from the passively watchful who gave short responses to those who were more relaxed in their story-telling. It was also noticeable that more men than women interviewees became emotional (and cried). To a large extent I attribute this to our common gender. Here too, there were cases where elderly men treated me paternally as if they were telling their stories to a little boy sitting at their feet.

There are many intersecting power relationships at play, and these can change from day to day. Portelli tells the story of the communist worker whom he interviewed twice, with a year between interviews. In the first interview Portelli presented himself in the so-called neutral researcher role. The interviewee assumed that since Portelli was a middle-class outsider it would be safer to convey conservative views. In the second interview Portelli adopted a more honest approach and was struck by the differences in the information conveyed. Far from being a fascist, as Portelli suspected from the first interview, the interviewee was in fact a communist. Portelli states:

I had thought I was not supposed to 'intrude' my own beliefs and identity into the interview, and they too had responded not to me as a person, but to a stereotype of my class, manner and speech. I had been playing the 'objective' researcher, and was rewarded with biased data.

(Portelli 1971: 31)

Herein lies the test: if the interviewer is mercenary or behaves like an one-dimensional research stereotype in approaching interviewees, they will sense it and access to layers of information will be closed off. The interviewee has to *feel* that the interviewer *is empathetic* to his or her experiences and feelings if, as Frisch puts it, 'a shared authority' is to be achieved (Frisch 1990). In developing an open oral history dialogue there is a mutual assessment of each other's identities. Within this mutual assessment there is potential for emotions and unconscious mechanisms to affect the shape of the interview dialogue, especially within volatile social circumstances. There is a transferential relationship, a dialogue of transference and counter-transference:

If transference is considered in terms of unconscious sets, one can identify what triggers this process. There is then an expectation that the present will be like a similar situation belonging to a previously formed unconscious set. . . . It is this *mis-perception of similarity as sameness* [my emphasis] that brings about the phenomenon of transference, whereby previous experience and related feelings are transferred from the part and are experienced *as if* [his emphasis] they were actually in the present. This is why the phenomenon of transference can have such a sense of reality and immediacy. There may be a similar unconscious overlap between the experience of 'self' and 'other'. What comes from whom, in any two-person relationship, is not always clear. This is because the processes of communication can either be projective (one person putting into the other) or introjective (one person taking in from the other).

(Casement 1985: 6–7)

In psychotherapy the transferential relationship between therapist and client provides unconscious material to be resolved within the secure containment of the therapeutic relationship. In the oral history dialogue, however, there is a need to be sensitively aware of the transferential relationship as far as possible, so as to guide the interview in appropriate ways. The oral historian cannot interpret the interviewee's unconscious on the basis of the limited interactions of an interview. However, interviewers need to 'listen' for unconscious cues in the interview dialogue. For example, when an interviewee attaches a disproportionate amount of emotion to certain events, people or issues, that might signal a projective identification. Alternatively, a lack of emotion expressed around events that were obviously traumatic suggests some form of defensive repression protecting the interviewee from disturbing emotions. It is the interviewer's job *not* to try to undo these unconscious defences, but to understand their impact on the construction of memories and identities.

Counter-transference also needs to be carefully monitored by the interviewer as this can provide clues to how his or her own unconscious is intervening. During the fieldwork I wrote post-interview notes describing the relationship context of each interview, my feelings and the feelings I 'sensed' the interviewee was grappling with. I experienced several instances of counter-transference. For example, I had interviewed a coloured man who had experienced violence from an abusive father and through his involvement in youth gangs in Windermere. The interviewee initially spoke with an aggressive macho attitude. This gradually softened as his feelings, especially sadness, emerged. I spent over an hour with him afterwards as he cried profusely. I kept an empathetic composure during and after the interview, but when I left, sadness overwhelmed me. Perhaps I had taken in too much of his sadness. Perhaps it was 'how he spoke about violence and especially *mes stekery* (knife stabbing) that triggered something in me' (interview notes, 21 August 1993). The emotions evoked by the transferential relationship can have a dramatic effect on the interviewer/interviewee relationship. In a therapeutic sense, there are often unexpected times when the interviewer has to be a safe container for the interviewee's emotions.

When aspects of the interviewee's past are associated with intense emotions such as pain, shame, guilt or fear, the interviewer treads on fragile terrain. Yeo argues that 'The problem of representation is experienced more often as private pain than as public problem' (Yeo 1988: 39). By initiating the interview dialogue the oral historian raises the issue of self representation. The following question is implicitly posed to the interviewee: Are your personal memories of any public worth? The interviewer's unequivocal response must be, yes.

It is not simply that all people have a past, but 'that you need a past of your own' (Grele 1991: 67). Therefore, 'People remember what they need to remember' (Tonkin 1992: 11). Oral historians can make a contribution towards meeting that need for a personal past, not as an isolated biography, but as a personal past meaningfully created and struggled for within a matrix of social and collective relationships. So, 'any life story, written or oral, more or less dramatically, is in one sense a personal mythology; a self justification' (Samuel and Thompson 1990: 11). It is at this critical intersection of self and identity *and* memories and stories that valuable interpretations can be made.

Portelli has argued that:

> memory is not a passive depository of facts but an active process of
> creation of meanings. Thus, the specific utility of oral sources for the

historian lies not so much in their ability to preserve the past, as in the very changes wrought by memory.

(Portelli 1991: 52)

Such change wrought by memory, however, 'directs our attention not to the past but to the *past present relation*' (Popular Memory Group 1992: 211). This relationship is crucial because for the life story narrator, Bertaux-Wiame argues, 'the first purpose is not to describe the past "as it was", or even as it was experienced, but to confer to the past experience a certain *meaning*: a meaning which will contribute to the meaning of the present' (Bertaux-Wiame 1981: 257).

The overwhelming majority of the fifty-four interviewees spoke of Windermere in glowing terms as a place of peace and togetherness, a place where young and old from different cultures lived happily together. For African interviewees, this romantic gloss on the Windermere past had a distinctly sharper, tenser edge because of its frequent comparisons with contemporary violence in Guguletu. The following sequence of quotes from African interviewees illustrates a series of past/present comparisons:

> We used to live in harmony. There were no *skollies* [hooligans], one could travel at any time of the night without fear of being robbed or stabbed. Neighbours were very friendly to each other. Everything was cheap that time. If we could be allowed to go back we'll be the first to leave.
>
> (Mr B. M.)

Other African interviewees made similar references to peace and violence:

> If they say we can move back to Windermere, oh, ja, I can move anytime. This place is a horrible place. I mean where we stay here now, what can we do? When we were young in Windermere we used to walk till midnight, but here in Guguletu, uh uh, you can't! We had a nice time in Windermere.
>
> (Mrs A. Q.)

> Play with the coloured children there. Ah, it was nice there, the coloured people. No fighting, nothing. All just one person. No, we stay nicely with the coloured people there. Anytime they can say to us, 'Go back to Kensington'. I can be the first one! Ah, ha, ha, ha. Mmm it was not so heavy like here.
>
> (Mrs M. Y.)

One of the African interviewees, who was born and raised in Windermere, said:

70

It was a sad story when everybody had to move out of Kensington. A sad story. Well those who were left behind were just lucky, because quite a few people are still there that we grew up with in Kensington. So we had to move out of the place man, hê! Even if, even if you can come back and say Babsie, they say, you can come back. I can be number one.

(Mrs S. D.)

The most powerful comparative message, interwoven with the peace/violence contrast, between the Windermere of the 1950s and the Guguletu of the 1990s, is the perceived loss of community:

Now these days, it's Guguletu where your neighbour is your enemy. Whereas in the olden days your neighbour was your sister. You can't ask your neighbour now please give me some sugar. No, she hasn't got it and the next thing the children fight, then the big people get involved. Now in the olden days if we used to fight with one another in our area [Windermere/Kensington], the big people just come and sort it out and take sticks and give us there. 'Now you fight!' [She bangs the table with her hands.]

(Mrs S. D.)

These passages refer to three related effects of apartheid: first, the damage to elder/youth relationships; second, the rupture of community and neighbourhood networks; and third, a deepening of the gap between politics and the private personal sphere. In a similar vein, Passerini has argued that Fascism 'accentuated the gap between the political sphere and daily private life, thus creating wounds in the tissue of memory, which could not easily recompose what had been forcefully separated' (Passerini 1992: 13).

In the above passages. I would argue we can hear interviewees making assessments of the painful effects caused by the social engineering of the apartheid system and the repression of anti-apartheid opposition. Furthermore, while all these interviewees were poor and lived under difficult conditions in Windermere, the limited material advances in their contemporary lives were overshadowed by the turbulent political and social conditions of township life from the 1970s onwards. A striking repetition in most of these stories is the longing to be the 'first one' to go back to the Windermere/Kensington area, and of course to go back to the 'youthful' days that can never be recaptured or relived.

The slum, for so many years a byword for poverty and deprivation, is transfigured into a warm and homely place, a little commonwealth where there was always a helping hand. The narrative of hard times becomes a record of courage and endurance.

71

The characteristic note is elegiac, saying good-bye to what will never be seen again, an affectionate leave-taking . . . the slum recaptures the symbolic space of 'the world we have lost'. Many, maybe most of the facts will be true. It is the omissions and the shaping which makes these stories also myth.

(Samuel and Thompson 1990: 9)

This kind of myth is not a common sense falsity or untruth: that is not the issue here. This myth-making contributes to the creation of memories which help people to live their lives in difficult times. Myths help to form complete stories about a personal past that will always be incomplete. Moreover, this 'Remembrance . . . in essence points to the incompleteness of the present' (Norval 1994: 12), an 'incompleteness' born of the unfulfilled needs, wants and desires that interviewees have lived with in their struggles to survive.

When interviewees tell their life stories, a tremendous army of emotions is evoked. Narrating one's life story is an emotional event Myth making, as an indelible element of story telling, is about pushing the limits of vocabulary and culture in order to express and understand the emotions of a traumatic past and present. It is all about putting into words and stories the diverse mixture of emotional experiences that is embedded in conscious and unconscious memory. As Bhabha suggests, 'Re-membering (sic) is never a quiet act of introspection. It is a painful remembering, a putting together of the dismembered past to make sense of the trauma of the present' (Bhabha 1987: 83). It is through this narrative 'putting together' of one's life stories that oral history has an implicit therapeutic value. Speaking the words, sentences and stories can offer containing form(s) to the terrifying formlessness of feelings and fragmentary life experiences.

In contrast to the above interviewees, there was a minority of Guguletu interviewees who did not paint a romantic gloss on the Windermere past and tended to focus more on the harshness of the present. The following dialogue with a male African interviewee reflects these patterns:

SF: And when you are at these meetings [burial society meetings] do you ever talk about the Windermere days?

BG: Not actually. We almost forget about the things of Windermere, Kensington.

SF: You almost forget?

BG: Mmm.

SF: Why?

BG: Ha, ah. What can I say? I, I don't know. There's a lot of problems here, that's why. You see?

SF: And that makes people forget?

BG: Yes, we've got no time for those old things now. We must look at this, what is happening now and these days.

72

For the following African interviewee there was anger and resentment at the violence (and poverty) in contemporary Guguletu. However, these experiences of hardship were additions to the horrors he saw in Windermere of the 1950s:

> We don't talk about the Kensington *dingus, besigheid* [thing, business]. Because it was too bad there. Nobody like it, anymore now. To talk about that *besigheid*, because was struggle in Kensington. Everybody know, was all the people was struggle at Kensington. Sometimes you will come from work in docks there, sometimes overtime late at night. We come home later past twelve, past one. Here come the, that fucken *dingus*. The band here. You know if you don't like this man, in midnight, I try to take a paraffin or petrol, we throw it over his house. Burn there. You know was *mos* [because] a shack was too close together, no space, passage between. If you are, you burnt, this *hokkie* [shack] here, that next door be burnt, then another one next door. All over. Now must wait, how many people inside there? Then you count how, one, two, you know how many people was burn inside? Ah Kensington, that place was no good there. The white people never take care, not a fucken *dingus*.
> (Mr B. R.)

In a similar vein a coloured interviewee who was involved in youth gangs in Windermere said:

> Let me tell you this, today, in this modern time of us living, you get black on black killing, to me it's a farce. Because this thing has been happening since I was a *laaitie* [small youngster]. Black and black killing was there, they were killing each other. Fingoes, Xhosas, Zulu and all today, but, years ago you know *pêl* [pal]. Let me tell you, *Here!* [God] We were standing on the stoep, and a guy would take out a chopper, and just chop a guy like that.
> (Mr G. M.)

There is little doubt that Windermere was at times a violent place. There is searing hurt expressed in these previous two stories, which are in direct contrast to the comforting tones of the earlier stories about Windermere. Life was tough then, and life is tough now. My sense is that for most interviewees there was considerable pain associated with the Windermere past.[12] For some that pain is managed by reconstructing their memories in a comforting way. On the one hand, memories of pain and hardship were suppressed (and repressed); on the other hand, happy memories were exaggerated and romanticized. Freud argued, 'As the indifferent memories owe their preservation not to their own content but to an associative relation between their content and another which is repressed, they have some claim to be called screen memories'

(Freud 1991: 83). In several instances the romantic memory constructions of Guguletu interviewees were possibly a form of screen memory, which concealed the displacement of significant memories laden with painful emotions.[13] In contrast, for other interviewees like those above, anger and aggression towards all this hardship, past and present, were openly expressed.

There were gender differences in these memory reconstructions. Male interviewees tended to recall present-centred, so-called 'reality-based' memories. However, my interpretations only partially support Hofmeyer's argument that men are more likely to tell 'true' historical accounts than women, who tend to use fictionalized narratives (Hofmeyer 1993). In so far as I focused on the reconstruction of memories to fulfil present needs, both female and male interviewees reconstructed their memories in fictionalized forms. The critical issue is not how much more or less men or women fictionalized their narratives, but that there were differing fictionalized images and patterns in men and women's storytelling. I would argue that the so-called 'reality-based' memories (of predominantly male interviewees) of the past were a defensive, at times avoidant, response to discomforting feelings of pain.

The various forms and degrees of pain experienced under apartheid must be dealt with, consciously or unconsciously, by both men and women. Moral judgments cannot be made about which coping mechanisms are most appropriate. In psychic terms, the personal need is about how best to cope with, manage and defend a fragile sense of self and identity, which always has to survive in the present, but bears the burden of the past. The interwoven micro-power struggles of day-to-day living construct the 'conditions for remembering' (Freud 1991: 87). It is through interpreting these discursive conditions for remembering *and* story-telling that more may be understood about the construction of memory, myth and identity.

For all interviewees Windermere was (for either positive or negative reasons) a very significant phase in lives of physical and social movement. In particular, rural to urban movements required a range of life strategies for survival. These life strategies were vital to organising consciousness (Bozzoli 1991). Both the physical movement of African people from Windermere of the 1950s to Guguletu of the 1990s and the movement of social memories between these places and times constituted a cultural dialogue. Apartheid destroyed Windermere, but the popular memories of Windermere still speak to individuals from within, through dreams, fantasies and feelings.

One African interviewee spoke of her parents appearing in her dreams at night to warn her of danger in Guguletu, and to tell her not to go out the next day. Another African interviewee spoke of the 'spirits' warning her of the dangers in the community. These past images of Windermere, parents and childhood interweave to form both a kind of solace to the individual and a defensive communication about approaching danger.

Windermere also speaks to individuals through the reminders of other Windermere people living in Guguletu. I frequently found interviewees who could point out several other former Windermere people next door, across the road and down the street. An African interviewee stressed that 'remembering is so good because we are helping one another. That's what, we are not forgetting one another, when we come together even here in Guguletu' (Mr A. Z.).

The splintering of communities like Windermere through apartheid laws was counterposed with remembering the Windermere past as a unified whole. In the process, remembering became an act of reaffirming social ties. Remembering the Windermere past, a time before apartheid, also became an act of solidarity against apartheid's separations and exclusions. As Lowenthal comments, 'we need other people's memories to confirm our own and to give them endurance. . . In the process of knitting our own discontinuous recollections into narratives we revise personal components to fit the collectively remembered past' (Lowenthal 1985: 196). Memories filled with harmonious images of Windermere created a mythical wholeness of 'our community' and 'us' as unified 'one'.

The active process of recalling memories in the present (as distinct from the memories themselves) simultaneously reflects an unfulfilled desire for community and the symbolic creation of a community-in-memory. African interviewees' frequent reiteration of the term 'Windermere people' affirms both their community-in-memory and their shared sense of community identity. The mythical wholeness of the 'Windermere community' was often contrasted with the ethnic fissures and 'racial' divisions of life under apartheid. An African interviewee said, 'We were sent away, we must come to Guguletu. They didn't want any black person around, that coloureds must be themselves and so on. That is apartheid. That is definite, it is through apartheid' (Mr A. Z.).

Both African and coloured interviewees had vivid memories of the Windermere days and both tended to romanticize those days. Where most of the African interviewees in Guguletu had a community-in-memory constructed through their popular memories and identification as 'Windermere people', this simply did not happen amongst coloured residents in Factreton. The following coloured interviewee said:

En die Africans wat hier gebly't daai tyd, was nou van die soort wat soe kaalvoet geloop't, kaalvoet soorte. Maar ek kan meneer sê, daai kaalvoet soorte, hulle respek vir 'n mens gehet. Hulle sul nooit met jou geinterfere't nie. As hulle jou kry in die aand en dit is laat, dan sal hul sê, 'Meisiekind waar bly jy? Jy moet huis toe gaan, jou Ma wag vir jou'. Nou soe was hulle, nie die geleerdes van vir dag nie, hulle maak jou dood. [And the African that lived here that time, were of the type that walked bare foot, bare foot types. But I can tell mister, those bare foot types, they had respect for a person. They would never interfere with one. If they get you at night and it is late, then they would say, 'Girl child where do you live? You must go home, your mother is waiting for you.' Now that was how they were, not the educateds of today, they make you dead.]

(Mrs D. A.)

The noble savage was cast within a romantic view of the peaceful past and contrasted with the murdering educated African of the violent present. A crude 'racial' othering and stereotyping dominates the passage. While all coloured interviewees remembered the Windermere days. they did not seem to have developed any collective identity around and through these social memories. The absence of these identifications revealed a silence. How coloured and African interviewees remembered the Windermere past, and how they used these memories in the present, are interconnected with historical patterns of cultural difference and identity. A coloured interviewee told the following story:

Windermere was a goeie plek gewies, dit was maar net die mense in Windermere gebly't, wat nie soe lekker gewies't nie, soos dit all over gaan nie. Die tenants kom nie met die ene, en die ene klaar nie, maar Windermere was 'n goeie plek. Ek sê maar elke dag, as ek nou nog kan 'n sink huis kry in Windermere, wat daar nou met sink huise gewies't, dat ek soentoe getrek, na my ou dorp toe. Dit was baie lekker daar. [Windermere was a good place, it was but the people that lived in Windermere, that wasn't so nice, as it goes all over. The tenants don't get on with the one or the other, but Windermere was a good place. I say every day, if I can get a zinc house in Windermere, as there were zinc houses, that I would move to my old village. It was very nice there.]

(Mrs C. S.)

Paradoxically, this interviewee denied a sense of community, but praised Windermere the place romantically. This ambivalent sense of community identity was evident amongst most coloured interviewees. They had remained behind in the same place while the space around them was being transformed by the apartheid state.[14] In the process, their sense of place and belonging must surely have been affected. In contrast, African interviewees spoke of their first-hand experiences of being forcibly removed to another space and place in Guguletu or Langa. Most coloured interviewees cast themselves in the roles of distant or close observers of these historical events. It was rare to find a coloured resident who acknowledged their social and emotional impact. It is therefore not surprising that coloured residents did not develop a sense of community-in-memory about Windermere.

There is little doubt that many coloured and African people lived together happily in Windermere, but a mixture of accurate observations and mythical truths was constantly shaped by an unfulfilled desire for peace, tranquillity and stable community living in the Guguletu and Factreton of the present.

This unfulfilled desire was unconsciously projected on to the past, which was reconstructed in the form of harmonious and comforting memories of the Windermere community. As Passerini argues, 'Hopes, fears and projections converge into shaping memory and its strategies' (Passerini 1992: 12). For African interviewees this need for peace and togetherness was partially met within a fragile sense of community identity, constructed through a symbolic discourse of Windermere, their community-in-memory. In contrast, coloured interviewees did not express a community-in-memory and in the process constructed a more ambivalent sense of community identity, shaped by the bewildering transformation from Windermere of the 1950s to Factreton of the 1960s and 1990s.

Finally, these memories and myths from Windermere still have considerable currency amongst a particular generation of African and coloured people living on the Cape Flats. Documenting these memories through oral history interviews has been a difficult process within a turbulent social context. While this context requires flexible and sensitive access strategies, it also amplifies the social *and* emotional significance of the oral history dialogue. The moving memories of former Windermere residents constitute one profound way of negotiating the strains of living within a culture of violence.

Notes

I acknowledge and appreciate the critical comments and questions provided by Paul Thompson, Mary van der Riet and the anonymous reader.

1   Note the term 'black' is used to refer to those individuals defined as 'African', 'coloured' and 'Asian' under apartheid laws. These terms and the term 'white' are imbued with a shifting mixture of positive and negative meanings from the apartheid era. These contested terms will be used in this study as they are the dominant labels used by the interviewees in referring to themselves and others.

2   'The present' unless otherwise stated, will in this paper refer to the January to September 1993 period. For further discussion on the Windermere community, and the theory and methodology developed, see Field 1996.

3   The term 'culture of violence' is used in a descriptive sense to characterize the context of violent conditions of day-to-day living in black townships. The term refers to both common law and political forms of violence. The historical roots of the culture of violence are to be found in the interwoven political, economic, cultural and psychological formations produced under colonial, segregationist and apartheid regimes. See Marks and Anderson 1990. For an overview of the historical literature on violence in South Africa see Beinart 1992.

4   The fifty-four interviewees consisted of twenty-five African, twenty-three coloured and six white individuals. Their ages varied from fifty to ninety-two, with the majority being between sixty and seventy-five. As this paper focuses on the impact of the culture of violence on black (coloured and African) interviewees, white interviewees are not referred to here. However, I do intend

exploring the differences and similarities between white and black interviewees' memories in a separate paper.

5 The spatial area on which Windermere once stood is also partly covered by the lower-middle-class coloured community of Kensington.

6 Official population figures in the 14,000–20,000 range are cited by annual reports of the medical officer of the Cape Town City Council (CCC), 1944–54. The percentage estimates are my speculative calculations, drawn from Western Cape Administration Board (WCAB) records and newspapers of the 1958–63 period.

7 'Shebeens' are usually venues for illegal trade in alcohol. While some shebeens sell drugs and sex, there are other shebeens that are part of ordinary family networks and constitute an important supplement to the household income.

8 The Windermere community of the 1950s was spatially situated in the middle of the area currently referred to as 'Factreton' and 'Kensington'. While the Factreton/Kensington area is spatially separate from the network of suburbs referred to as the 'Cape Flats', due to a common history of forced removals, it is nevertheless symbolically a part of the Cape Flats.

9 Gossip in this instance opened up access, but it can just as easily close off access to the researcher. For an analysis of the structure and significance of gossip, see Bergmann 1993.

10 I initially thought that my white presence was having a specifically negative bearing on the interviewees. This was dispelled when the black African research assistant noted that in his previous interviewing experience with African interviewees these kind of responses were also typical.

11 Within the interviewing context it is sometimes difficult to distinguish between 'silences' and 'refusals'. Subtle indirect questioning can be used, but ultimately the interviewee has the right to withhold information.

12 A small number of interviewees expressed pain and sadness explicitly through crying (six out of fifty-four interviewees). A few interviewees were also on the verge of crying at different stages in the interviews.

13 I have not applied any psychoanalytic model but rather I have used psycho-analysis as a 'sensitising theory' (Ian Craib, personal communication, 1994). See Gay 1985.

14 By the term 'place' I mean a socially constructed sense of feeling that one 'belongs' or is at 'home' within a specific physical location. The term 'space' is used as a political, social and geographical term to mark the juxtapositioning and relationships between people within a particular physical terrain. These terms have blurred boundaries.

References

Beinart, W. (1992) 'Introduction: political and collective violence in Southern African historiography', *Journal of South African Studies*, vol. 18, no. 3.

Bergmann, J. (1993) *Discreet Indiscretions. The Social Organisation of Gossip*, New York.

Bertaux-Wiame, I. (1981) 'The life history approach to the study of inter-racial migration', in D. Bertaux (ed.), *Biography and Society. The Life History Approach in Social Sciences*, London.

Bhabha, H. (1987) 'What does the black man want?', *New Formations*, vol. 1.

Bozzoli, B. with Nkotsoe, M. (1991) *Women of Phokeng. Consciousness, Life Strategy and Migrancy in South Africa, 1900–1983,* Johannesburg.

Casement, P. (1985) *On Learning from the Patient,* London.

Field, S. (1996) *The Power of Exclusion: Moving Memories from Windermere to the Cape Flats,* unpublished Ph.D. thesis, University of Essex.

Figlio, K. (1985) 'Oral history and the unconscious', *History Workshop Journal*, vol. 26.

Foucault, M. (1976) *The History of Sexuality. An Introduction,* London:.

Freud, S. (1991) *The Psychopathology of Everyday Life,* London.

Frisch, M. (1990) *A Shared Authority. Essays on the Craft and Meaning of Oral History and Public History,* New York.

Gay, P. (1985) *Freud for Historians,* New York.

Grele, R. (1991) *The Envelopes of Sound. The Art of Oral History,* New York.

Hofmeyer, I. (1993) *'We Spend Our Years as a Tale That is Told',* Oral Historical Narrative in a South African Chiefdom, London.

Lowenthal, D. (1985) *The Past is a Foreign Country*, Cambridge.

Marks, S. and Anderson, N. (1990) 'The epidemiology and culture of violence', in N. Manganyi and A. Du Toit (eds), *Political Violence and Struggle in South Africa,* Johannesburg.

Norval, A. (1994) 'Images of Babel: language and the politics of identity', *Journal of the Southern African Studies Conference,* York.

Passerini, L. (1987) *Fascism in Popular Memory*, Cambridge.

—— (1992) 'Memory and Totalitarianism' (*International Yearbook of Oral History and Life Stories, vol. 1*), Oxford: OUP.

Popular Memory Group (1982) 'Theory, politics and method' in Centre of Contemporary Cultural Studies, *Making Histories, Studies in History – Writing and Politics*, London.

Portelli, A. (1991) *The Death of Luigi Trastulli and Other Stories. Form and Meaning in Oral History*, New York.

Samuel, R. and Thompson, P. (1990) *The Myths We Live By*, London.

Scott, J. (1990) *Domination and the Arts of Resistance. Hidden Transcripts,* London.

Swart, C. (1983) 'Windermere, from the peri-urban to suburb. 1920s to 1950s', Honours dissertation, University of Cape Town.

Tonkin, E. (1992) *Narrating Our Pasts. The Social Construction of Oral History*, Cambridge.

Yeo, S. (1988) 'Difference, autobiography and history', *Literature and History,* vol. 14, no. 1.

4

OPPRESSION, RESISTANCE AND IMPRISONMENT

A montage of different but similar stories in two countries

Jan K. Coetzee and Otakar Hulec

Introduction

At the beginning of this decade, remarkably similar transitions began in different parts of the world and under very different social, economic and political circumstances. It is important to focus anew on those regions, where comprehensive oppression has had a devastating effect on the lives of the majority, as the experience makes it clear that more humane political and social systems will enable people to become more than they are.

Much has been written on the authoritarian and totalitarian structures which had been put into place by the perpetrators of injustice and the masterminds of comprehensive systems of oppression. Less attention has been given to the experiences of individual victims of human rights abuses. In an attempt to redress this imbalance, this essay focuses on some of those who were on the receiving end of the social, economic and political violence that these tyrannical regimes unleashed.

Our information was obtained by recording the life histories of a selected group of political activists who were charged, stood trial and were incarcerated in prison or in labour camps for lengthy periods during the post-Second World War era as a result of their opposition to authoritarian rule.[1] It provides an account of aspects of the experiences of former political prisoners in South Africa and in the then Czechoslovakia.

Not only does this essay touch on the nature of repressive measures employed by the governments concerned, but more importantly it also provides an opportunity to testify to past injustices. The testimony of traumatic experiences during long periods of incarceration highlights the human capacity to oppose authoritarian and totalitarian rule, to resist techniques and strategies employed by repressive states, and to reorder their way of life in such a way that survival is possible. These testimonies of the immense trauma experienced by victims of oppression become living proof of the human ability not merely to survive, but to work towards personal growth and moral strengthening in the face of the most abhorrent humiliation, suffering and hardship.

Different but similar: the suppression of human rights

In South Africa as well as Czechoslovakia, years of authoritarian and totalitarian rule were marked by a range of human-rights abuses. This essay does not purport to deal with the way in which these governments operationalized their rule. Above all, this is an account of individual struggles, not those of organised political movements. As part of the broader context we will, however, refer briefly to aspects of legislation, economic and social structuring as well as repressive machineries introduced to maintain power and control.

In South Africa the political situation changed dramatically in 1948 when the National Party gained a narrow parliamentary majority. The Nationalists, more determined and more confident of state power than their predecessors, started to introduce what would become one of the most notorious forms of social engineering, apartheid.[2] In order to crush any opposition, major restrictions were placed on democratic political activity. Various legislative measures were enforced by harsh action to end the various defiance campaigns, including bannings and imprisonments.[3] After several confrontations, the regime announced the banning of the ANC and the PAC (the two most important liberation movements) with effect from April 1960.[4]

In Czechoslovakia the disillusionment following the 'betrayal' by Western allies such as France and Great Britain towards the end of the Second World War enabled communist leaders to emphasize the support coming from the Soviet Union during the same period. This enabled several communist politicians to enter the provisional government, and gave rise to stronger pro-communist sentiments among Czechoslovakian intellectuals, workers and small farmers. In many ways people felt more optimistic about a future linked with the Eastern Bloc.[5]

At the beginning of 1948, during preparations for a new election in May, activities among all political parties began to increase. Expecting defeat at the elections, the communists mounted a political *coup d'état* during February 1948 and the new government began to 'build a socialist country'.[6] The new regime instituted political persecution which led to the restriction and sometimes the destruction of political freedom and civil rights (Kaplan 1993). Strict censorship over newspapers, magazines and books was imposed to silence opposition. Repressive measures against perceived opponents of the regime were followed by various forms of structural violence.[7]

After the deaths of Stalin and the communist President Gottwald, the political situation improved somewhat, leading to a new era of 'socialism with a human face', and the short-lived 'Prague Spring' of 1968. But the violent crushing of the reformers by the Soviet Army in August 1968 unleashed a new wage of political oppression. From 1948 to 1989 more than a quarter of a million people in Czechoslovakia were officially convicted of opposing the regime and given sentences of various forms (Kaplan 1993: 19).

Resistance

Hardly any part of the lives of people who lived in South Africa and the former Czechoslovakia was left untouched. Within both states the authoritarian and totalitarian systems sought to control and impose norms on all the social dimensions of human life. The final aim of these comprehensive systems of oppression was to force people to 'finally succumb to the insidious process that continually undermines hope and subverts the desire to "become"' (Goldberg 1978).

This was indeed the case with millions of South Africans classified by acts of parliament as non-white, as well as with large numbers of people in Czechoslovakia. They were caught up in a comprehensive range of oppressive entanglements that influenced their daily lives. Most of those who lived under these conditions accepted, almost passively, the institutionalised socio-political domination under which they found themselves. To many the yoke of oppression became part and parcel of an internalised definition of reality, a self-evident fact of life. But this was not the case for those who told us their stories; those who eventually stood trial and were sentenced to long-term incarceration, whether it was on Robben Island (home of one of the world's most notorious penal institutions) or in prisons and labour camps scattered all over the then Czechoslovakia. These were the people of resistance.

In South Africa upsurges of resistance against the apartheid system received much more direct support among the masses of oppressed people than was the case in Central Europe. The keystone of the system was forced separation on the basis of race. Living together as an oppressed group developed a strong awareness among blacks of belonging to the same category. This factor constitutes the most important explanation for the difference between the experience of political imprisonment in South Africa on the one hand, and Czechoslovakia on the other. The everyday situation of non-white South Africans constantly called for the use of mass struggle through boycotts, strikes and other forms of civil disobedience. The fact that the regime managed to maintain control over the entire way of life of the majority was due to its monopoly of military power, its financial and mineral resources, continued support by many of its Western allies and the way in which it used law as an instrument of total oppression.

We referred earlier to the way in which the South African legal structure determined where you could stay, who you could marry, what jobs would be available and even what kind of education you would receive. The law not only determined all aspects of the social structure and what people were allowed to do; it also prescribed how and what they should think.[8] The fierce legal penalties imposed on those who deliberately challenged laws forced the dissenters to abandon the Defiance Campaign of the 1950s.[9] Other forms of struggle were subsequently introduced.[10]

All the former Robben Island political prisoners who told us their life stories related aspects of the social functioning of the law, indicating their experience of the formal characteristics of the law as an instrument in keeping the authoritarian regime in place. The law gradually and systematically became an ever-more powerful instrument of '"dark" social engineering' (Podgorecki 1993: 83). The massive use of force against people during the 1950s and early 1960s compelled the leaders of the liberation movements to look for alternative forms of struggle. It was felt that without the use of violence the African people could not succeed in their struggle for liberation. In November 1961 the ANC's *Umkhonto we Sizwe* (Spear of the Nation) was formed. Its plan was to sabotage state installations without taking human lives. In contrast the militant underground movement *Poqo* (We Go It Alone) of the PAC turned to tactics of intimidation and did not shrink from taking lives (Davenport 1987: 400–5). Eventually the law was used to deal with those not prepared to accept the social structuring of South Africa.

In Czechoslovakia, as in South Africa, the whole of the legal system and the security establishment were guided by the political sections of the criminal code. The most important issue there, however, was the fight against the enemies of socialism and communism. Anyone seeming to offer even the slightest support to the 'subversive elements' in society was regarded as belonging to the enemy. The guardians of the system often applied merciless interrogation, and would even occasionally resort to the supreme measure of capital punishment. Under this regime it was impossible for the oppressors to rule without prison confinement, while the ordinary people were constantly made aware of the fate awaiting them should they step out of line.

The inner experience of incarceration: humiliation and degradation

Oppression (and in particular political imprisonment) is above all an exercise in power, an attempt to instill or maintain authority. The agents of the state used many technical and psychological strategies in attempts to enter the world of the private self of the political prisoner without having much personal contact with the prisoners. By compelling them to behave in a certain way, and exposing them to degrading practices (such as regular strip-searches, forcing them to wear particular clothing, addressing them in demeaning terms, and setting the non-political prisoners against them), an attempt was made to dehumanize them. The state and its agents were aware that if people lose their integrity, they are headed towards the destruction of their personality and of their uniqueness as individuals.

On arrival at Robben Island it was made clear to the South African political prisoners that they were in for hard times. Almost all the warders were Afrikaans-speaking white men (coming mainly from the lower socio-economic strata of the South African white population). They were highly prejudiced against what they would often refer to as 'communists, terrorists, barbarians, and uncivilised hordes'.

> He was saying, 'This is prison, it's not going to be with the police, so you are going to shit here. This is prison, you are no more in the location. You are going to shit here.' That fellow [warder] was not saying any other thing than that. . . .
>
> Even the language they were using. When talking to us, saying that we must eat, they would use the language they use when the eating is done by animals: 'Vreet, vreet, vreet!' 'Hou jou bek' (shut your trap) when they wanted you to keep quiet. You know you were so degraded, honestly.
>
> (Former Robben Islander 2)

> No, they were ruthless [the warders on Robben Island]. They treated us more ruthless than they treated the criminals. I suppose the intention was – the aim was for us to die on Robben Island, all of us, you see. One was saying, 'You dogs, do you think you can rule South Africa? You want to become cabinet – who are you? You want to take over.' And they they would tell us a lot of things about the African states and so on. 'You want to mess up this country too. And that you will never achieve.' They would call us by all names and beat us. . . .
>
> Thereafter we would go out with the span to work – work at the quarries, chopping stones and so on. And then in the afternoon we would go back to the cells . . . there was that thing which was very bad. This thing of 'ukuthawuze' – you go naked and then they start searching you.'
>
> (Former Robben Islander 1)

> You know it is so cold on Robben Island, almost throughout the year. We would be given jerseys, say in April, by September they were taken away because they say it is summer. Whilst it is bitterly cold. They say, 'How can you wear jerseys in summer? It is summer.' . . .
>
> And initially we were not allowed to take sandals and shoes inside the cell. Before you enter the cell you park them next to the door along the wall. You get your shoes tomorrow morning – not in the cell. Then in the morning they rush you to such an extent that

you take anybody's shoes – size ten and size six this side. Then you become so confused and in the process what else can you do but to keep those shoes or sandals and then you put them on your shoulder and they would shout, 'Hey, look at them. They don't know shoes from outside. Look, this is exactly what they do outside: they go into the shoe shop, they only point out the shoe that they want without considering the size. This is a typical example of what they do outside. *Hulle ken nie skoene nie! Kyk hoe dra hulle hulle skoene!* . . .

We were people with aspirations and with a mission. They knew that. That is what they wanted to break.

(Former Robben Islander 6)

A major difference between South Africa and Czechoslovakia was that political prisoners in the latter were normally kept together with criminals. Just as on Robben Island, any form of mutual social empathy between the political prisoners and the warders (who represented the state) was deliberately reduced to the minimum. Not only did the warders see this lack of empathy as a logical part of their task as overseers of the punishment, they also often deliberately turned to humiliation and degradation as part of this role.

We were not looked at as political prisoners. There were murderers and thieves and people like that with us. And they looked at us as something much worse than these murderers. They were saying that on our hands there was blood of their mothers and I don't know whatever. So, you see, we were really class enemies.

(Former Czechoslovakian prisoner 2)

The real psychological oppression was in Leopoldov. There the guards kept telling us that from here you will leave only with your feet first. And we were in terrible physical condition, so that we saw that they are really going to ruin us physically because of lack of food. . . .

Yes, the first line or the first limit was reached after three years because when you have spent in prison such a long time, the civilian in you evaporates somehow. The monotonous life somehow drives the civilian out of you. We used to call it brain-leaked. You had a leaking brain like a MUKL – a man destined for liquidation. [MUKL is the acronym for the four Czech words literally meaning 'man destined for liquidation'] . . .

We started not to care for health, not to care for life. We were somehow proud to be prisoners. I heard prisoners saying, 'If we ever get out from here we will shoot even the geese on the pond.'

We hated the system. I started to hate the civilians, because they were part of the enemy. 'You are keeping your mouths shut and you live here peacefully and we are suffering the hell there.'

(Former Czechoslovakian prisoner 1)

I had no experience of exposure to physical pain or torturing but we experienced something of it. A young woman (it was winter) was called to the basement of the prison. She had to stand there for hours without any dress – naked and without shoes. She had to stand on cement. After some hours steam was released – it was hot and there was no air to breathe. Then it was cold again. And so it went on for a fortnight. The woman was also without necessary tampons and she could not wash herself. Voices behind the door would sound, 'Has she already died?' . . .

Her twelve-year sentence was later lowered to six years and she could go home earlier. Later, all her woman organs had to be removed. She could not have children.

(Former Czechoslovakian prisoner 3)

The inner experience of incarceration: working towards strength and solidarity

From a very early stage the leaders on Robben Island realised that what a person believes others think of him is a precious value cherished by anyone. Therefore, one of the most powerful mechanisms to assist their comrades in dealing with the abnormal conditions of long-term incarceration was to instill a feeling of solidarity and belonging. Any prison term carries with it a strong element of condemnation, censorship and punishment – emphasised by the phenomena of iron-bound captivity, exposure to humiliation by warders, and extreme isolation. It was therefore essential to build group solidarity, to demonstrate approval of the cause and to ensure that each individual experienced acceptance by the group. This could only be done by stubbornly adhering to the principles and policies of the struggle, and insisting on debating and preserving them, creating a collective courage and strength.

You know what the prison warders used to say: '*Poqos* [initial name of the PAC's militant underground movement, used indiscriminately to refer to any 'terrorists'] they don't care for your tobacco, they don't care for your money – you can leave your fifty rand or what not. They don't care for it. But if there was a newspaper . . . (and in fact they were correct) . . . if there was a newspaper – that newspaper you would never get. You can do whatever – you won't get the newspaper. The *Poqos* will make it a point that they take the

86

newspaper with them to the prison cells.' And I say to you – limited as those newspapers used to be, we used to keep all those things in our memories. We would discuss those newspaper items for days and nights and months.

(Former Robben Islander 2)

We were struggling for clothing, struggling for food, struggling for many other things. We would discuss, every time. Each and every cell would discuss our complaints and then after discussing the complaints we would decide on a delegation to go to the authorities and put forward these complaints. . . .

In prison if you were not constructive it was very dangerous. You could become mentally deranged because you were sentenced maybe to sixteen or twenty years. It was no use thinking about your wife, girlfriend or your children outside. There was nothing you could do. So in order to avoid that, you must get very busy in studies and in sport. You must do some constructive things. You must not have the chance of thinking of a lot of things.

Another advantage in prison [at a later stage] – it is a question of having enough time to study. To concentrate on studies. You discussed many things. You read a lot. Something that one cannot afford outside here. But the main thing is that you have no contact with the outside world. You are a human being. How to be in prison, sometimes you think about this thing – that, well, I am going to stay here for so many years, when I go out I will be old and so on. But you have to accept that. . . .

You see in every cell there would be a study officer who is going to declare studies, and close the studies too. Then after closing the studies, they start reading cuttings.

(Former Robben Islander 1)

A lot of us were illiterate; couldn't read or write. Then we devised a system whereby if you had a standard eight then you must teach standard six right from standard one or sub-A. Each one teach each other. The prison authorities never had a hand in helping us in that. That time there was another section which was being built [it was under construction]. So we used to take those cement pockets and convert them into books. There were very skillful people there who would bind them together in book form. So we would take this into the cell and that is where it started – even on the floor. Sometimes you were not supposed to sweep the floor, we needed that dust. Once the sun gets into the cell then the starters wrote the five vowels, 'a e i o u', they must read that and then the technique of writing on the floor. But as well as these cement pockets helped us, there were not enough to cover the whole population of the prison.

(Former Robben Islander 6)

Congregating a uniquely selected group of people with exceptional insight and leadership qualities inevitably established an extraordinary community on Robben Island. Despite the brutal crushing of periodic outbreaks of resistance among South Africa's non-white groups, the victims of the oppressive regime managed to constitute their own way of survival. Despite the degrading character of long-term incarceration, under the guidance of true leaders the political prisoners were able to maintain a set of binding principles. Opportunities were created for them to contemplate inner thoughts and feelings, to identify with the values of the group and to experience growth in their own lives. More than anything else this contributed to survival amidst an effort to reduce life to its primordial mechanism: merely staying alive. And it brought about much more than a mechanism of survival. The accolade 'University of Robben Island' was indeed an apt description of the formative effect incarceration had on the alumni of this institution.

The camaraderie between fellow political prisoners, the feeling of belonging and the sharing of common ideals which guided the entire period of imprisonment on Robben Island, were almost totally absent from the situation in which political prisoners found themselves in Czechoslovakia. It was largely up to the individual to delve into his or her own inner resources to find the strength so necessary for survival.

The moment you decided to wait for something, it was already a death sentence for you. Those were abnormal situations, but you had to adapt to it. It was a part of your life, whether normal or not, and it was your duty to go through it somehow.

(Former Czechoslovakian prisoner 2)

These years in prison were the worst years of my life, but I am not sorry for it. I am a baptised Christian, but so as I started to trust in God in the prison, can nobody who wasn't imprisoned. There is an old proverb that the man who wasn't on the sea cannot pray. I would change it now: the man who wasn't in the prison cannot pray. Because so as you pray in the prison, you never pray in civilian life. . . .

During the first two or three years we still lived in the hope that something will happen, that the regime will fall. But nothing was happening. Step by step we became dull, became primitive. The thing that we were most interested in was food because we never ate enough. . . .

Some of us had photographs of our family. So in the evening we went to bed and put the photographs on the blankets and watched the wife and children and so on. The evenings were very sentimental. . . .

But in Leopoldov gathered priests, professors, scientists and other members of the intelligentsia. Although we had to be liquidated there slowly by hunger, the prisoners started to study foreign languages. We were allowed to smoke there and we rolled cigarettes. So we had cigarette papers and from a whole bunch of cigarette papers you made something like a copy book. You could sew through. By a sharp and hard piece of pencil you could make notes there. So for instance, I remember, Rudla Vašata who was plucking feathers with me in Leopoldov, he was sitting beside me. He had under his shirt a roll of toilet paper and it was full of English irregular verbs. So each morning before we started to work, we met there, and we started to repeat all irregular verbs.

(Former Czechoslovakian prisoner 1)

Survival against all odds

From the accounts above it is clear that the price of dissent was indeed a heavy one. The history of opposition in both countries is a tragic one, consisting of endless numbers of crippled and ruined fates. As well as those who lost their lives in the struggle for liberation and democracy, every single person who spent time in a prison or a labour camp suffered permanent damage in terms of opportunities, lost youth, disruption to family life, health, as well as material and spiritual welfare in the broadest sense of the word.

In many ways it was easier for those who spent long periods of political imprisonment on Robben Island to manage their frustration, anger and lust for revenge. The remarkable way in which the leadership on the island managed to channel the potential for frustration and aggression that might have been directed against fellow prisoners and even warders needs mentioning. It was only by developing special ties that strengthened the values of human solidarity that a potentially dangerous and destructive situation could have been avoided.

The Robben Islanders managed in various ways to contribute towards mutual bonds of reinforcement and to keep alive a sense of meaningful existence. By combining values beyond the boundaries of their imprisonment (appreciation of the moral support outside; keeping alive the ideological beliefs) with a strong maintenance of discipline, they created a moral environment which carried them through the long years.

The Disciplinary Committee (DC) was very strict and it would not allow people to be loitering in the yard becoming engaged in corruption and other things. Everybody must go out with a span and go and work.

(Former Robben Islander 1)

To be taken from everyday life to the extremities of long-term incarceration means to be shorn of the elaborate systems of relationships: not only the directly visible ones such as the home, family and friends or work environment, but also the abstract ones such as culture and tradition. Even if it was not intended to deprive prisoners from their culture and tradition, long-term imprisonment could easily have led to this happening. But by being kept together on Robben Island, with ample opportunity to discuss issues, the South African political prisoners were given the opportunity to devise strategies and to uphold aspects of their culture. One such aspect was the traditional rite of circumcision (particularly important in the Xhosa tradition – the strongest one represented on Robben Island).

We realised that those who came in as young prisoners were going to stay in prison for a long time and then circumcision was necessary for them. [On the question whether the ANC organised this:] *Haai!* No, the ANC pretended as if it did not know anything. It was done clandestinely. We did not know about it. We would only discover it the following day when we were going to play soccer that most of our youngsters were not there. They had been circumcised by [Former Robben Islander 4]. They were staying in the cell – getting pains there. You know this thing of circumcision – no water, no what. Very strict.

(Former Robben Islander 1)

I was an *ukwaluka* – the man who performs the circumcision.[11] . . . Yes, with Schoeman. Then these young boys of the Western Cape, Transkei, Border, and the Eastern Cape [Xhosas] had a better chance now. That was April/May 1974. I started circumcising right until July of that year then I stopped. Then I started again in December. The total number: 361. I stopped in October 1981. . . .

I saw trouble between prisoners and warders where the warder was carrying the gun and he wanted to shoot the prisoner. I know what the cause of that was that this young boy never reported to anybody because he was supposed to be circumcised before time. It is the time now when he is supposed to be a man. By a certain time (when a boy reaches eighteen) he must be circumcised.

I know in jail there is only one committee to discipline the people. It is our custom. That is why I said: 'Let me circumcise these boys here to put them into the correct line.' Because government can't put them in the correct line because they don't know that it is a question of circumcision.

(Former Robben Islander 4)

The political prisoners in Czechoslovakia did not have a support and social structure as was the case on Robben Island. Although many religious leaders found themselves in Czechoslovakian prisons and labour camps, the prison authorities were ruthless in preventing them from performing any counselling role. They indeed engaged in religious activity, serving midnight masses in the cells or in some cases down mine shafts, but it was not possible to contribute to a sense of belonging or to assist those who experienced anxiety. A former prisoner, who was her mother's only support, said the following when asked about possible effects of her imprisonment:

There were no physical scars. But I certainly had and still have emotional scars. Even now I dream several times a year of being imprisoned again and what is more, my mother being there with me, or she alone, without me. I wake up with fear that she won't survive it. These nightmares are very unpleasant. They still come after thirty years. I did not fear that I might die in prison but I was terribly afraid that my mother might die. Such thinking was returning to me almost every evening when the light was switched off, when we were left to ourselves. In the first three years it was not so bad but every following year it was heavier and heavier. Then the fourth came, the fifth, the sixth, the seventh . . . and the idea struck: will this go on as long as the twelfth?

(Former Czechoslovakian prisoner 2)

In conclusion

Our comparative analysis began by emphasising the similar way in which oppressive legal systems underpinned authoritarian and totalitarian regimes. We found similar accounts of the humiliation and degradation suffered by those who took a stand against the oppression. All of those who told us their life stories had to make special efforts to strengthen themselves – physically as well as emotionally – during their endeavours. But that is where the parallels end.

In South Africa the system of apartheid has been destroyed and a new government represents the majority who were previously forcefully and structurally oppressed. This achievement has naturally affected and affirmed the memories of those who were imprisoned as a result of their fierce opposition to these injustices. The authoritarianism practised in South Africa was less all-pervading, and in the end, less effective than the full-fledged totalitarianism of the Eastern Bloc countries. The racial divide in South Africa brought immeasurable pain and humiliation, but at the same time it created the opportunity for solidarity and the establishment of an united resistance against the oppressor. The political victory of the ANC provided the ex-Robben Islanders with a basis they could use to recover from their experiences. Success in the struggle created an ability to integrate into a coherent life story the hardship and humiliation of their incarceration with the accomplishment of the victory. Most of the former Robben Islanders would echo the following words:

> I had become very proud of my incarceration. Even if I can die, I know that I had fought for the betterment of my people and that has been realised. We voted and now we are busy with the second stage of our struggle – nation-building. I bear nobody a grudge.
>
> (Former Robben Islander 6)

On the other side of the globe the assessment of their suffering and treatment is starkly different. Notwithstanding the political changes in the former Eastern Bloc countries, those who went through the ordeal of long-term incarceration do not recontextualise their traumatic experiences into purposive life stories in the same way as the former Robben Islanders. They do not reinterpret their suffering as being for the collective good of others. Asked whether she regarded what she had gone through as worth while, one elderly lady proclaimed:

> On the contrary, I lost everything that I had. And what was worst, my mother lost her flat which was given to her. If I had the opportunity to do things over, I would never ever, never ever do it all again.
>
> (Former Czechoslovakian prisoner 3)

The preceding narratives teach us important lessons about the nature of memory. There is undoubtedly a tendency to incorporate current conditions when evaluating past experiences. People's interpretations of past experiences of long-term imprisonment are tinted by their current political and material conditions. The ethos, values and esteem of their movement (and now political party – the ANC) have changed the very lives of former Robben Islanders. They tend to reflect on the objective circumstances of the actual periods of incarceration against the background of the political victory which culminated in the first democratically elected South African government. The distinction between broad social, political and economic factors on the one hand, and individual understandings and interpretations of both present and past circumstances on the other, is however not unique to the life stories on which this research is based. Many researchers have highlighted the tendency of respondents to over-emphasise current situations as opposed to past experiences when relating their account of events. [12]

In the case of the former Czechoslovakia, those who told us their stories were not convinced that the political structure in their country had changed dramatically. Although the present situation was different from that of the past, they did not regard the change as being a victory for their own struggle. On the contrary: a degree of isolation and alienation from the prevailing social and political structure is reflected in their life stories. The injustices and trauma that they had experienced remained strong when they looked back on their lives. The former Robben Islanders indeed experienced the outcome of their struggle as a victory. Political empowerment became the fulfilment of what they had always striven for. The emotional and physical trauma became meaningful and gave dignity to their experiences.

Notes

1   Most of those who told us their life histories were imprisoned from the 1960s, commonly for periods exceeding ten years. The South African political prisoners were mostly charged with acts of sabotage and furthering the aims of banned organisations such as the African National Congress (ANC) and the Pan Africanist Congress (PAC). Those in the former Czechoslovakia mostly stood trial as 'enemies of the state'.

2   Central to apartheid was the racial classification of the population (Population Registration Act 1950). The aim was the separation of the races as much as possible in all spheres of life (Pampallis 1991: 179–190) and a systematic banishment of the country's black majority to the rural periphery. The Mixed Marriage Act 1949 and the Immorality Act 1950 prohibited marriage and extramarital sex across racial boundaries; the Group Areas Act 1950 and the Prevention of Illegal Squatting Act 1951 allowed racial zones to be defined and people to be moved between them; the Reservation of Separate Amenities Act 1953 ensured separate and unequal public amenities, while the Bantu Education Act 1953 provided for a separate and highly discriminatory education system for Africans.

3   For example, the Suppression of Communism Act 1950, the Public Safety Act and the Criminal Laws Amendment Act of 1953.

4   Including the killing of sixty-nine people and the wounding of a further 180 at Sharpeville on 21 March 1960 (as a result of protests against the pass laws).

5   Russians were looked upon by the Czechoslovaks as liberators and heroes, but the communists did not seize power in Czechoslovakia immediately (Kurland 1974).

6   Factories and workshops were nationalized; the collectivization of farming took place; and groups of armed 'working soldiers' (*delnicke milice*), deployed by the new government, began action against the 'enemies of socialism'. Special 'action councils' (*akčni vybŏry*) were formed to eliminate the 'bourgeois enemies' and all political rivals.

7   '(T)o have been arrested . . . and expelled from Communist Party membership . . . has meant a loss of one's job, apartment and social position' (Kurland 1974: 13–14).

8   The Unlawful Organisations Bill 1950 (later renamed and passed as the Suppression of Communism Act) forced the Communist Party of South Africa

to go underground; the Public Safety Act and the Criminal Laws Amendment Act threatened extremely harsh action against people who defied the law.

9   A strategy of mass resistance to laws such as the pass laws, stock limitation laws, Bantu Authorities Act and Group Areas Act.

10 See Pampallis 1991: 189–213. These forms of struggle included opposition to Bantu Education, attempts to revitalise African trade unions (leading to the South African Congress of Trade Unions – SACTU), various community issue-based struggles, the Women's Movement, an upsurge in rural resistance and, above all, the protests against the pass laws in the late 1950s and early 1960s.

11 The authorities allowed former Robben Islander 4 to continue performing circumcision with assistance from the warder-in-charge of the hospital on Robben Island.

12 See Arrow and Hankopolija 1985: 24, Skocpol 1984: 378–9, Weinstein 1990: 84, Clausewitz 1968: 188–9 and Sayer 1992: 22 as examples of arguments for the incorporation of subjective factors into interpretations of and reflections on past experiences.

References

Arrow, K. and Hankopolija, S. (1985) *Frontiers of Economics,* Oxford: Basil Blackwell.

Clausewitz, C. von (1968) *On War,* Harmondsworth: Penguin.

Davenport, T. R. H. (1987) *South Africa: A Modern History*, Basingstoke: Macmillan.

Goldberg, I. (1978) *Oppression and Social Intervention*, Chicago: Nelson-Hall.

Kaplan, K. (1993) *Politická Persekuce za Komunistického Rezimu v Ceskoslovensko*, Prague: Institute for Contemporary History.

Kurland, G. (1974) 'The Czechoslovakian crisis of 1968,' in *Events of Our Times* 15: 1974.

Pampallis, J. (1991) *Foundations of the New South Africa*, Cape Town: Maskew Miller Longman.

Podgorecki, A. (1983) *Social Oppression*, Westport: Greenwood Press.

Sayer, A. (1992) *Method in Social Science,* London: Routledge.

Skocpol, T. (1984) *Vision and Method in Historical Sociology,* Cambridge: Cambridge University Press.

Weinstein, E. (1990) 'Simmel and the theory of postmodern society', in B. Turner (ed.) *Theories of Modernity and Postmodernity*, London: Sage.

5

THE UNENDING WAR

Social myth, individual memory and the Malvinas

Federico Lorenz (translated by Gabriel Ozón)

> One dies of war like any old disease.
> Wilfred Owen, *A terre.*

> Time the destroyer is time the preserver.
> T. S. Eliot, *The Dry Salvages*

The Malvinas War of 1982 meant the loss of more than 600 Argentinian lives.[1] The battle was tough and intense. Although the conflict was short, the Argentinian death rate (equivalent to 1,000 soldiers per year) was more than treble the rate of American deaths during the Second World War, and almost ten times greater than in Vietnam, showing both the concentration of British fire-power and the ferocious character of the combat (Ceballos and Buroni 1992: 93).

The most recent figures estimate that since the war almost 300 veterans have committed suicide. In addition, according to figures from a September 1996 survey, out of 4,000 veterans living in Buenos Aires and its outskirts, 851 are unemployed.[2] It is hard to conceive of more forcible evidence to back up my interpretation: that for its participants, the Malvinas War remains an unresolved double trauma of, first, the war itself and, second, the shock of post-war return, above all due to the gulf between social and individual myths.

If, in a veteran's words, 'recollections are the eternal tenants of memory' (Rogido 1994), oral history can be extremely helpful in making them sufferable. Of course, we must never forget that 'it will help nobody to confuse listening as a therapist with listening as a historian' (Samuel and Thompson 1990: 6). We cannot resolve traumas, but we can study them and show how they originate.

My aim has been to study the relationship between individuals and collective mental structures in the Malvinas War and the way the social image of the war developed. Source materials included personal interviews with thirty veterans and civilians (*no combatientes*) of different age-groups between 1994 and 1995, and research on bibliographic and journalistic sources.

There is an 'official' past that enables a society to recognize itself as both heir and participant in a specific historical process; a past that feeds off (and modifies) *collective memory*, 'the area of social appropriation of the past, of collective retrospection, of management and control of the past' (Robin 1989: 69). This official past draws on elements from the cultural background of the community which it seeks to interpret, in order to find previous references from within its target social group, so as to provide both foundations and confirmation to support its subsequent imposition. Hence the government, or the dominant social class, may search for consensus by staging some elements that belong to the social imagination, that 'mixture of ideas and images' (Passerini 1990: 54) which constitute (to adapt the title of an outstanding book) the myths communities live by.

It is worth noting that such a myth − even if it draws on relatively stable structures and judgements − is essentially dynamic in its response to realities that dispute the validity of a certain social pattern. Thus, every social myth can at the same time include some individuals and exclude others, depending on their social standing. The attempt to impose a consensus on imagination causes individuals to try to fit their personal histories within the social image that is meant to be shared. Of course, 'every mythical corpus . . . divides by joining, both separates into ranks and creates interdependence, thus playing a direct and efficient role in keeping collective life alive' (Ansart 1993: 98).

This approach suggests the need to study the relationship between the individual and the social at their exact meeting point: to investigate 'how each individual story draws on a common culture: a defiance of the rigid categorization of private and public, just as of memory and reality' (Samuel and Thompson 1990: 2). But what happens when the collective imagination so distorts or suppresses a past event that it neither includes nor contradicts the personal experiences of those who played a role in it? Such a disconnection in memory can be seen as in itself a trauma, for 'our memories are risky and painful, if they do not conform with the public norms or versions of the past' (Thomson 1996: 11).

I believe this to be the case with Argentinian veterans of the Malvinas War.[3] This was the only Argentinian war during this century, and it has left deep scars in our society:

> I believe the military didn't collapse down during the *Proceso*. . . . [4]
> Although we now talk about the Mothers [of Plaza de Mayo] and stuff . . . that was not the key to it. Malvinas was: because it affected the structure of the Army itself, and its relation with society. . . .
> Malvinas triggered the return of democracy.
>
> (la Greca, interview)

Moreover, the war was lost, and that has influenced its social assimilation: it is far more logical for a society to search for explanations in defeat than in victory. Defeat also requires scapegoats: it is easier to put the blame on a minority group than to own up to a collective responsibility. Thus the forging of the Malvinas myth helped soothe the hurt that defeat inflicted upon national pride.

In his study of the relationship between the diggers and the Anzac legend, Alistair Thomson (1996: 11) came across some similar contradictions. However, it was a positive view of Anzac performance in the Great War that shaped collective identity. The mythical virtues of the Anzac soldier developed into a cornerstone of the Australian national character. Gallipoli was construed as a decisive turning point in the making of Australian nationhood, for it was the place where the performance of its soldiers was put to the test, and became a source of collective pride. In Argentina, on the contrary, since social identification with the soldiers was not widespread, the collective memory of war stemmed from a strongly *negative* posture connected with the Malvinas.

The fact that, in the eyes of Malvinas ex-combatants, the real truth about the war is not known is the main reason why they feel unable to fit their own experiences of the war into the socially constructed image of it. As a result, they not only bear the trauma caused by war as such, but also the frustration produced by the contradiction between the social explanations of Malvinas and their own histories.

The name 'Malvinas' is strongly present in Argentinian social imagination. Every Argentinian – nuances notwithstanding – is moved by the sound of it. In 1982, when he knew he was going to war, Omar Olsiewich remembers feeling 'happy then . . . because you've read about them at school, but . . . from a distance' (Olsiewich, interview). One lecturer on recent Argentinian history, although critical of the war, nevertheless agrees that '[The Malvinas] have this value for us. . . . I think our *Argentineness* is connected with them. . . . Malvinas is . . . like an open wound on the people . . . Maybe that's why [the military] exploited them' (la Greca, interview). In a similar spirit Ernesto Sábato, writing on the tenth anniversary of the battle said: 'I'd . . . again be on the side of those guys who . . . were dying to defend some rocky islands, which were in reality useless. For they were, and still are, a symbol' (Sábato 1992).

After the landing on 2 April 1982, the Argentinian people enthusiastically supported the recapture of the islands. Money was raised, and the scale of volunteering recalled 1914 in Europe:

> Joy, not war was in the air. . . . Not a big difference between the atmosphere of the World Cup and that of Malvinas. . . . Couldn't understand our fanaticism. . . . People giving stuff for the soldiers reminded me of some documentary of Mussolini, the Abyssinian War.
>
> (la Greca, interview)

97

The press was heavily censored throughout the conflict, and that brought about the paradox of a widespread belligerent euphoria together with a striking lack of news from the islands to support it. In that situation, 'the Argentinian people, deeply moved . . . forgot about unemployment, misery and everyday tragedies to uphold a cause without asking for anything in return', as a later, self-indulgent view put it (Montenegro and Aliverti 1982: 20).

After the surrender of the national troops on 14 June 1982, Argentinian society exchanged its patriotic euphoria for bitter disappointment and a sense of having been cheated: 'Lots of credulous readers of official information believed we were winning the war. When they were faced with defeat, they couldn't take it' (Esudero 1995: 24). *The Names of Defeat; Malvinas: the Secret Plot; The Outrageous War; Heroic Deed or Shameful Defeat?* are some of the titles of books published immediately after the war. They reflect the astonishment of a society searching for explanations of a war that they were winning – up until only 'four hours before defeat was made official' (Montenegro and Aliverti 1992: 20).

The most obvious culprits were the military. One of the first explanations was to hold the *de facto* president Leopoldo Galtieri responsible for the defeat. He is still considered a 'messianic mind who decided to get us all involved in a useless and inordinate war' (Roldán, survey). This contributed to the self-exculpatory *myth*: that we were *led* into war.

The organizational mistakes by the High Command were confirmed in the *Rattenbach Report* (an *ad hoc* Military Committee which established the specific responsibilities of the various Commanders), which amounted to an acknowledgement of the High Command's failure. In the aftermath, the very same media which had once echoed official propaganda started denouncing blunders and oversights during the war.

It was at this moment that the veterans entered the scene. Called 'the boys of war' (*los chicos de la guerra*) because of their youth – they were eighteen- or nineteen-year-old conscripts – they were now regarded as victims and passive actors in the conflict:

> They should've sent trained, able people to war, not those *innocent boys* who knew nothing about it. . . . We must be really thankful to them, because they went and fought for the country and some were killed in a war with no purpose at all . . . some *little Argentinian soldiers* lost their lives and some were shocked for good, that's the Malvinas for you. . . . It was good just for fucking up those *poor kids'* lives.[5]
> (Gomez, survey, my emphasis)

Such is the view that Argentinian society has constructed in order to be able to deal with ex-combatants. Does it match the view that they themselves have built to try and understand their experience? No: and that is the source of the double trauma of the veterans. They were seen as innocent and inexperienced victims of the conflict. But do they see themselves like that? Or is that how they want to be seen? As veterans, what relationships do they really want to build with their fellow countrymen?

There were two stages in the explanations of the Malvinas War on offer in the post-war period. The ex-combatants returned to a society in shock, which at first tried to ignore them. But before long society constructed a comfortable explanation which placed responsibility away from itself and, at the same time, transformed the veterans into victims. This enabled Argentinian society to play a paradoxical role, offering inclusion at the price of excluding compassion: for it had to label them in order to help them.

In the immediate aftermath, the returning veterans found themselves returned to a society too dumbfounded to relate to them: 'I think there are two guilts, that of the state and that of society. . . . Society's guilt is not . . . to have taken them back . . . disengagement from their problems. . . . We forgot about the war and about everything else' (la Greca, interview). The state initially sought to deny the existence of veterans, a bitter experience for them, by means of the same propaganda apparatus used throughout the conflict: '[Talking about the Malvinas] was forbidden. We had to sign a form before being demobbed. . . . "What happened there is *your* experience, and only yours"' (Ayala, interview). The term coined by the press to refer to this isolation of the veteran within society was 'demalvinization' (*desmalvinización*).

Now what experiences were these veterans really 'bringing back home'? What had happened on the islands? We must remember that recollection remains traumatic for many veterans: 'I don't like to talk about it – Many vets went loony. Questions, questions, and you still remember the Malvinas – I don't talk much, don't like the memories' (Morel, interview). In general, I conducted the interviews without any questionnaire, thus making the recall itself the pivotal force in the story. The pattern which emerged is in some respects similar to that found in the interviews carried out by Gabriele Rosenthal with veterans of the Great War: on the one hand, a precision in terms of space and time; on the other, a reluctance to speak of the experience of war (Rosenthal 1991a: 123).

On the first point, the amount of precise detail about time in veterans' accounts is striking:

> The 14th. It was over – Monday. We'd gone under fire Friday 8 p.m. We were there – until Saturday – noon, I think. We stopped there 'cause they took the position held by B Company on the 7th. I was – in C Company.
>
> (Morel, interview)

On the second point – the war experience – in general accounts are rather laconic. Occasionally, some personal anecdotes are told, but even then there is a tendency towards comparison, analogy and third person narrative:

It was something – like – something – not fantastic, 'cause a war is not fantastic. Some fireworks, from New York, the 4th of July, those celebrations at a time when everything is bombs! – that was from 6 p.m. to 7 a.m., fire, fire and fire.

(Diego, interview)

Where war experiences are described, they do not involve any reference to death, whether those of friends or foes. In general, the accounts of battles are painfully simple: 'They were crushed like bugs. It was terrible, screams everywhere, really ugly' (Ayala, interview). Only rarely are casualties mentioned. Veterans never talk directly about deaths at their own hands, preferring euphemisms: 'When they [the British] arrived, we did what we had to do' (ibid.).

Most of them solve the contradiction in the concept of 'legalized death' by stressing that they had no possibility of choice:

Right then, I'd say that the first shot was the hardest to fire. . . . I felt awful, I'd never killed anything, let alone a man. . . . Then, well, I thought if I didn't fire I was dead meat and – was never coming back. . . . Right then, that thought was common among us. . . . Seems stupid, killing a bloke [but] you are a pawn, you're placed there and, 'OK – you did OK, keep on playing'. Now if they played you wrong, you're dead meat.

(Olsiewich, interview)

A further reason why death is excluded from many different recollections is that very often it was comrades who died:

Sometimes speaking about it . . . isn't as hard as going through it . . . terrible. You can bear hunger, thirst, or whatever – but you can't bear the sight of your mates – lying about. . . . One badly injured – another in pieces – it's terrible. . . . It happened to me. . . . We were close friends, really thick.

(Ojeda, interview)

Indeed, the violent death of close companions has carved the deepest wound in the hearts of most veterans. Their feelings range from helplessness to guilt for not having been able to help them:

I just remember losing him – lost his body, it slipped from my fingers. In my mind I wanted to save him . . . wanted to get him out. . . . That's my guilt. Lacking . . . the strength, dunno, being a doctor, or something – to build a stretcher and drag it. I couldn't. Just couldn't! I blame myself for that!

(Diego, interview)

100

Some even reflect on the unfairness of their having returned while others are still lying on the islands: 'Why comrades with families and all, and not me?' (Morel, interview). This kind of self-inflicted reproach increased after their return in the face of the 'reception' they were given. It was fuelled not only by the feeling of having been involved in a useless effort, but also by the hardships many veterans continued to experience in finding their social place: 'Why didn't I die in the Malvinas?. . . What was the use of coming back if I'm gonna be mistreated?' (Diego, interview).

The Malvinas War had much in common with earlier trench warfare. For Argentinian troops, the war meant waiting for the British assault in fixed positions on the barren hills surrounding Puerto Argentino. They also experienced frequent raids and constant bombardment from air and sea, ensuring a situation of permanent tension. Some of the patterns noted by Rosenthal (1991b) can also be found in the veterans' interviews. For example, she remarks on the 'break in the iterative structure of daily time, that is, a break in routine: you did not know when the attacks would take place, nor whether you could sleep at night. . . . You don't think about tomorrow but live day by day.' A Malvinas veteran similarly recalls:

> There, in that place . . . days go by, one, two days – they gave us hell, planes flying over, it was a hellish barrage. The navy was gunning us . . . real loud shit. . . . You couldn't sleep – hellish. . . . Shelling in the morning, shelling at night. You – couldn't rest, sometimes not even eat.
>
> (Diego, interview)

Tension increased still further as rumours spread: 'We made heavy jokes. "Don't fall asleep tonight 'cause they will get you." There was a whisper that they cut the throats of soldiers in their positions. And the night was so black you couldn't see your hand' (Ayala, interview).

Listening surreptitiously to neutral radio stations gave information about the real situation, but at the same time raised anxieties about families 'in the Continent':

> I heard something, not clear . . . how the Pope was coming, to bring a letter to the President saying something, didn't know what then. . . . We found a radio station, Uruguayan, I think. . . . There were two nuclear submarines . . . ready to fire an atom bomb.
>
> (Diego, interview)

All this anguish strengthened the desire in most soldiers for things to come to an end, one way or the other: 'There we had nothing to lose. People said: "Well, let them come – they are taking me prisoner, or I'm leaving some other way, but I'm leaving." . . . We were tired. . . . We had had enough of that place!' (Olsiewich, interview). They faced an invisible enemy with:

passive resistance – you can only look for shelter. . . . Our desperation was seeing them, almost face to face. . . . It drove you mad . . . 'cause they shelled you every day and you could never see them. . . . We couldn't wait for the end of it. Stop – they, or us! . . . And waiting there for your last breath! . . . You didn't know if you would make it, if you would be free.

(Ayala, interview)

Another veteran recalled:

the constant repetition of similar situations, altering routine and then turning into routine. . . . That first night sure was rotten. Later, not really – just as the cold, the bombardments. . . . The first time we didn't even count the bombs they were dropping on us; then we did . . . We bet on on the number of bombs we were getting.

(Olsiewich, interview)

To make matters still worse, the Malvinas War was literally an insular conflict, so that the Argentinian troops felt like prisoners in the battlefield, and not only because of the British blockade. Throughout the interviews, references to Argentina as 'the Continent' are particularly significant: the veterans saw it as something quite distinct from their reality, as a synonym both for lost peacetime and for social indifference to their situation, which thus added psychological to geographical isolation: 'six hundred kilometres away from the Continent, we were being riddled, we were dying, lots of us, and here many people were fooling around' (Diego, interview). Another remembered how:

Sometimes it was sentry duty on the radio-station. . . . We could listen to some shows here. . . . So, you started talking of what you'd heard. . . . 'Oh, if I were there, now I'd be doing this.' . . . You felt like dirt. So you tried not to – talk of what was going on here, as if it didn't exist . . . but of what we could do here to get out.

(Olsiewich, interview)

As the situation deteriorated, the Malvinas soldiers increasingly took on a fatalistic attitude towards death. The constant bombing and deaths of comrades and mates strengthened the belief in the inevitability of immediate death: 'I *knew* I was gonna die. Who was I to say: "No, I'm gonna make it"? . . . My mates were dying, why not me?' (Rogido 1994).

War also reshaped personal relationships. In adversity, comrades were the only support and shelter available. Individuals were measured against solidarity in a common war. This is noticeable in the accounts of relationships between conscripts and officers and NCOs: 'We were lucky too. Our captain was quite cool. . . . He was military all-over, though . . . but when the shit hit the fan, he was a good man – no-shit attitude' (Olsiewich, interview). This is not an isolated appraisal; and there are also examples of the reverse attitude. For example, it was common to refer to the similarity in how soldiers were treated in the battlefield and in the barracks:

> If they caught you unshaven . . . field punishment. . . . In two and a half months you haven't seen a bathroom, how come you are supposed to have a smooth face? It didn't seem to be a war. It happened to one of my mates. . . . We all had to stand up against [the officer] and told him that either he set him free or else.
>
> (Ojeda, interview)

For many, the shared conflict and experiences on the islands created a new kind of solidarity built at the cutting edge; and when they returned, most veterans clung onto it, as opposed to sliding into social indifference:

> Among the conscripts (we got on) very well. There were no divisions between Class '62 and Class '63. . . . Groups developed . . . like small worlds within every Company. Small families. . . . If one was down, then everybody . . . tried to cheer him up, to stop him thinking shit.
>
> (Olsiewich, interview)

Very often too, the British adversary is recalled as if an equal. Many soldiers thought of them as men under the very same circumstances as themselves: 'I don't bear any grudge against them. 'Cause they . . . were doing their duty, just as we were' (Ayala, interview).

War introduced many decisive changes in the lives of veterans. On the one hand, they endured a reality where there was no distance between life and death. On the other, they experienced the emergence of new feelings of solidarity resulting from experiences impossible in peacetime. Also, they came to question social authority as represented by the Army after its evident failure in the war. The Malvinas altered the 'normal' view of life and social order shared by young individuals, for it was this very order that had led them to the war. For them, defeat meant the *failure of a social myth*.

A new myth would be born after 14 June, when the veterans were back in their communities. This myth emerged from the interaction between the experience of veterans and the image society which was already building of them.

Malvinas was a limited, if intense, war in terms of the number of troops engaged in combat. By 27 May 1982, there were 7,135 Argentinians on the islands (Official Report of the Argentine Army 1983). Hence only a small part of the Argentinian population was directly affected by the conflict. It took place in the extracontinental area, thus threatening only Patagonia. It was also a short conflict that did not create any kind of wider social commitment beyond an awareness of 'the existence of a war'. Although it was labelled a national war by the government, people did not experience it as such, even in something as basic as productive effort. The Malvinas were 'far away':

> On 18 June 1982 . . . lots of Argentinian young people were coming back as prisoners on the *Canberra*. . . . I heard a show host saying with a shameless smile that 'today it's a great day for the Argentinian people: the national squad plays today, and all our hopes are with them in Spain' [World Cup 1982].
>
> (Kon 1982: 9)

Argentinian society sought explanations but ignored the facts, and received veterans with mixed and contradictory feelings. Most of them were brimming with joy and pride at being alive and 'in one piece': 'Coming back – such a good thing! . . . Wanted to share my joy with everybody – I was so happy. . . . My feelings? Terribly proud of defending my place – my country. . . . Wanted people to hug me, kiss me; hug and kiss them too' (Cano, interview). Those feelings were mixed with sorrow for dead comrades: 'I thought . . . about those that lay there, and about their relatives coming to meet them – and the news that their sons were lying . . . there in the Malvinas' (Morel, interview).

The reality of return proved quite different from their expectations. The amount of time spent in the interviews in recalling it shows that disappointment in that longed-for return was as traumatic as the shock of war, if not more so. One of the most vivid memories involves the way in which they returned; sometimes they see in it a token of times to come:

> When I came back from the Malvinas . . . it was night when we got to the barracks. Night everywhere and hiding from people's eyes. If I went 'I'm in the Army', that was it. . . . 'Watch out, he's a soldier and been in the Malvinas too!' Watch out, they'd say! And then I'd be cold-shouldered, left aside, as if I were – shit, I can't find the words.
>
> (Diego, interview)

Or as another put it: 'Got home 2 a.m., had to leg it forty blocks from the railway station. Didn't even come across a poor dog on the way!' (Morel, interview). At the same time, the veterans' behaviour on the islands started to be questioned. They had to *account for it:*

> I've argued with people. . . . "So, you've been there, but not much of a performance 'cause we lost them." And I'd go "Look, I don't know: I was there, for good or bad. What did *you* do? Turn on the telly? I did all I could." You lost so you have to take shit.
>
> (Olsiewich, interview)

Thus a common feeling among veterans was of having been left to their own devices in a war that had been waged by everybody: 'Galtieri appeared on the balcony in Plaza de Mayo. . . . People said OK, get them back, and they packed the square. . . . Both the people and the soldiers are responsible for what we did' (Diego, interview).

Their war experience thus not only drove a wedge into the lives of veterans, but also alienated them from many of those closest to them:

> When we started to talk [my mates and I], my mom was washing up. We had entered our world. . . . When we came out of that microworld she was still there – the same plates in her hands – standing – and listening. There I realized that . . . *somehow* we had to start to talk. We had to tell us what had been going on with us.
>
> (González 1994)

This rupture caused some of them to withdraw into themselves, choosing not to talk as a reaction to what they experienced as lack of sympathy and solidarity. This only served to exacerbate the psychological consequences of the war:

> Fifteen days . . . I was under fire – not much, but it kills you. . . . Your mind works away . . . a lot faster – doesn't sleep, doesn't get enough rest, see things it should not see. That stays there, and you are really bitter. . . . People telling you 'your fault'. . . . Instead of soothing you, it folds you over . . . you don't speak . . . aching inside, you cry, go mad at night – because of the dreams.
>
> (Diego, interview)

In this context, I have identified three pathways followed by veterans in attempting their social reintegration. I have called these three ways those of the Veterans Association members; of regular soldiers; and of the reintegrated veterans.

Veterans' association members

This group has anchored itself to the image of the veteran. At present, these men are those most closely concerned with the war, to the extent that their appeal to their fellow countrymen for charity and solidarity is criticized by other veterans who do not share their views. Faced with discrimination, they have fallen back on their traumatic past. This reaction stems from their urge to 'make sense of the past', since:

> most of all for the excluded, collective memory and myth are . . . constantly resorted to both in reinforcing a sense of self and also as a

source of strategies of survival. In this context it is often persecution and common grievance which define belonging.

(Samuel and Thompson 1990: 19)

The social image of veterans corresponds in the main to this first group, which has solved the contradiction of return by traumatically reaffirming its veteran character and accepting its marginal status. They perceive society as indifferent to them, and this usually triggers a similar response. Paradoxically, since they are a minority, paying back in kind in fact increases their exclusion: 'Their [civilians'] shitty things are their problem, not mine!' (Morel, interview).

The particular age of most veterans adds to the difficulties of postwar reintegration. As Rosenthal remarked in another context, 'The time to raise a family and the time to build a professional identity in peacetime were replaced, for this generation, by wartime' (Rosenthal 1991b). Many veterans had hoped for social appreciation in the form of a steady job. Before the war, half of the interviewees lived in rural areas, while the rest had come from a working-class background.[6] Members of this group, mostly unemployed or underemployed, resorted to selling Malvinas stickers on trains and buses: 'I expected something different. . . . Maybe a welcome party, a job. I'll be fifty and still peddling stickers. . . . Some will be eighty and this will still go on' (Ayala, interview). It is this image of men in green jackets and decorations selling stickers which for most of the general population symbolises Malvinas veterans: 'The veterans are stuck in my mind as on the bus. . . . I see it as a kind of social debt. . . . People never give to anybody, but when the vets get on, they're given some money: . . . conscience money, guilty conscience' (la Greca, interview).

Veterans reacted against this 'guilty conscience' and against the pitiful light in which they were seen. Thus they built a counter-image in which 'the narrative of hard times (became) a record of courage and endurance' (Samuel and Thompson 1990: 9). In their view, compassion for their suffering during the war is considered to be negative; and charges against the Army are interpreted as further worsening the already noxious image of soldiers:

They see us: 'Poor guys – terrible experience'. . . . By debasing the Army, vets were debased too. No distinctions were made, so the bravery of soldiers could never stand out. . . . If it had been hot, we would've been dead hot. It was cold – so we froze to death! . . . In a war you go through hunger, hot and cold weather and the like.

(Cano, interview)

Moreover, this group considers that fighting in the Malvinas enables them to claim their *Argentineness* on stronger grounds. They were, before and after the war, deeply convinced that the war was fought for a just cause: 'I went there for our flag. We went there in search of something which was, which is ours' (Morel, interview).

This group is trapped in a vicious circle: post-war alienation and their response from within that alienation. They conclude that 'only your comrades can understand you' (Ayala, interview). As they see it, they have been left to their own devices, which only contributes to deepening their introspection: 'When I'm down, sometimes – I feel bad sometimes, like many of us – just by being alone. . . . If you don't find a way out – there's no one else out there to help you' (González 1994). Although they take pride in their self-sufficiency, there is a note of desperation in the need for it:

> We'll be famous, we'll be great. The day they die us (sic), when they build a monument to us. . . . What's the use of all that? What we need is their support now. . . . They think we're wandering about 'cause we like it.
>
> (Cano, interview)

This was the context in which they turned for support to the veterans associations:

> When I came [to the Veterans House] and saw lots of guys who had been in the Malvinas with me. . . . Unbelievable. . . . The rapport with the others, knowing you're talking about the same things – that everybody is going through the same problems – all of these things brought me here: knowing that my problem is not just mine.
>
> (Diego, interview)

On the other hand, in their eyes their alienation itself implies the discredit of the social system and its values: 'If I ever go stark raving mad, I won't kill myself. . . . Not necessary. . . . Wanna get killed? Choose a politician and shoot him. . . . Big fish: then politicians would care about the vets' (ibid.). After the war, from fighting the British they have turned to fighting indifference: 'People . . . don't know – a war veteran. . . . I see people as the enemy we have to defeat' (ibid.).

Regular soldiers

Since regular soldiers were reluctant to be interviewed, we have chosen one life-story which illustrates the differences between the memories of the conscripts and those of regular members of the army (whether on service or not). Regulars were blamed by their comrades for the defeat, which coincided with the transition from dictatorship to democracy (1982–4). It was also during this period that charges started to be raised against the army over its excesses during the Dirty War (*Guerra Sucia*).

FEDERICO LORENZ

'Diego' was a lance corporal in the Fourth Infantry Regiment. He states
he still cannot 'put together' his 'civil' experience and his career up until
1984, when he was discharged from the Army. In this most interesting
account the ideological military frame is retained throughout, allowing
'Diego' to take a critical stance from within the very institution he describes
and, at the same time, to adopt a similar attitude towards civil society, but
in this case from his veteran standpoint. Moreover, his individual story can
stand for a multiple of possible war experiences. 'Diego' was wounded, lost a
friend on Mount Two Sisters, was taken prisoner and, when repatriated had
no chance of an immediate social reintegration because his career as a professional soldier prolonged his experiences until his discharge. In addition, he
has endured the traumatic destruction of his family environment. Following
an argument *about his bravery in the Malvinas*, his pregnant wife and her
parents were killed in an accident.

'Diego' maintains categorical differences between the conscripts and
himself: 'All of us who went to the Malvinas felt them in our hearts. The
NCO's, that is: not exactly the other ranks' (Diego, interview). He feels the
charges made against the army as if they were charges against himself. But
in his view, if the army failed, if supplies were deficient, the rank and file
should also take their share of the blame. This assertion recurs strikingly
throughout his account:

> Some soldiers accused me of not checking the weapons . . . and they
> knew . . . we had them tested a million times. . . . But they don't say
> 'I dropped the rifle in the mud . . . didn't clean it up, it was always
> dirty', they don't say that. Whose fault is it, then? The NCO's, of
> course.
>
> (Ibid.)

Also, some of his brothers-in-arms had proclaimed that only those soldiers
who had been to the Malvinas were responsible for the defeat: 'the whole
burden of defeat. . . . Our own comrades threw it all on our backs' (ibid.).

'Diego' felt that the institution which had ruled his life had turned its
back on him just when he most needed it. Then a questioning attitude crept
in: 'Galtieri or anybody: you hold fast, motherfucker! You're sleeping tight
in your warm bedroom. . . . There I do admire the British, their generals in
charge were knee-deep in shit' (ibid.). 'Diego's' break with society also meant
moving away from the Army: 'I'm sick and tired of the Army! . . . I'm sick
of being commanded! . . . The way they deal . . . with some of us who've been
in the Malvinas is something shitty. . . . "No, sir", "Yes, sir", "sir", "sir", "sir"
– I'm sick of "sir"!' (ibid.) His present tense account mirrors the actual
immediacy of the pain in his life. His frequent underscoring of the way he
dealt with his soldiers is also interesting. My interpretation is that he is
trying to detach his personal behaviour from the social image of the army.

Reintegrated veterans

The reintegrated veterans are those who have incorporated the Malvinas experience into their lives, understanding it as an addition to their own history as well as a new starting point. Generally speaking, they are able to speak freely about the war, have found a place for themselves in society and, in many cases, a steady job. In achieving this, their families and friends played essential roles when they came back from the war. I have chosen Omar Olsiewich as an example because his life-story illustrates all these characteristics. He tells it with relative ease. He compares his brain to a house full of chests, which he has been moving about: 'Don't know whether it's all neat and tidy, but there is some room left. . . . That's why . . . I don't mind talking about it' (Olsiewich, interview).

Omar acknowledges how his social environment was supportive from the first moment of his return: 'People got me on my feet again. . . . In the neighbourhood, they tried to keep me busy – And I was never alone!' (ibid.). He got a steady job rather quickly, which made it easy for him to distance himself from the 'military' image: 'Saying I'm a vet. . . . I don't really say it. I don't want to be given money out of compassion.'

His answer to the question, 'Would you go back to the Malvinas?' is particularly revealing when compared with those of the other two groups. They often state that they 'would go back with better equipment', regardless of the chances of a new war. But Olsiewich is emphatic:

> You do these kind of stupid things once in your life. . . . It's easy: go to any regiment. . . . Someone without an arm, some other with just one leg – kids that went nuts. . . . At that price what could I get from going back? Destroying more people?
>
> (Ibid.)

He even has a strongly negative view of 'militariness', distancing himself from the army which took him to war. In his account, expressions like 'they say or do military stuff' often come up. Moreover, defeat had undermined his belief in the authority of the Army:

> There were no more . . . sergeants, nor non-coms. . . . Lots of them had torn off their stripes before boarding the *Canberra* – the rank and file were taken there first . . . and you'd tell them: 'And now you give commands. . . . When you'd ripped off your stripes, you didn't use to shout so loud.'
>
> (Ibid.)

In the case of this group alone, there is a *positive* turning point after the Malvinas War:

When we went up on the deck [of the *Canberra*] . . . when we saw the blue sea, we were overwhelmed . . . as if it was all over now. . . . We're back! A peaceful sensation. . . . Just the wind and the sea. . . . A feeling of – relief. . . . *As if you were feeling OK with yourself.*

(Ibid., my emphasis)

The obvious contrast between Omar and those in the the first two groups can be accounted for if we consider that, from the very first, he enjoyed everything that the others were asking for: support from their social environment and a job. That has allowed veterans like Olsiewich to consider the Malvinas War a traumatic, but nevertheless surmountable, experience.

Conclusion

Other factors have also played a role in shaping the attitudes which I have outlined. Too much generalization would overstate the case, but most of the Veterans Association members who were interviewed had experienced especially hard and painful situations; in addition, most of them were soldiers from the inland provinces who never returned to their homelands. However, it would be necessary to study more cases before reaching a firm conclusion about how these factors affected their responses.

Studying how social myths – the food of the collective imagination – are reshaped and accommodated to different realities is just one aspect of this task. A veteran can say: 'The telling is good for me, 'cause it's something historical and you've been there, it's good they know. . . . I want people to know what happened there' (Ayala, interview). The oral historian, gripped by the social imagination he or she tries to study, can tell the veteran in return of the changes which can be perceived in the evolution of the social myth of the Malvinas: of a transition from a jingoist nationalism to an infinitely more human and less blindfolded position:

Instead of remembering our territorial claims, we should particularly remember our youth [because] Argentinian territory is not marked merely by a waving flag. . . . In that ludicrous war, we recovered nothing, but lost a great deal; and we can say they are 'our Malvinas', but only because their land has been stained by Argentinian blood'.

(Vega, interview)

Notes

1 The official figures are 615 dead (Moro 1985).
2 Figures provided by the National Committee of Veterans.

3   It is worth noting that when talking about themselves, Malvinas soldiers seem to use the expression 'ex-soldier' (*ex-combatiente*) or 'veteran' at random. Although we have chosen the latter for the purposes of translation, the different nuances of these two terms remain significant.

4   This refers to the so-called *Proceso de Reorganización Nacional*, the last military dictatorship in Argentina (1976–83).

5   The label '*los chicos de la guerra*' became extremely popular as the result of a book with the same title by the journalist Daniel Kon. The first Argentinian film on the Malvinas was based on this book.

6   Official figures could not be obtained.

References

Ansart, P. (1993) 'Ideologiás, conflictos y poder', in E. Colombo, *El Imaginario Social*, Barcelona: Altamira.

Army Report (1993) *Official Report of the Argentinian Army.*

Ceballos and Buroni (1992) *La Medicina en la Guerra de Malvinas*, Buenos Aires: Circulo Militar.

Esudero, L. (1995) in *Clarín*, 5 March, p. 24.

González, W. (1994) in *Veteranos de Malvinas*, América TV.

Kon, D. (1982) *Los Chicos de la Guerra*, Buenos Aires: Galerna (references are to the 13th edition, 1984).

Montenegro, N. and Aliverti, E. (1982) *Las Nombres de la Derrota*, Buenos Aires: Nemont.

Moro, R. (1985) *La Guerra Inaudita*, Buenos Aires: Pleamar.

Passerini, L. (1990) 'Mythbiography in oral history', in R. Samuel and P. Thompson (eds), *The Myths We Live By*, London: Routledge.

Robin, R. (1989) 'Literatura y biografia', *Historia y Fuente Oral*, vol. 1.

Rogido, W. (1994) in *Veteranos de Malvinas*, América TV.

Rosenthal, G. (1991a) 'German war memories and narrability', *Oral History*, vol. 19, no. 2.

—— (1991b) 'Narración y significado biográfico de las experiencias de guerra', *Historia y Fuente Oral*, vol 4.

Sábato, E. (1992) 'Con pena y sin gloria', *Clarín*, 29 March, p. 20.

Samuel, R. and Thompson, P. (eds) (1990) *The Myths We Live By*, London: Routledge.

Thomson, A. (1996) *Anzac Memories: Living with the Legend*, Melbourne: Oxford University Press.

Survey respondents and interviews

Ayala, Ramón, 5th Marines Battalion, interview.

Cano, Alejandro Ramón, 4th Airborne Artillery Group.

'Diego' (pseudonym on request), lance corporal, 4th Infantry Regiment.

Gómez, Gabriel (15), survey.

La Greca, Frances, interview.

Morel, Domingo, 7th Infantry Regiment, interview.
Ojeda, José Omar, 3rd Brigade, interview.
Olsiewich, Omar, 3rd Mechanized Infantry Regiment, interview.
Roldán, María Eugenia (54), survey.
Vega, Patrica (46), interview.

6

LYNCHING STORIES

Family and community memory in the Mississippi Delta

Kim Lacy Rogers

In 1996, Mrs Myltree Adams, a native of Coahoma County in the Mississippi Delta, recalled her childhood in an African-American farming family near the small town of Coahoma. Her parents and grandparents told her cautionary stories about the prevalent white supremacy of the South, and the racial segregation that was a fact of life in the 1930s and 1940s. One story Adams remembered 'quite vividly': her father's brother 'was mobbed and killed by white people, and that stayed with us a long time'.[1]

Why had the mob done this?

> My father's brother's wife was a maid, chief cook and bottle washer in [a white] man's house, and somehow or another they started a [sexual] relationship. They [the whites] first told her husband that he had to leave. My uncle and aunt had two children already, and he'd slip back to see them. They conceived another child, and when he came home to see the youngest girl, the whites mobbed him and shot him up. They said there wasn't a place on him big as your hand that didn't have a bullet hole in it. The men were on horses, and they just ran him down and shot him down like a dog.
>
> (Adams 1996)

The shooting was traumatic for Adams' family:

> As a result of that, my father didn't allow white people in our house. He didn't allow no white man near us, and we could not even work for white people. My daddy didn't allow white men to come in our house, in our yard. He didn't like no peddlers, nobody to get around us.
>
> (Ibid.)

113

Myltree Adams' interview is part of the Delta Oral History Project (DOHP), which tape recorded 116 oral interviews with African-American community leaders in Bolivar, Coahoma, Sunflower, and Washington counties of the Mississippi Delta between 1995 and 1997. These counties had majority black populations for most of their histories, and were developed as cotton planting regions in the late 19th century. All of these counties produced strong civil rights movements in the 1960s, and have also experienced the mechanization of cotton agriculture, a decline in farm tenancy and sharecropping, and massive out-migrations of African-Americans since the 1940s (Cobb 1992).

Myltree Adams' interview contains several themes that are emblematic in the narratives of Delta activists. Her story features a contrast between the brutality of the past, a participation in protest and political activities in the 1960s, and personal achievement in the post-movement years. Adams' story also features an element that was chillingly commonplace in the Delta: white violence could strike any African-American male, it seemed, with suddenness and fury.

Adams' family was fortunate and extremely unusual: her father owned a 200-acre farm, and could remain relatively independent of white people, as sharecroppers and tenant farmers – who worked shares on white planters' lands – could not.[2] Myltree Adams herself finished high school in Coahoma, married, and had three children. After she and her husband divorced, she moved back to her parents' farm to help with the crops, and worked part-time as a cook, seamstress, and hairdresser to support her children. She also became involved with Dr Aaron Henry's historic efforts to organize and sustain a local branch of the National Association for the Advancement of Colored People (NAACP) in Coahoma County. During the 1960s, Henry, Adams, and other black activists organized their communities in an effort to register black voters and to overcome the fear that African-Americans in the Delta felt about challenging white supremacy.

Organizing black voters in Mississippi in these decades was a sometimes fatal effort. Adams' family received death threats, her phone was tapped, and NAACP members escorted her home 'many a night'. The treats and harassment 'kept my daddy and mama and family kind of afraid, and my other kinfolk, because I kept doing it. You know, somebody had to die.' In fact, a number of black Mississippians did die in terrorist murders and bombings in the 1950s and 1960s. The most famous murders made their way to the national and sometimes international news: Emmett Till in 1955; Medgar Evers in 1963; George Lee of Belzoni in 1955; Vernon Dahmer of Hattiesburg in 1966; and James Chaney, Andrew Goodman, and Michael Schwerner in 1964 (Dittmer 1994; Payne 1995). Many other African-Americans had their homes bombed and their livelihoods threatened, or were forced to leave the state for attempting to vote, for participating in demonstrations, or for acquiring too much money or property.

Even though her parents and extended family were frightened of white reprisals for her work, Myltree Adams contended that she:

> was not scared. . . . I guess I thought I could help bring about change, and I wanted to see a change. I knew it couldn't stay that way forever. Nothing remains the same. And you would run across some people who wanted to change, who were willing to change.
>
> (Adams 1996)

Adams continued her NAACP and voter registration activities, became active in the coordinated efforts of the Council of Federated Organizations (COFO) in the civil rights movement of the 1960s, and began working for Project Head Start in Coahoma County in that decade. As a community service worker for the agency, she persuaded parents to register to vote while she recruited toddlers for the educational program. In these efforts, she was supported by Henry and the NAACP, and also by the very few enlightened leaders of the white community, like planter Andrew Carr.

Through her work with the NAACP, COFO, Head Start, and other community organizations, Myltree Adams became a power in Democratic Party politics in Coahoma County between the 1970s and 1990s. In 1996, she worked as an administrator in Head Start, maintained personal contact with voters and organizations throughout the county, and considered running for a position on the Coahoma County Board of Supervisors when she retired. Her story, though dramatic, is one that she shares with a number of African-American women community leaders in the Mississippi: a movement from voter registration and civil rights activism to Head Start employment to politics.[3] Yet her narrative also links her journey of change and growth to the dark and bloody history of Mississippi's past – a history written in the blood of lynching victims.

Myltree Adams' narrative links two stories that are prevalent in interviews conducted with African-American activists and community leaders in the Mississippi Delta by researchers from the Delta Oral History Project (DOHP). The first story is a community, and sometimes family, trauma narrative: the lynching story. As an example of the extremity, the arbitrariness, and the violence inherent in the system of racial segregation and white supremacy, the lynching story has achieved a central place in African-American literature, and has come to represent the joined spectres of racist evil and savagery in African-American history and folklore.[4]

Yet this story of terror, humiliation, and destruction – and its communal memory – are most frequently linked by our narrators to life stories that emphasize family resourcefulness, self-sufficiency, sacrifice, and personal agency. The Delta narrators link the narratives of community and family trauma to longer and more comprehensive dramas of family and personal self-assertion and efficacy.[5]

As told by family members or by community elders, the lynching story was a graphic and ghastly warning of what could happen if a black – particularly a black man – was perceived by whites as transgressing his 'place' according to the assumed standards of racial segregation and white supremacy. Such transgressions might include 'sheltering a fugitive, disputing a white man's word, dating a white woman, testifying or defending [oneself) against whites, or just acting "troublesome"' (Zangrado 1980, White 1969). In this role, the lynching ritual served as an effective method of deliberate terrorism and social control of African-Americans in heavily-black counties.[6]

Yet the lynching story also seems to have had contradictory effects in the racial socialization of the women and men who emerged as community activists in the 1950s and 1960s. First, the terror, brutality, and sadism of the white mobs thoroughly discredited the system of white supremacy and the state which maintained it in the eyes of the African-American women and men who matured between the 1930s and 1950s. In doing this, lynching stories reinforced the claims of national NAACP leaders and local and state leaders who pushed for anti-lynching legislation from the 1920s onwards. Continuing brutality against African-Americans in the 'modernizing' South from the 1940s through the 1960s underscored the need for equal rights, voter registration, and equal opportunity under the law.[7] The activists who heard lynching stories as children had absorbed the behavioural warnings that the stories conveyed, while they were simultaneously given a high sense of personal worth by parents who struggled to maintain some independence from white control, by strong teachers in segregated schools and in historically black colleges, and by a religious socialization that stressed righteous action and community service. By the 1950s and 1960s, these women and men were prepared to fuse these diverse influences into civil rights activism (Morris 1984).

As mature community leaders interviewed in the 1990s, the Delta activists appear to have made yet another use of the 'southern horrors' of the past. Telling the lynching story documents a community and sometimes family trauma, as narrators recall the reality of terrorism. The same story also affirms the agency of the victim, as narrators recount his life and actions. These acts of testimony in turn restore agency to the surviving family and community, as narrators portray the process of surviving the culture of violence and segregation as an act of self-assertion, resilience, and courage. Further, testifying involves naming the person or group responsible for the lynching, and holding those individuals – and their social system – responsible for their deeds. Thus the lynching story has become part of the historical memory of generations of Delta blacks.

Narrators link communal survival of terrorism to their own families' survival strategies, and emphases on self-improvement and education. Recollections of family efforts to achieve independence from white control, and of parents' sacrifices to ensure that their children received an education, are among the stories that link the survival of terrorism in the past to the struggle for civil and political rights in more recent years. The lynching story also links the narrator to the memory of the victim: in telling this tale of trauma and loss, the narrator gives back to the victim his agency, his body, and his history – all of those attributes that were to have been obliterated by the rope, bullets, and/or fires of the mob ritual. This trauma narrative thus becomes a narrative of witnessing and commemoration, a narrative that connects acts of victimization and resistance across decades and worlds (Caruth 1996).

This same narrative contains even another imperative: it provides a historic documentation of the necessity for federal protection from lynching, for movement activism and protest, and for national intervention in the racial practices of Southern states. Over the long history of 'Southern horrors' against African-Americans, the lynching story serves as a powerful moral justification for personal narratives of activism, protest, and community leadership (Schecter 1997).

Yet among these mature community leaders, the lynching story also seems to serve as a reminder of the fragility of the gains of the Civil Rights movement and of black empowerment. For it is a narrative of personal assertion and disaster, of independent action, and horrible retribution. It is a narrative that creates expectations of violence and death, a history that worries its narrators into a constant, edgy vigilance and distrust of their present successes. The lynching story remains a corrosive and bitter memory of pain and fear.

The reality of lynching in Mississippi

Lynching stories have appeared in at least fourteen of the eighty-three interviews conducted by the Delta Oral History Project between August 1995 and July 1996. Many of our narrators have asserted that their families protected them from the knowledge of such brutality, but could readily recall other stories of whites' exploitation and mistreatment of African-Americans. Stories of beatings, tar-and-featherings, evictions, and 'covert lynchings' or 'disappearances' were common, as were stories of men – sometimes family members -who were forced to leave the state temporarily or permanently due to a conflict with whites.

Between 1889 and 1945, 'Mississippi accounted for 476, or nearly 13 per cent, of the nation's 3,786 recorded lynchings', according to historian Neil McMillen (1989: 235). Since lynchings were often not reported, the death toll from this form of vigilante justice was probably much higher. Sunflower and Coahoma Counties counted nine lynchings each in this period; Washington and Bolivar had thirteen each. McMillen asserts that some 70 per cent of lynchings occurred in 'the plantation districts with the greatest density of black population' (McMillen 1989: 229–30). Part of lynching's terror in African-American communities resulted from the barbaric practices of lynch mobs, which had as their aim not just the execution of black victims, but the torture, mutilation, and obliteration of black bodies. Lynch mobs frequently castrated, flogged, dragged, and burned their victims in addition to shooting and/or hanging them (Turner 1993). According to McMillen, 'Between 1900 and 1940 at least fifteen blacks died in public burnings', which one newspaper described as 'NEGRO BARBECUES' (McMillen 1989: 234). Such cruelty and sadism suggest that the mobs sought to obliterate the very existence of the victim, and hence the possibility of remembrance and mourning. The awful destruction of bodies, and the mobs' explicit and implicit threats to family members frequently prevented relatives from seeking justice, prosecuting the killers, or even honouring the dead with a proper wake, funeral, and burial. The lynching story is thus as much about erasure as it is about violent retribution and terrorism, as much about not knowing, secrecy, and the ultimate control and denial of information as it is about maintaining white supremacy.

Trudier Harris, who views lynchings as the ritualized 'exorcism' of blackness by white communities, contends:

> lynching and burning rituals reflect a belief on the part of whites, in their racial superiority. Simultaneously, such rituals reflect a belief in the inferiority of Blacks as well as denial of anything white, especially white women, or representative of 'whiteness' (education, clothes, social status) to Blacks. To violate the inviolable, as any Black would who touched a white woman or became mayor of a town, is taboo. It upsets the white world view or conception of the universe.
>
> (Harris 1984: 11–15)

While pro-lynching Southern whites commonly defended the practice – well into the 1940s and 1950s – as a necessary defence of white Southern womanhood from the depredations of black rapists, contemporary researchers and later scholars reported that relatively few lynchings – as few as a third, according to anti-lynching activist Ida B. Wells – involved even the accusation of rape. Wells believed that lynching was 'an excuse to get rid of Negroes who were acquiring wealth and property' (Carby 1987: 107). McMillen cites NAACP estimates for the years 1889 to 1935 that indicate only '19 per cent of all blacks lynched in the United States – and 12.7 per cent of those lynched in Mississippi – were accused of rape' (McMillen 1989: 235).

Lynching stories as trauma narratives

Among Delta narrators, lynching stories as trauma narratives commonly contain several elements or motifs. The first is a perceived violation of norms, contractual agreements, or prerogatives of whites by an African-American. Whites – usually a mob – then seek vengeance. The nature of the violation is sometimes shrouded in mystery and secrecy: families are frequently left without real knowledge of the final fate – or manner of death – of a loved one or friend.[8] Narrators sometimes contrast the self-assertion and dignity of the 'offending' African-American male with the viciousness and cowardice of white mobs. Finally, the lynching story juxtaposes the positive example of the victim's self-assertion or insistence on dignity against the craziness and unpredictability of whites.

The prevalence of lynching stories and other accounts of the physical, emotional, and psychological abuse of African-Americans in the Delta suggest that the violence that maintained white supremacy produced a pervasive sense of communal trauma among the black population. The Mississippi Delta is a football-shaped region bordered by the Mississippi River on the west, the Yazoo River on the east, and by the cities of Memphis, Tennessee to the north, and Vicksburg, Mississippi to the south. Much of the labour in its cotton fields was performed by black sharecroppers and tenant farmers who laboured for as little as three dollars a day through the mid-1960s. A few wealthy planters and bankers have owned most of the lush black acres that bloom with white cotton bolls in the spring, which has meant that a majority of whites and African-Americans in the Delta were poor farmers until recent years. The land itself has a dark, brooding, dramatic quality: fields stretch into copses of trees on a horizon, streams and swamps line two-lane roads that link towns like Alligator, Shelby, and Ruleville. Thunder storms explode with terrifying force out of a wide, volatile sky. In these counties, where relatively few whites controlled and exploited thousands of African-Americans, fear and fantasy sometimes determined life or death for any targeted black male.

L. C. Dorsey, who grew up in Sunflower County, recalled a widespread fear of the 'mob crew' among African-Americans in the Delta:

There was a tremendous amount of fear in the community and in almost every house of this faceless group of people who arrived at your home at night, on horses and in cars, to drag you out and kill you for any little infraction of rules you didn't always know about. People worried tremendously about their sons and the menfolk in their families. People worried if a white man looked at a black girl, and they tried to keep them in the background because they couldn't protect them, They couldn't protect their wives and stuff. . . . What you remember about it was the fear, that there was no way to be protected, and this was really driven home with the death of Emmett Till.[9] It was all this fear that these people had of white folk, that they would come and get you in the middle of the night and kill you. I understood the fear so strongly that it wouldn't even let them [the adults] talk out loud.

(Dorsey 1996)

Worries for their young sons made many African-Americans very protective towards their children, especially in Mississippi. Preston Holmes, whose father worked as a contractor in the all-black town of Mound Bayou in Bolivar County in the heart of the Delta, recalled that his parents were very strict and kept their children close to the house (Holmes 1996). Roberta Martin of Boyle in Bolivar County told of being shocked and frightened by the murder of young Emmett Till in 1955. Said Martin:

It was terrible, because I had two sons; one was born in 1956, and one in 1958. I never allowed my boys to go out and walk anywhere. When they'd go to see their friends, we'd always carry them, because white people were bad about seeing you walking – they'd throw [things] at you, or run out the road after you. After they killed that boy, I was afraid for my boys to walk the road.

(Martin 1996)

Pervasive feelings of dread and fear haunted many families. Sollee Williams, who was born in Sunflower County in 1912, remembered a story that her father told:

There was a man, a black man that had supposedly killed a white fella. And this group [of whites] was out looking for him, and my dad heard them coming. He was so afraid that they would do something to him that he put us [her mother, Sollee and her siblings] into a big box. He was so afraid of what they'd do to him.

(Williams 1995)

The whites did come to the door, questioned her father, and then rode away. 'We just stayed for hours in that box. He was afraid they'd double back. He was just sweating . . . it was just so much tension. You were afraid to do anything that might cause a scene' (ibid.).

Bernice White, also from Sunflower County, recalled some of the stories that her aunt told her:

whenever there was a killing, like a lynching or a rape scream, she said that everybody would go in, close their doors. In the community, they didn't walk the roads, they didn't sing. Like a lot of people at that time, when they walked a lot, they would sing. [But if African-Americans heard that] something had happened, they would try to take to the back fields and go the back ways, not to be seen, because if anyone was caught, especially a black male, that meant he might be accused. If not, he probably would be assaulted some type of way before they would let him go. Usually they [whites] would find someone who they said would have done whatever they thought had happened.

(White 1995).

Such terror and dread within a population are symptoms of communal trauma. According to sociologist Kai Erikson, societal trauma can emerge from 'a *persisting condition* as well as from acute events'. Contemporary experiences of societies ravaged by war or terrorized by dictatorial regimes demonstrate that 'damage can be done to a whole people by sustained dread and dislocation'. Communal trauma, writes Erikson, appears in two forms, one of which creates 'social climates, communal moods, that come to dominate a group's spirit'. Especially devastating are those collective traumas 'that have been brought about by other human beings' because these 'not only hurt in special ways but bring in their wake feelings of injury and vulnerability from which it is difficult to recover'. Members of a victimized community or population may come to feel that 'the environment . . . has proved to be brittle and full of caprice', and may develop a 'sense that the universe is regulated not by order and continuity but by chance and a kind of natural malice that lurks everywhere' (Erikson 1994: 228–41). This seems especially the case among groups whom Robert J. Lifton has termed 'designated victims': 'the Jews in Europe, and Blacks in this country' (Caruth 1995: 128–47).

Reports of lynchings and rumours of lynchings and murders haunted the memories of many narrators. Johnny Lewis, who grew up in Simpson County in the south-eastern Mississippi, recalled that he learned early 'how you should act to prevent certain things from happening to you. Particularly, being a black male. You definitely had to know your place.' As a boy, he heard of black men being lynched in adjoining Smith County, which had a notorious white settlement named Sullivan's Hollow. 'Black folk used to say that there was a sign there that said, "Read, Nigger, and Run. If You Can't Read, Run Anyway."' Lewis remembered that as a boy, he heard of the execution of Willie McGee, a black man in Laurel, Mississippi, in 1951.[10] After this, 'we used to play execution . . . and one of us would *be* Willie McGee and try to visualize an execution' (Lewis 1996).

African-American families and communities dealt with this fear by seeking to avoid all contact with whites, and to 'crunch down and lay low and stay in your place, or you left the South and went North, and both things happened regularly', according to L. C. Dorsey (1996). While economic transformation and the mechanization of cotton agriculture spurred much of African-American exodus from the Delta counties since 1940, discrimination, white violence, and oppression have also been cited by migrants as reasons for leaving the region (Griffin 1995). Blacks who left the Delta 'never came back', said Dorsey:

> They wrote letters and they sent for their relatives to come up there or visit, but they never came back here. They never wanted to live in that environment. It was accepted. The level of killing that went on on plantations, the beatings, [were] all part of life in that situation, and the choices were presented as being quite clear.
>
> (Dorsey 1996)

African-Americans who remained in the Delta, particularly those who were mired in the endless toil and indebtedness of the sharecropping system, were often plagued by an exhaustion and weariness that Dorsey later described a 'just chronic fatigue, where these people worked so hard they were just rundown, and constantly tired and needing sleep. I'm sure some of them were also depressed' (ibid.).

In contradiction to the white segregationist mythology of lynching-as-justifiable-punishment-for-rape, our narrators recalled lynching stories which began as conflicts between whites and blacks over real resources and prerogatives. Both parties tended to view the initial conflict as caused by a racial and/or personal violation. Whites became angry if African-American tenants or sharecroppers did not stay 'in their place', work as they were told to, or resisted white authority in some way, such as keeping their children in school rather than taking them into the cotton fields when quite young. Whites also attacked blacks who were considered to be uppity, or who tried to vote and act politically, or who didn't take a planter's or boss's 'advice': like Myltree Adams' uncle, who returned against 'the man's' orders to visit his wife and children.

African-Americans attributed such conflicts to whites' presumption of total authority and control, which conflicted with the desires and prerogatives of black men and their families. African-American tenants and sharecroppers could expect to be cheated out of their earnings annually by white landowners because 'there was absolutely nothing that the white person who he [a black man] was working for was bound to honour in this whole business of keeping records', according to L. C. Dorsey, who grew up near Drew in Sunflower County. She believed that her father expected to be cheated annually of his profits by the planter he worked for: 'he had lived during the Joe Pullum experience, where Pullum had died standing up for his right not to be cheated out of his labour.' In 1925, Pullum, a World War I veteran, had insisted on his right to the returns on his labour, and had then been attacked by a mob of white men, with whom he fought a gun battle. Pullum managed to kill some thirteen whites before his capture. After the mob killed Pullum, 'they tied him to a car and drug him through the streets of Drew, cut off his ears, I think, or castrated him . . . and put it in jars in the city (Dorsey 1966, Mills 1993).

Dorsey's story recounts the violent death, mutilation, and display that marked the most savage lynchings. Other narrators stressed the elements of secrecy and the unknown which shrouded many disappearances and deaths, Daisie Conwell of Winstonville in Bolivar County recalled that she had 'a cousin down there at Belzoni that a white man killed'. She didn't know why the man was murdered, but 'It was a group of them. I don't know whether no group shot him or not, but it was a group of them that was mad with him' (Conwell 1996). Mary Tyler Dotson recalled the murder of her brother in Jonesboro, Arkansas, in 1931 – for unknown reasons: 'White folks'. The brother had been riding the rails home after working in St Louis. He was killed in Jonesboro: 'They claimed he was out there in the [rail] yard playing and ran into the train. He didn't have no scar or nothing but on his cheek. That's what our boss man told.' When Dotson's father tried to borrow a planter's truck to drive to Arkansas and recover his son's body:

> Jimmy Heathman [the plantation boss] said, "No, I'd advise you don't go up there, Frank. I'll advise you, don't go to Arkansas." . . . They was going to kill my daddy if he went up there. Some of them white folks [that] did it.
>
> (Dotson 1995)

Robert Love of Indianola told a family lynching story that stressed a mob's scapegoating, and the long-term mystery of his grandfather's disappearance. Love's grandfather was a carpenter by trade, but in the late nineteenth century, he found himself having to sharecrop in Sugarlock by Meridian in eastern Mississippi. While roofing his house, Love's grandfather was approached by the planter on horseback. The planter told him to come get his wife and children to do some work. The carpenter said he would come after he had finished, but that the planter hadn't hired his wife and children. The planter cursed the grandfather, rode away, and later returned, asking Love's grandfather for a talk. When the carpenter approached the planter's horse, the planter began to beat him with a chain. Following this beating, the grandfather took his shotgun to a store where the men of the community gathered every night. When the planter rode up to the store, the carpenter fired two shots and killed him. Love's grandfather then disappeared. Later the Klan picked up one of the grandfather's friends, castrated him, and lynched him. The grandfather was not heard from until his death in Birmingham, Alabama, many years later (Love 1995). His family – like the families of Daisie Conwell and Mary Dotson – was left without knowledge of his final fate, and any inquiry would have been dangerous to those concerned.

Of all of the traumatic features of the lynching story, surely this absence of knowledge is one of the most devastating, because it denies closure to the survivors and friends of the victim or the missing man. As critic Cathy Caruth has written, 'Through its very missing [such a story] . . . bears the impact of trauma', because trauma is not simply the effect of destruction, but also, fundamentally, an enigma of survival' (Caruth 1995: 40, 68–72). Why does one survive when a loved one has disappeared or been murdered? Why is one left alive – except, perhaps, to tell the tale and bear witness to the loss, including the loss of not knowing what, in fact, occurred.

Lynching stories recount the violence and grief that African-Americans experienced during the age of segregation. These same stories discredit the system of white supremacy by exposing the calculated barbarism of the mobs. As trauma narratives, these stories contained warnings and generated anger and resistance. They gave women and men a moral and psychological imperative to oppose segregation and to demand equal rights in the years following the Second World War.

Robert Love had 'learned to speak up for myself' from his parents: 'my daddy was a quiet man, but he didn't take anything off anybody.' In the 1950s, Love, a Second World War veteran and public schoolteacher, joined the local branch of the NAACP, even though the members were regularly harassed and threatened by the local White Citizens' Council, a segregationist organization devoted to blocking racial integration. Love kept working with the NAACP because:

> when you've made up your mind you're going to do something, you go ahead and do it. We just made up our minds that if it meant getting killed, we were going to try to take some of them with us, too.
>
> (Love 1995: 44–5)

Like many Mississippi blacks of these years, Love and his friends were armed. Many African-American veterans like Love 'felt like "This is my country, I put my life in danger for, and I'm going to get treated the way I should be treated." . . . Most of the men who went into the war returned back, and then started going to school on the GI Bill' (ibid.: 7–9). These men were a determined force in African-American protest and community organizations in the post-war years.

Sollee Williams of Sunflower County graduated from Tuskeegee Institute in the 1930s, and worked for many years in Chicago. In the 1960s, she returned home to Indianola and began work in voter registration drives. She became politically active because of 'seeing conditions here, and seeing conditions up there [in Chicago], and seeing that it wasn't fair anywhere. I thought I could help change things' (Williams 1995). Williams, Love, Myltree Adams, and many other Mississippi blacks were convinced that the South's racism was unjustifiable and ripe for change, and took calculated risks to bring about the political transformation of their state.

Mississippi was transformed politically between the 1950s and 1960s, but only with the determined actions of local African-American community leaders, a few daring state-wide leaders, and only tardily-engaged national organizations. A combination of local insurgence, 'outside' organizations like the Student Non-Violent Coordinating Committee (SNCC), the Congress on Racial Equality (CORE), the NAACP, and the state-wide Council of Federated Organizations (COFO), in concert with a largely unwilling national government, brought basic rights of citizenship to black Mississippians. This political transformation ended the reign of terror and the era of lynching that white supremacy had long imposed on black people. When young civil rights workers from SNCC, CORE, and COFO came into communities in Sunflower, Bolivar, and Coahoma Counties in the early 1960s, they found numerous local citizens and leaders who were ready to launch a full-scale assault on segregation and white supremacy. Local leaders like Amzie Moore of Cleveland, Aaron Henry of Clarksdale, and Fannie Lou Hamer of Ruleville (in Sunflower County) welcomed the assistance that the young people brought between 1961 and 1966 (Dittmer 1994, McAdam 1988). Women and men like Daisie Conwell, Mary Dotson, Robert Love, Johnny Lewis, Myltree Adams, and L. C. Dorsey transformed the legacy of lynching stories into the agency of social movement activism, which is now recognized as a proactive process of healing and recovery from the devastations of personal and social trauma (Herman 1992).

It is not surprising, then, that narrators like L. C. Dorsey, Sollee Williams, Johnny Lewis, and Robert Love link lynching stories to personal narratives of agency and activism. In telling the lynching story, they bear witness to both a thwarted search for self-assertion and dignity in the past, and to the horror of white violence and mob savagery. These stories provide a sense of continuity and coherence between the successful activism of recent years, and doomed acts of self-assertion by those who perished in the age of segregation. In the long memory of African-American history, lynching stories are acts of testimony and resistance that restore the lives and traumatic deaths of the victims to a tragic history of racial violence and oppression. Narrators were warned by these stories, but were not immobilized by them: the political changes they launched ended the pervasive fear of lynching and terrorism among Mississippi's African-Americans.

Memories of lynchings and other forms of racial violence have, however, left their mark on many narrators' life-stories. If the cumulative story of most of their lives has been that of survival, achievement, and community leadership, it is a story that has been constructed and reconstructed from often painful experiences. Thus, many narrators acknowledge the sometimes corrosive effects of remembering the segregated past, even as they assert that their experiences of fear and dread must be transmitted to younger generations.

Roberta Martin of Boyle, Mississippi, said, 'I don't trust people, white people. No, I don't trust them. I can't.' Martin's own experiences in Bolivar County had generated much of her distrust, but television dramas about slavery and race exacerbated her feelings. She recalled asking her daughter, 'Why do they keep showing those kinds of pictures? They're not helping. . . . They're talking about race relations, trying to do something about race relations, and they keep showing those kinds of pictures, and they don't do nothing but cause hate.' Further, the public furore over the fall 1995 not-guilty verdict in the O. J. Simpson murder trial seemed proof to Martin that white racism had not changed much:

> You look at all the black people that have been murdered, lynched, killed, and in this country, these people [whites] like to have gone crazy because they found O.J. Simpson not guilty. Now, I'm not going to say he was guilty or not guilty, but I'm just thinking about how sick and unfair they are. How do they think we felt about all the killing and stuff that has been done to us? It'll show you, they don't think we're nothing. We don't supposed to care about ours.
>
> (Martin 1996: 36–7)

For Martin, the changes brought by the civil rights movement and federal intervention had not significantly altered white Mississippians' racial attitudes. 'Some of [the whites] have changed because of the federal government making things happen', she said. But Martin believed that most Mississippi whites wanted to 'go back to the way it was' in the days of segregation (ibid.: 50–3).

Myltree Adams attributed the continuing distrust and fear that many African-Americans felt towards whites to their bitter historic experiences. 'A burned child feels fire – regardless. . . . You don't stick your hand on a hot iron if you got burned the last time you put it up there.' Many older blacks in Coahoma County did not pass on their memories to their children and grandchildren. They kept their silence, Adams said, because 'some of them are ashamed, and then some of them are still kind of fearful of what might happen, because we still haven't come from a very, very, very long way . . . We have blocked it out' (Adams 1997: 7, 8).

Adams herself continued her family tradition of not allowing white people inside her home:

> I don't let white people in my house. I usually go outside and talk to them. And I don't allow no salesmen, or insurance people, unless they're black. People I don't know don't come in my house, no white folks hardly at all, because I was raised like that. My daddy did not allow white people in our house, because of his

brother and the way his brother got shot. They shot him up, about
his own wife.

(Adams 1997: 18–19)

A long-dead social thinker wrote that 'fear is the memory of pain'
More recently, writer Janet Malcolm wrote: 'Time heals all wounds,
smooths, cleanses, obliterates; history keeps the wound open, picks at it,
makes it raw and bleeding' (Malcolm 1995: 62–3). Both statements can
be applied to our Delta narrators' necessary and painful mission of
remembering and telling their histories of fear, oppression, and pain. To
forget this traumatic past – as at least one Mississippi state official
recently urged – would necessitate a wilful abandonment of the record
of struggle and loss that has, over generations, enabled our narrators to
struggle and achieve. Many of our narrators see their duty to remember
as a moral obligation to ancestors, parents, and to the children and
grandchildren who will survive them. But these memories have a cost:
our narrators cannot relax and fully enjoy the changes they have helped
to produce. Like many survivors of collective traumas and disasters,
their narrative expectations of the present and future and shaped by a
story of suffering, fear, and the random and terrible explosions of terror
and violence. And so they view post-movement Mississippi with a
wariness and distrust, half-expecting the virus of racism to erupt in new
places and in different forms.

Notes

I would like to thank Albert Broussard, Jerome Bruner, Graham Dawson, Tom Dent, Susan Rose, and Julius Thompson for their generous comments on previous drafts of this essay.

1   Mrs Myltree Adams, interviewed by Owen Brooks and Kim Lacy Rogers, Clarksdale, Miss., 19 April 1996. This interview was conducted as part of the Delta Oral History Project (DOHP), a collaborative effort of Dickinson and Tougaloo Colleges. This project was funded by the Collaborative Projects programme of the National Endowment for the Humanities.
2   Sharecropping and tenant farming developed after the Civil War (1861–5) between land-rich but often cash-strapped white planters and their landless black and white labourers. In sharecropping, the most dependent tenant arrangement, a planter furnished a farmer with a cabin, land and 'provisions' – seed, foodstuffs, a mule for ploughing – in return for a specified amount of the cotton crop, usually one half. The planter also charged the sharecropper for any provisions he and his family received above the minimum allotment. These charges were levied against the sharecropper's remaining share of his family's crop. Over years and even generations, many sharecroppers fell into debt to the planters. See Cobb 1992: 101–13.
3   Adams' trajectory was shared by many women community leaders in Sunflower,

Bolivar, Washington, and Coahoma Counties between the 1950s and 1990s (see Dittmer 1994, 363–88; Rogers 1996).

4 See Harris 1984; Gunning 1996; Carby 1987; Fry 1991; Griffin 1995.

5 I am grateful to Jerome Bruner for his analysis of agency in the formation of life stories and personal narratives (Bruner 1994: 40–54; see also Bruner and Kalmer 1997).

6 According to W. F. Brundage, 'Lynching was a powerful tool of intimidation that gripped blacks' imagination whether they lived in a mob-prone part of the South or in the relative safety of a border state' (Brundage 1997: 2).

7 Such de-authorization and self-authorization are critical cognitive steps in preparing individuals to engage in mass movement political activism (McAdam 1982).

8 See Harris (1984) for the ways in which such rituals functioned as affirmations for the ideology of white supremacy and the legitimacy of such punishment.

9 Emmett Till, a teenager from Chicago, was visiting an uncle in Money, Mississippi, when he was murdered by two white men in 1955. The men dragged Till from his uncle's house in the night, shot him and dumped his body in a river because he had allegedly whistled at a white woman. Although the Till murder became a national and international example of the tyranny and violence of white supremacy and racial segregation, an all-white Mississippi jury acquitted Till's murderers (Dittmer 1994).

10 Willie McGee was accused of raping a white Laurel housewife in 1945. McGee's initial trial lasted less than a day. The judge sentenced McGee to the electric chair. Three trials followed, and the Mississippi Supreme Court upheld the third conviction – despite testimony from McGee and his wife that he had been having an affair with his accuser for a number of years. McGee was executed in 1951 (Dittmer 1995).

References

Brundage, W. F. (ed.) (1997) *Under Sentence of Death: Lynching in the South,* Chapel Hill.

Bruner, J. (1994) 'The remembered self', in U. Neisser and R. Fivush (eds), *The Remembering Self: Construction and Accuracy in the Self-Narrative,* Cambridge.

Bruner, J. and Kalmer, D. A. (1997) 'Narrative and metanarrative in the construction of self', in M. Ferrari and R. Sternberg (eds), *Self-awareness: Its Nature and Development,* New York.

Carby, H. V. (1987) *Reconstructing Womanhood: The Emergence of the Afro-American Woman Novelist,* Oxford:.

Caruth, C. (ed.) (1995) *Trauma: Explorations in Memory,* Baltimore.

—— (1996) *Unclaimed Experience: Trauma, Narrative, and History,* Baltimore.

Cobb, J. C. (1992) *The Most Southern Place on Earth: The Mississippi Delta and the Roots of Regional Identity,* New York.

Dittmer, J. (1994) *Local People: The Struggle for Civil Rights in Mississippi,* Urbana.

Erikson, K. (1994) *A New Species of Trouble: Explorations in Disaster, Trauma and Community,* New York.

Fry, G. M. (1991) *Night Riders in Black Folk History,* Athens, Ga.

Griffin, F. J. (1995) *'Who Set You Flowin?' The African-American Migration Narrative,* Oxford.

Gunning, S. (1996) *Race, Rape, and Lynching: The Red Record of American Literature,* Oxford.

Harris, T. (1984) *Exorcising Blackness: Historical and Literary Lynching and Burning Rituals,* Bloomington.

Herman, J. (1992) *Trauma and Recovery,* New York.

McAdam. D. (1982) *The Political Process and the Development of Black Insurgency,* Chicago.

—— (1988) *Freedom Summer,* Oxford.

Malcolm, J. (1995) *The Silent Woman: Sylvia Plath and Ted Hughes,* New York.

McMillen, N. (1990) *Dark Journey: Black Mississippians in the Age of Jim Crow,* Urbana.

Mills, K. (1993) *This Little Light of Mine: The Life of Fannie Lou Hamer,* London.

Morris, A. D. (1984) *The Origins of the Civil Rights Movement: Black Communities Organizing for Change,* New York.

Payne, C. (1995) *'I've Got the Light of Freedom': The Organizing Tradition and the Mississippi Freedom Struggle,* Berkeley.

Rogers, K. L. (1996) 'The Movement and Mobility', unpublished manuscript.

Schecter, P. A. (1997) 'Unsettled Business: Ida B. Wells Against Lynching, or, How Antilynching Got Its Gender', in W. F. Brundage (ed.), *Under Sentence of Death: Lynching in the South,* Chapel Hill.

Turner, P. A. (1993) *I Heard It Through the Grapevine: Rumor in African-American Culture,* Berkeley.

White, W. (1969) *Rope and Faggot: A Biography of Judge Lynch,* New York.

Zangrando, R. L. (1980) *The NAACP Crusade Against Lynching, 1909–1950,* Philadelphia.

Interviews

Adams, M. (1996) interviewed by Owen Brooks and Kim Lacy Rogers, Clarksdale, Miss., 19 April (DOHP).

—— (1997) interviewed by Jerry W. Ward, Jr. and Kim Lacy Rogers, Clarksdale, Miss., 26 June (DOHP).

Conwell, D. (1996) interviewed by Owen Brooks and Kim Lacy Rogers, Winstonville, Miss., 27 February (DOHP).

Dorsey, Dr L. C. (1996) interviewed by Owen Brooks and Jerry W. Ward, Jackson, Miss., 21 June (DOHP).

Dotson, M. T. (1995) interviewed by Owen Brooks and Kim Lacy Rogers, Indianola, Miss., 2 October (DOHP).

Holmes, P. (1996) interviewed by Owen Brooks and Kim Lacy Rogers, Mound Bayou, Miss., 21 February.

Lewis, J. (1996) interviewed by Owen Brooks and Kim Lacy Rogers, Clarksdale, Miss., 3 April (DOHP).

Love, R. (1995) interviewed by Owen Brooks and Kim Lacy Rogers, 27 September 1995 and 7 October (DOHP).

Martin, R. (1996) interviewed by Owen Brooks and Kim Lacy Rogers, Boyle, Miss., 15 April (DOHP).

Williams, S. (1995) interviewed by Kim Lacy Rogers, Indianola, Miss., 21 August (DOHP).

White, B. (1995) interviewed by Kim Lacy Rogers, Indianola, Miss., 21 August (DOHP).

7

CONTAINING VIOLENCE

Poisoning and guerilla/civilian relations in memories of Zimbabwe's liberation war

JoAnn McGregor

Introduction

Civil wars anywhere involve not only divisive and traumatic violence but also lasting and troubling memories. My subject here is one specific and acute example of such violence: that of the Rhodesians' covert poisoning of guerrillas in Zimbabwe's liberation war and the witch-hunts of accused civilians that followed. By exploring different actors' recollections of the witch-hunts, and the moral and political issues they raise, I hope to convey something of the moral complexity of living through and with the memory of such traumatic events. But I am also concerned with the events themselves, and from the various, often contradictory accounts, I reconstruct a plausible version of what happened in order to illustrate the devastating effects of this counterinsurgency strategy.

The Rhodesian poisoning tactic involved infiltrating guerrilla supply lines with poisoned clothing and food. It was a deliberate attempt to exploit the popular association between poisoning and witchcraft and to break the relationship between guerrillas and civilians on which successful guerrilla warfare depended. Though political and military leaders often managed to find the source of the poisons, changed supply routes and disciplined guerrillas and youth who threatened violence, at times the death of poisoned guerrillas provoked devastating witch-hunts in which scores of civilians lost their lives.

Guerrillas often dwell on the mysterious and troubling deaths of poisoned colleagues and the ensuing reprisals in personal accounts of wartime operations that are otherwise little concerned with the experience of violence and tend to focus on military strategy and tactics. For civilians too, the experience of witch-hunts provided some of the most persistent and painful of memories (Alexander *et al.*, forthcoming).[1] As Jeremy Brickhill has noted, the Rhodesian poisoning tactic did not ultimately affect the outcome of the war, but it 'poisoned the future' (Brickhill 1992–3).

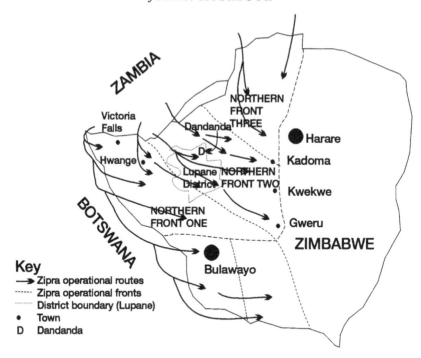

Figure 7.1 ZIPRA incursions and operational areas, 1979

The Rhodesians used poisons against both of Zimbabwe's liberation armies (ZANLA, the armed wing of ZANU, and ZIPRA, the forces of ZAPU), but in this article, I focus on one notorious witch-hunt which occurred in the ZIPRA operational area of Lupane District, Matabeleland North. It features so strongly in wartime memories partly because it was exceptional. In general, ZIPRA managed to contain violence in their operational areas more successfully: lines of guerrilla command were well developed, standards of discipline were often high and commanders could also rely on the authority of the ZAPU party committees.[2] The party structures were commonly headed by trusted people of seniority and respect

Table 7.1 Glossary of terms used in the chapter

ZANU	Zimbabwe African National Union
ZANLA	Zimbabwe African National Liberation Army
ZAPU	Zimbabwe African People's Union
ZIPRA	Zimbabwe People's Revolutionary Army
Inyanga	Traditional healer, diviner
Sangoma	Spirit medium associated with the Ndebele. Often also a traditional healer (*inyanga*)
Muti	Herbs used as medicine, poison, charms or spells

who provided continuity in local leadership and mediated dealings between guerrillas and civilians. So where violence spiralled out of control it became notorious, a point of moral reference for how things should not be. Such violence provides a powerful symbol of the vulnerability of both guerrillas and civilians, the fears and dependencies of both sides. As a point of comparison, it also helps illuminate why and how violence was more successfully contained elsewhere.

My emphasis on containment may seem misplaced in talking about a situation in which violence spiralled out of control. However, as Andrew Apter has pointed out in the very different context of Nigeria, witch-finding should be understood not just as a 'symptom' of tension and instability, but as a drama that seeks to comprehend and control it (Apter 1993: 113). In the context of the elevated insecurities of the liberation war in Matabeleland, a remarkable range of individuals and institutions were involved in efforts to understand and control the guerrilla deaths and reprisals against civilians. These included the guerrillas themselves, party youth, ZIPRA commanders, senior party officials, and other prominent members of the local community such as traditional healers and Zionist prophets.

Their accounts of violence are not just about the pain of lives needlessly lost, but about heroic acts of bravery. Civilian leaders risked their lives in their endeavour to control unruly youth whilst guerrilla commanders faced greater insubordination over this than over any other issue.[3] In trying to contain violence, the different actors used a range of arguments and appeals, relating to military strategy, to ideas drawn from pre-war practices of divination and other means of dealing with witches. In finding a solution, they built alliances that bridged the division between guerrillas and civilians which poisoning had so fatally widened.

The first part of the paper describes the particular wartime context of ZIPRA's Northern Front. It then turns to the existing body of literature on witch-hunts in the liberation war. The main part of the paper explores moral debate over guerrilla deaths and witch-killings in Lupane District, focusing on recollections of a series of notorious events which are infamous all over the Northern Front.

The military context: ZIPRA's Northern Front and Rhodesian counterinsurgency

The notorious witch-hunts that concern this paper accompanied Rhodesian use of poisons in the final year of the liberation war, particularly after 1978. Guerrillas had entered Lupane in serious numbers in 1977 and by late 1978, much of the district was semi-liberated and under the control of ZIPRA guerrillas operating through ZAPU party structures. Government authority in the rural areas was increasingly restricted to garrisoned district offices. In terms of ZIPRA's military strategy, 1978 marked the 'turning point' in the insurgency after which ZIPRA aimed to consolidate control over areas which the Rhodesians had lost, by deploying regular forces in their defence and preparing attacks on the government rural garrisons and major towns (Brickhill 1995). This strategic change was important in relation to the poisoning discussed below, as it strengthened lines of military command.

Of the three divisions of the Northern Front created at this time, Northern Front Two (NF2, which encompassed Lupane) was the most severely affected by poisoning. This was because NF2 was particularly important in strategic terms as it gave access to some of the main towns of the highveld and had the largest number of guerrillas concentrated within it (Nkomo and Dube, interview).[4] When NF2 guerrillas were assembled after the ceasefire, suspect items of guerrilla clothing were sent for forensic testing, and the tests provided confirmation of the use of poisoned clothing (ibid.). This knowledge did not, however, reach many of the communities affected, who have received little information to either confirm or discredit their wartime beliefs about the causes of the mysterious guerrilla deaths.

ZIPRA's war strategy in Matabeleland built on ZAPU's long history of nationalist activism and highly organized party structures. Jeremy Brickhill's work has brought attention to the significance of the network of rural ZAPU committees in facilitating guerrillas' entry and operations in rural communities: he explains that 'guerrillas did not need to build a new support base or establish their legitimacy. They could simply say they were "Nkomo's boys" and seek out party members in the community' (Brickhill 1995: 70). Our research has basically confirmed his arguments.

In the early and mid-1970s, ZAPU prepared for guerrillas' penetration: committees paralysed after the wave of arrests in the 1960s were reactivated, the geographical scope of rural party structures was extended and contact between centre and periphery was improved by increasing the number of provincial-level party officials. Where party committees were inoperative at the time the guerrillas arrived, guerrillas resuscitated them. The party structures organized food, supplies and other support to guerrillas and mediated relations with civilians. They provided for some continuity in authority in the rural areas during the war, though the relationship between guerrillas and civilians nonetheless remained fragile. It was this fragility that the Rhodesians sought to exploit.

The Rhodesian army and CIO created the Selous Scouts to operate in areas where regular troops could no longer move. They used the credo that the 'means justify the ends'. Their 'all-important task' was to 'improve the kill rate and they were not too fussy about how this was achieved' (Ellert 1993: 142).[5] Knowing that guerrillas depended upon civilians for the supply of clothing, equipment, foodstuffs and other supplies inside the country, they endeavoured to infiltrate these networks and poison the goods that passed through them (ibid.). Various poisons were used including a type of organophosphate known as parathian:

> impregnated into the fabric of clothing so that poisons would be absorbed through soft body tissue . . . where prolonged contact could be achieved. . . . After exposure to the poison . . . the victim would experience symptoms which included bleeding from the nose and mouth and a rise in temperature.
>
> (Ellert 1993: 142, 144)

Thallium and a rat poison called warfarin were used in food and drink.

The Rhodesians claimed significant success from their poisoning operations: Stiff notes that within the Rhodesian CIO, 'It was said that there were some months when Sam Roberts [responsible for designing the poisons] had killed more terrorists than the Rhodesian Light Infantry' (cited in Ranger, forthcoming: 12). ZIPRA commanders also claimed that 'Rhodesian poisoning was the most effective' strategy (Nkomo and Dube, interview). Nicholas Nkomo, commander of the NF2 forces, claimed that more guerrillas were lost through poisoning than in battle (Nkomo, Ms.). Of course, poisoning was not the only tactic of the Selous Scouts: they also specialized in 'turning' captured guerrillas, and sending them back to stage horrific killings of civilians designed to alienate guerrillas' popular support.[6]

Violence and guerrilla/civilian relations: the literature

The existing literature on the war has dealt with witch-killings in different ways. For anthropologist David Lan, working in the ZANLA operational area of Dande, witches epitomized all that was evil and constituted the illegitimate and 'cognitive antithesis' of *mhondoro* spirit mediums, the latter being the source of moral authority and goodness. His structural analysis symbolically opposes witches and sell-outs on the one hand, to guerrillas and spirit mediums on the other. Lan argues that killing witches was popular and legitimate in the eyes of civilians: it was 'universally agreed' (Lan 1995: 36). He elaborates how some people were pleased to see witches killed, and regarded this as 'good work the guerrillas had done' (ibid.: 168). Lan goes as far as to argue that it was the killing of witches that clinched civilian support for the guerrillas: 'The guerrillas' explicit and aggressive policy against witches was the final turn of the key in the lock. The doorway to legitimate political authority was opened wide' (ibid.: 170).

In contrast, most other authors, amongst them Norma Kriger, Richard Werbner and Michael Bourdillon, analyse guerrillas' killing of witches by trying to understand social tensions rather than cognitive structures (see Bourdillon 1987). They tend to emphasize the role of local jealousies and hatreds, the killing of innocent people and the trauma it entailed for civilians. Richard Werbner's 'social biography' of a family in a ZIPRA operational area in Matabeleland South documents the immense and lasting pain witch-killing caused to the families who lost members. Werbner sees violent wartime witch-killings as the replacement of more benign peacetime accusations:

> In place of the controlled, everyday argument in peacetime about moral character and sorcery came something uncontrollably monstrous in wartime: a campaign against sorcery that was brutal and often arbitrary. This anti-sorcery campaign, imposed by youths as strangers, if in the guise of 'children', was out of the control of elders bound by the passions and responsibilities of close kinship.
>
> (Werbner 1991: 150)

In Norma Kriger's (1992) study of the war in ZANLA's operational area of Mtoko, witch-hunts feature as one of many examples of guerrilla coercion and terror used against peasants. She uses such cases to support her broader argument that civilian support was not readily forthcoming but was elicited only through guerrilla coercion. She also uses descriptions of witch-killings during the war as evidence of what she calls 'struggles within the struggle' and how the guerrillas were pulled into entirely local disputes based on the social cleavages of gender, generation and stratification (Kriger 1992, Chapter 5). She specifically exempts ZIPRA operational areas from the conclusions of her study because of the critical importance of the ZAPU political structures (ibid.: 45).

These three texts' treatment of the topic of wartime witch-killings is constrained to some extent by their broader parameters and goals.[7] Lan's much criticized use of structural symbolic opposites frames his discussion of witchcraft, obscuring non-consensual views and debate over the legitimacy of individual cases. His assumption that political struggle was good and would bring a release from suffering precluded a consideration of its traumatic memory (Lan 1997). Werbner focuses on testimonies from one family whose members were themselves victims of accusations of selling out and witchcraft. Though their testimonies are diverse and are contextualized with regard to neighbours' views, they cannot, indeed are not intended to, represent a broader range of actors. Kriger tends to draw on fairly standard social categories in discussing the patterns of jealousies in such accusations, so that youth are pitted against parents, women against men, outsiders against chiefly lineages and so on.

This chapter will show that although guerrillas did become implicated in local disputes, the alignments and structures set up to deal with witch-hunting were often far more complex than sociological oppositions allow. I emphasize the range of perspectives and individual agency, albeit in the context of the institutions in the semi-liberated areas. However, a discourse on youthful overzealousness, uncontrollability, criminality and degeneration is a feature of my material as much as Kriger's and other authors on the war.

The literature also agrees on the conflation of the categories 'sell-out' and 'witch' during the war. Lan, for example, argued that, 'Anyone who is opposed to the altruistic and benevolent *mhondoro* and their protégés, the guerrillas . . . was placed in the category to which the ancestors are structurally opposed, the witch' (Lan 1985: 170). But symbolic opposites and cognitive categories need not be invoked. Werbner notes that sorcerer and witch 'were not easily separated: the sorcerer and the sell-out were often equated in practice or were labels different people used for the same victim of suspicion' (Werbner 1991: 150).

Though the terms are often used in a conflated way, I think it is none the less important to draw some distinctions. I shall argue that both with regard to moral discourse and with regard to formal military and political strategy, witches and sell-outs were not always treated as the same category.[8] Of course, much moral debate over the killing of witches and sell-outs focused on the way individual cases were handled, whether sufficient evidence existed, whether warnings were issued and so on. But the legitimacy of killing witches was also the topic of moral debate at a normative level and in terms of military strategy in a way that the killing of sell-outs was not. Killing proven sell-outs after they had ignored a warning to discontinue was a necessary wartime act. In contrast, members of the ZIPRA High Command and senior party leaders argued that neither ZIPRA strategy nor ZAPU's constitution endorsed killing of witches as part of the war effort. After witch-killings got out of hand, all suspicions about civilians were supposed to be referred to the ZIPRA Command. These arguments impinged on village-level acts, debate and reflection. The issue was not whether or not witches existed and were practising during the war – on that there was universal agreement – but whether it was appropriate to devote military effort to hunting and killing them.

Witchcraft and its control before the war

Witch-finding efforts in the war drew on the stock of cultural and historical resources related to understandings of, and means of dealing with, witches in peacetime. The many and varied practices for dealing with witchcraft in the decades before the war informed the content, though not the violence, of subsequent wartime acts. Wartime witch-hunts therefore can be seen as drawing selectively on familiar performative acts and bodily practices. At the same time, they changed both the acts themselves and their meaning by incorporating them into a new context and stimulating renewed questioning of their moral validity, not least due to the introduction of unprecedented levels of violence.

The decades before the war were marked by massive and disruptive forced removals into Lupane from the highveld around Bulawayo. The social tensions and instability created by the evictions, the process of forging new communities, the subsequent nationalist activism and political repression provided the context for a surge in witchcraft accusations in the 1950s and 1960s.[9] The social cleavage between evictees and early settlers seems to have been particularly salient for accusations of witchcraft, at least initially. Ndebele-speaking evictees stereotyped early settlers (many of whom were of Tonga origin, and spoke Tonga), as backward and possessors of fearful herbs and charms, particularly a charm known as *ulunyoka*. *Ulunyoka* was used by men to protect their womenfolk and caused genital ailments to any man who slept with a woman so protected. Evictees were often Christians who had accumulated considerable wealth prior to the evictions and were regarded with suspicion partly for these reasons.[10] Nationalist mobilization gave rise to a new political leadership drawn mainly from the ranks of the evictees while youth had a new role and status in the rural and urban sabotage campaigns. The schools that had opened after the evictees' arrival in the late 1940s provided the younger generation with both aspirations and frustrations.

Practices of divination and witch-eradication in the decades prior to the war did not entail killing witches. As Werbner has described, *sangoma* spirit mediums were particularly important in dealing with witches: associated with the Ndebele, 'they enacted a counter-aggression to attacks by sorcery by dancing, costumed as warriors and brandishing spears' (Werbner: 201).[11] They divined and prescribed herbs, blood sacrifices and other ritual acts of therapy (ibid.). Chiefs for their part were prevented from dealing with witches under the Witchcraft Suppression Ordinance of 1899. In the context of the evictions, they lobbied unsuccessfully to have these powers reinstated. However, there is some evidence that their courts continued (illegally) to deal with cases of witchcraft through a combination of divination and compensation.[12]

Famous itinerant witch-eradicators passed through and cleansed the communities of Lupane before the war. Those of most repute were outsiders, often Malawian or Zambian. Chikanga, for example, is famous over a large area of east and central Africa. Detailed accounts exist of Chikanga's activities, and those of other itinerant witch-cleansers.[13] As Mark Auslander has described, itinerant witch-eradicators aimed not to kill witches but to 'cure them by confiscating their magical paraphernalia and by medicinally rendering them incapable of doing evil', promising 'the wholesale eradication of witchcraft while making it possible to reincorporate the accused back into the community' (Auslander 1993: 177). The day-long performances they staged entailed long queues of people filing past the witch-finder, and a hasty judgement of cleanliness or guilt. This was followed by humiliation and condemnation of the accused. As these were generally figures of seniority, wealth and authority, this appealed to youth and others excluded from the powers and respect they held. Attendance at the meetings was compulsory in the sense that non-attendance could be taken as a sign of having something to hide and lead to castigation as a witch. Identified witches would be told to fetch their charms and herbs which would be burnt, medicine would be rubbed into incisions in the skin and witches were threatened that future resort to witchcraft would bring death. Mark Auslander has argued that although the ritual of such meetings appealed to youth because old men and women were humiliated and berated, off the stage, little in the way of actual power was delivered through these events (ibid.: 189).

Zionist churches also grew in influence in this pre-war period, and were associated with powers against witches (ibid.: 175). They were also loosely associated with the itinerant witch-cleansers, both in terms of the careers of individual witch-cleansers and prophets, and by association between their practices.

No wartime witch-eradication meetings were conducted by pre-war itinerant witch-identifiers. One influential *sangoma* medium who was in the ZAPU youth in the 1960s, however, later presided over wartime witch-eradications, spoke with respect about Chikanga and others and staged events resonant in their performance with their peacetime precursors (C. N., interview). Though the means of identifying witches during the war drew on these pre-war practices, the violence that accompanied them during the war had no peacetime precedent. Nor can it be explained by invoking nineteenth century poison ordeals. The violence against witches during the war was a product of the context of war and not of pre-war norms of handling witches.

Wartime violence in Dandanda

With this historical context in mind, I turn below to the accounts of a particular series of violent events that occurred in the final year of the war in Dandanda, northern Lupane. Because the ZAPU structures had in general enabled guerrillas to enter and operate with as little disruption to rural society as possible, events in Dandanda gained notoriety all over the Northern Front and became much recounted wartime stories. As such they have been subject to a good deal of elaboration, exaggeration and distortion. Events in Dandanda were in no way characteristic of ZIPRA's operations over the rest of the Northern Front, nor was the violence characteristic of all groups of guerrillas in the area. The stories about violence in Dandanda are revealing about power and control in the semi-liberated areas, danger and fear on the part of civilians and guerrillas. The events are memorable for the way violence escalated and for how it was eventually brought under control.

The series of events were divisive and complex, and hence it is to be expected that individual accounts conflict. Even those directly involved often only knew part of the sequence of events from direct observation. Eighteen years have elapsed since these events took place and estimates of the numbers killed in Dandanda have been exaggerated out of all proportion. Some guerrillas claim up to one hundred guerrilla deaths, and civilians sometimes similarly inflate the numbers of civilians killed. My aim in what follows is both to establish a plausible version of what happened and to explore how individuals involved reflected on and explained the violence and discussed their attempts to contain it.

The bare bones of the story are as follows. Violence in Dandanda began with mysterious guerrilla deaths. This was attributed by guerrillas to a Rhodesian-sponsored poisoning ring and numbers of civilians were killed in subsequent witch-hunts. Two key women in the executive of the local ZAPU women's committees were among those killed, and became the focus of much subsequent moral debate over witchcraft. They were killed in a large public meeting, attendance at which was compulsory: the first was a young woman accused of being a Rhodesian agent at the head of a poisoning ring involving a network of young girls who poisoned guerrillas' food. She confessed and identified a second older woman as an accomplice. As the latter was being killed, she threatened that all guerrillas who had participated in her killing would die, as would their comrades. After her death, guerrillas did continue to die, and in escalating numbers. Witch-hunts continued on a new and larger scale, involving several mass witch-eradication meetings resulting in civilian deaths. Other suspects were taken individually from their homes and killed without ceremony by guerrillas and youths.

This basic history was not interpreted in a uniform way. Views on the causes of guerrilla deaths and efforts at control were wide-ranging. Below, I tease out the different strands of argument in the accounts I was given in interviews. Though I treat these threads separately, the various explanations frequently overlapped and were often not regarded as exclusive: those who emphasized the role of a ring of Rhodesian collaborators, for example, could also elaborate on the role of witches. Nor can the explanations be matched neatly with different social actors.

Many guerrillas, party officials and others explained the cause of guerrilla deaths partly in terms of a Rhodesian poisoning ring.[14] They elaborated on its means of operation in various ways. Some said the woman at its head travelled frequently to Hwange town, where her husband lived and where the Rhodesian CIO had its nearest headquarters (T. S. M., interview). This alone would have made her subject to much suspicion. One claimed she got her poison via the auxiliary forces operating in neighbouring Gokwe, where poisoning was also rife (C. N., interview). Others focused on her own later confession of acting for the Rhodesians: one guerrilla, for example, explained:

There was a young lady who came to the area with that poison, she was sent by the Rhodesians to recruit youths to bring clothes and

poisonous tablets . . . she told us everything about it . . . Then we
killed the young lady and another person.

(O. D., interview)

Some said she not only brought clothes and poison into Dandanda, but also
imported beautiful women. Selected for their youth and beauty, these women
would lure the guerrillas to a death by poison (Nkomo, interview).

Although understandings of a Rhodesian poisoning ring were common,
they were not incompatible with interpretations of guerrilla deaths which
emphasized the role of witchcraft. The two strands of argument were
incorporated in various ways. Many accounts tended to merge the two
women central to the story into a single person, so the woman at the head of
the Rhodesian-sponsored poisoning network and the woman who laid the
curse on guerrillas became one person in popular memory. This made her
both sell-out and witch.

Labelling witches as sell-outs was also a means of legitimizing killing
them. Retrospectively, some guerrillas justified their actions in terms of the
wartime context. 'We were using military means to deal with witches', said
one (E. S., interview). This in effect reverses Lan's argument that it was
legitimate to kill sell-outs because they were in the same category as witches.
No one invoked an historical memory of nineteenth century witch-killings
as a justification for wartime acts. However, this argument should not be
pushed too far: the means of finding, interrogating and killing the two key
women in this story as well as others in the alleged 'poisoning ring' was
informed by their identification as witches, beliefs about witches and
practices of identifying witches. For example, the two women were
questioned not only about poisoning for the Rhodesians, but about their hold
over matters of fertility, their predation on children and the suspicious deaths
of women in their families during childbirth (S. M., interview).

The techniques used to identify witches and sell-outs involved in the
Rhodesian poisoning ring were varied. They often drew on the expertise of
diviners, but were sometimes said to be founded on no more than local
rumour and hatred. Guerrillas and local leaders sometimes emphasized the
attempt to institute checks, for example, by consulting more than one
inyanga. The NF2 commander, however, was dismissive both of the use in
this context of standard divining methods and of the reliance on rumour; he
pressed guerrillas repeatedly for concrete evidence, which was not
forthcoming. His demand for proof was met by threats on his own life: he
recalled 'on my insistence on proof, they were angry enough to tell me that
it was only a matter of time before I found myself in the same situation'
(Nkomo, interview). I shall return to High Command efforts to control
killings later.

Attempts to understand guerrilla deaths were, therefore, far from simply
a question of investigating the evidence for Rhodesian poisoning. Much

attention came to focus in addition on the woman's dying curse. Even those who suspected she was a sell-out also recounted stories of her supernatural powers as a witch. These supernatural powers generally related to how difficult she was to kill. She was said to have survived bayonetting and gunfire before burning plastic was wrapped on her naked body and she was hurled into a fire. Some said charms had to be broken (by jumping over an ammunition belt) before guns would fire at all (T. S. M., interview). Others described how even in the fire, she could be heard talking and singing for some time. Some said that her body swelled and swelled in the fire, and when she finally died a black bird emerged from the smoke (C. M. and C. N., interview). The nature of her threat as she died was also elaborated in various ways: some held that she had threatened with death those who had touched her body or participated in the bayonetting. Others said the curse also affected anyone subsequently touching those guerrillas or their guns.

Everyone concurred that she had supernatural powers of some sort. There was almost universal agreement among all but her family that she was a witch. The evidence for her being a witch was not only in the length of time she resisted death, but also in the fulfilment of her dying threat of subsequent guerrilla deaths. She was also held responsible for two other deaths in her own family, of women in childbirth. Her ability to continue killing after her death was generally attributed to a type of 'doctoring' known as *uzimu* that protected her and caused her spirit to continue to seek retribution after her death. Many *inyanga* and prophets were consulted in coming to this conclusion.[15] A local ZAPU branch official and *inyanga*, for example, recalled:

> We ran around . . . using both traditional and Christian ways of trying to find out about what were the causes of this disease which led to death. Our findings . . . were that they had . . . killed certain witches. According to our traditional belief, some people are medicated traditionally, so then when he or she is being killed, that person will defend herself, even if she is dead, by means of revenge.
>
> (M. N., interview)

As a result of further debate and divination, guerrillas, local party leaders and other civilians came to the conclusion that her killing was wrongful. Some had held this position from the outset. It was commonly said that such a person should not be killed. This understanding led to a range of strategies to try to pacify her spirit.

The means of appeasing the vengeful woman's spirit included compensating her husband in the form of a young girl and cattle. A ZIPRA guerrilla who was also an *inyanga* recalled:

> when the dying got really bad, nine, five, three [guerrillas] would die each day. We knew there had been a mistake. So we went . . . to

get cattle to pay for the damage we had done . . . to compensate the husband of that woman . . . the local people went to me with some ZIPRAs and I threw bones. I said that they had wronged by killing that woman.

(C. N., interview)

He claimed that the strategy of compensation came to him in a dream and that he successfully appeased the spirit. Most accounts, however, do not attribute any degree of success to the compensation.

Some guerrillas came to blame the husband for avenging his wife's death, rather than the woman's own spirit. According to one guerrilla, the husband confessed to having placed the charm himself and demanded six head of cattle and a virgin from the guerrillas as the means of breaking it (O. D., interview).

To her family, however, the woman was not a witch, though they do not dispute that she was difficult to kill or that she foretold subsequent guerrilla deaths if she was killed. They explained her death threats and subsequent efforts at compensation in very different light. They explained that she was difficult to kill because she was possessed by an ancestral *ihumba* spirit which came out when she was on the fire. *Ihumba* spirits are secretive lion spirits that affect women of Kalanga descent. They trouble the women possessed by them but are not evil or vengeful to others.[16] Her family emphasized her innocence, and her honour and bravery in not naming others to die when instructed to do so under torture. Her threats were not malicious in intent according to her daughter-in-law, who explained them in the following way:

As she was about to die, guerrillas had asked her to name another person who also bewitches. She said, "No, I don't know any, I don't want someone to lose their children because of me. I want to die alone. If you kill me, like this, you will carry your guns in twos or threes or fours." It was a saying, and she meant that guerrillas would die, and those who survived would be carrying their dead comrades' guns. She was just threatening them to try to preserve her life . . . she wasn't an *inyanga* or a witch . . . she had an ancestral spirit [*dhlozi*], an *ihumba* spirit . . . You could hear her talking in the fire as she was burnt, singing in the flames . . . it took her a long time to die in the fire. They couldn't kill her quickly. She took time to die because of that *dhlozi*.

(S. M., interview)

The consequences of the significance attached to the dying woman's threat were horrific for other members of her family. As the woman was being killed, relatives were warned not to show any emotion, as this would indicate that they too were witches. There was intense suspicion that other female members of the family were also witches. The daughter-in-law recalled guerrillas saying to her 'the child of a snake is also a snake', and 'you failed to tell us we were staying with witches, that is why you are thin: you also are a witch' (ibid.). Neighbours refused to greet them or enter their home. Youths and guerrillas put the whole family under constant observation. The daughter-in-law explained that even the debates over compensation to the family were a worry and ended in threats to kill the husband and son:

> What [X] said when she was killed became a problem for us. They told her husband: 'We'd better give you a small girl to pay back that we killed your wife.' They talked lots and lots of things. 'Maybe we'll try cattle' was another suggestion. But my father-in-law was very worried. 'I know nothing' he said, because he was faced with their constant questions. 'I know nothing, I didn't say those words.' They tried all those things, all that compensation, but in the end they wanted to kill him as well.
>
> (ibid.)

Husband and son were detained and interrogated by the guerrillas. The husband was killed and the son went mad on his release: he refused to sleep with his wife, talked incessantly and nonsensically about war and the guerrillas, and became obsessed with washing, going every few hours to the river to wash and try to clean himself. Because the daughter-in-law was also on the district level ZAPU women's executive, she was in constant contact with guerrillas, and the family turned on her, blaming her for selling her mother-in-law (ibid.).[17]

Efforts to prevent ongoing guerrilla deaths did not only involve this one family. Guerrillas called mass meetings in the forest to which the community as a whole was obliged to attend. The youths were sent to round everyone up and hundreds of people attended each meeting. Failure to attend these meetings would itself indicate guilt and one recalled being told: 'if you see the dawn before reaching the gathering point, kill yourself' (S. M., interview; see also Chitete elders, interview). Accounts agree that the guerrillas were in charge of these mass meetings. The youths encircled the gathered masses to prevent anyone escaping.

The pre-war precedent for these meetings can be found in the acts of itinerant witch-cleansers. In wartime, though, they did not involve performances symbolic of aggression towards witches or symbolic of the power of youth, but rather direct acts of violence and very real displays of the power of those who held the gun. They were provoked though by anger and an extreme sense of vulnerability and powerlessness in the face of guerrilla deaths.

ZIPRA guerrillas brought renowned *sangoma* mediums and Zionist prophets from outside the immediate vicinity to these meetings and thus gave the role of witch-identifier to an outsider of some repute. This may have been an attempt to avoid community members just identifying their neighbours, and so to enable the identification of real witches. Similarly, involving more than one identifier may have been an effort to prevent false identifications. As one guerrilla explained: 'Mostly when people were grouped, then the witches were smelt. The person would be brought in from a different area who couldn't know that thing. Because he didn't know people, he might identify the real thing' (C. N., interview). At one meeting, a sole *sangoma* presided (who was himself a ZIPRA guerrilla from a neighbouring operational area). People were forced to sing traditional songs until the *sangoma* was possessed, then they would file past and kneel at his feet for identification, which usually took the form of a rapid judgement. At the end of the meeting fourteen were shot and buried in a mass grave (Chitete elders, interview; H. K. and H. M., interview). At a second meeting where five seem to have died, *inyanga* and Zionist prophet presided together: individuals had to be vetted by both, and only when there was mutual agreement was the person killed.[18]

People confessed to acts of witchcraft and poisoning at these events. The ZAPU branch chair who was also an *inyanga* gave the following account of one of these mass meetings, in this case presided over by both *inyanga* and prophet:

> It was so difficult at that gathering because people would be sniffed out by those two people. They'd tell a person, 'you have been doing x, using these things against this person at such and such a time'. And people would agree to that. Others, when accused said they did that unknowingly. . . . Others were asked 'Do you remember I caught you bewitching a person on that day?' Then people would agree. That was all out of terror. Me, as an individual, I can say that fear penetrated my body . . . the *inyanga* and the Zionist were seated and all the villagers would file past.
>
> (M. N., interview)

Initially, the meetings and witch-killings were endorsed by the ZIPRA detachment commander, desperately trying to find the cause of the guerrillas dying. But later, when guerrilla deaths continued, even when suspected civilians were also dead, his attitude changed. The following account reveals his change of outlook and subsequent strategy of initiating a dialogue with civilians to understand and try to control guerrilla deaths:

> [The commander] X . . . was there [at the mass meeting] . . . at that time he was active in that, in identifying people to be killed because guerrillas were dying. He said to us 'villagers, you say giving birth is the same' (this is a saying, *ukuzala uyafanana*, meaning there should be no discrimination between your own child and someone

else's), 'but it is not the same because you are killing us' . . . he told us that at the meeting. He told us that a hundred would die for one dead guerrilla . . . only later, he called a different meeting and asked the parents to help. 'I can see we are lost,' he said. 'Please, what we are doing must stop. Guerrillas and civilians are dying. Let's work out a solution together.' [X] tried to stop everything very late. It was too late. He realized only late that killing the parents was not the solution to the guerrillas dying.

(S. M., interview; see also M. N., interview)

Members of the local community often recall the deaths from these meetings as horrific and arbitrary, and portray the guerrillas who organized them as wild and uncontrollable. They recall violent acts perpetrated by guerrillas outside the mass meetings in support of this, such as disrespectful behaviour when asking for food and abuse of women. One explained how the ZIPRA guerrillas were 'totally out of control, they didn't care who was who' (G. S., interview). Others referred to that group of guerrillas as 'that wild group' (S. T., interview), they were 'out of hand' (Dardanda elders, interview). Certainly, at the witch-eradication meetings, a wide range of senior authority figures were killed: members of the party district executive structures, respected rainmakers and other elders. The local ZAPU branch officer recalled:

A ZAPU official at district level was identified as being a big snake which was eating children in the area. He is one of those lying in the mass grave created at that meeting . . . there was another party chair who was engaged in trapping guerrillas with *ulunyoka*, he was a Tonga and was also killed . . . A famous [Tonga] rainmaker was also killed.

(M. N., interview)

ZAPU authority figures felt guerrillas were turning against them, and one branch executive member explained: 'It was a period when even our own children, together with their brothers were not behaving in a proper manner . . . our own guerrillas were now behaving in an improper way, turning their guns on us'. The youth were also blamed to a considerable extent, and elders recalled, 'some of us were killed by our own children' (Chitete elders interview).

The guerrillas' violence was motivated by their sense of vulnerability and anger over their comrades' deaths, a sense of powerlessness despite their guns. One talked of the mass meetings as a final resort because 'there was no way out of the situation' (C. N., interview). Some tended to downplay the number of civilians killed, emphasizing the guilt of those who admitted to poisoning as Rhodesian agents (E. S., interview; O. D., interview; C. N., interview).

Others admitted witches were killed and explained how they lost control of the youth who took things into their own hands. The *sangoma* presiding at one of the witch-eradication meetings emphasized the pain of the guerrilla deaths for their comrades:

> In cases where witches identified others, then a whole string of people would be killed. It was a bad thing that so many were killed in one day at some of the meetings, but because it was war and revenge for guerrilla deaths, it was possible. It was painful that guerrillas died because their families didn't know and didn't know [their son's] pseudonym, so who was going to inform their families?
>
> (C. N., interview)

The hunting of witches was finally brought to a halt when ZIPRA and ZAPU, having set up their own high-level investigation of events, strongly condemned the hunting of witches and exerted their authority. The commander of the NF2 forces, who was a member of the ZIPRA High Command, was also based in Lupane, albeit at some distance from Dandanda. He was clear from the outset that military strategy did not endorse the killing of witches as they were not military targets. He further condemned all killing of civilians without proof. He explained to guerrillas in one of the meetings held to sort out this issue:

> Witches have been with us since the beginning. In the places you come from and where you grew up, there are also witches. Some of you are the sons and neighbours of witches. In independent Zimbabwe we will also have witches. . . I was clear that we had no instructions to kill witches. So I gave these instructions to lower commands – no one can die because they are accused of being a witch.
>
> (Nkomo, interview)

He reached an understanding of what had happened on the basis of reading about French actions in Algeria and discussed this idea with others:

> The French used some kind of chemical to kill guerrillas, we all agreed that perhaps there was a secret weapon used by the Rhodesians to kill us and that it was done in such a way as to cause mistrust between us and the locals, because the enemy knew that our strength had its roots in the masses of the people. We then met with the senior regional commanders to work out means of stopping the rot . . . We decided . . . to stop the rot once and for all, and told guerrillas not to take the law into their own hands. No killing of civilians by guerrillas was to be witnessed, and any incident was to be reported to the command before taking action.
>
> (Nkomo, Ms.)

The guerrillas' response was initially one of fury. They threatened their commander, who recalls:

> Guerrillas were furious and were absolutely convinced that it was the locals who were responsible . . . I had trouble with some guerrillas who said we are dying not you . . . we are the ones who know about witches. So I said it is a High Command order.
>
> (Nkomo, interview)

With this order, they were brought into line. One guerrilla recalled: 'The High Command said not to deal with witches' (O. D. interview). Some subsequently apologized to civilians: 'Initially, we thought it was witchcraft, but later we apologized to the locals for what we had done', one remembered (E. S., interview). Others were disciplined and disarmed. But controlling witch-killing was a huge task: 'It really affected the war effort. Sometimes we found ourselves doing no operations. It affected morale terribly', the commander of the Northern Front forces recalled (Nkomo, interview). For civilians too, it took time to rebuild trust. The local ZAPU branch officer in Dandanda explained: 'When guerrillas came to our homes, they'd say "you're now used to killing us". It took us a long time to amicably have discussions. Both sides were dying' (M. N., interview).

Senior ZAPU leaders who endorsed the ZIPRA High Command position that witch-killing was outside the goals of the war also claimed success in halting it: 'We called meetings to tell them that's not the aim of the struggle', a senior ZAPU leader recalled:

> The boys had lost their direction, went into domestic affairs until it led to deaths. . . . That's where I personally stood up very strong. I told the boys, stop this rubbish, your guns won't shoot me. A lot of guerrillas died because of *muti* . . . many people were killed in this area, but then the guerrillas began to realize I was correct, but those deaths could have been avoided. . . . We had two or three of those big meetings then I defused the whole thing.
>
> (N. K., interview)

Though the senior ZIPRA Northern Front commanders in alliance with senior ZAPU leaders were responsible for halting the killing of witches, civilians often attributed the final success in halting guerrilla deaths to a Zionist prophet of considerable repute. He was called in as a result of meetings between ZAPU and ZIPRA. Known locally as 'Papa' (Pope), he was Vice Bishop of the New Holy Full Gospel Church in Zion of Zimbabwe, and was also a ZAPU district executive officer. He appeased the vengeful spirit of the wrongfully killed woman by conducting a cleansing ceremony at her grave. In his own account, he described a performance symbolic of pinning her spirit down and breaking its hold:

> The guerrillas had killed a person who was not supposed to be killed. She was a person, that if you kill her, you too will die. She told them as much . . . [and] all who touched those who died also died. I went there and prayed and prayed for those guys not to die. I prayed on the grave of the lady . . . so that she would not cause havoc killing people . . . I told [the ZAPU chair]: 'we have to pray here so that that woman can go to her grave. I can see her standing on top of her grave. We need to cool her spirit down.' I took a coin, the old type of coin used here with a hole in it and a new knitting needle. So the knitting needle was put into the ground with the money, the needle was pinning the money into the ground. On the grave we took the needle with the money and inserted it at the side where there was the head. Than at the end of the grave where the feet were, we inserted a horseshoe. The district chair asked me to walk along the top of the grave. So I walked straight across . . . four others had failed to do that. Then we prayed . . . this signified the end of deaths of guerrillas.
>
> (T. S. M., interview)

Though there was considerable certainty regarding the role of senior ZIPRA and ZAPU leaders in halting the killing of civilians, moral debate over the responsibility for the violence is often remarkable for its unwillingness to attribute blame. There is a sense in which everyone was involved. Deaths are sometimes described as a product of the situation, of civilians inevitably caught 'in-between'. As one group of kraalheads recalled:

> People appreciated the guerrillas, appreciated the idea of freedom, that was a good thing. Everyone accepted. But during their operations, this is what happened. We lived in fear. . . . Now people are troubled by this, they can't forget. You have to excuse the guerrillas though, you can't blame them; war kills particularly those who are not armed.
>
> (M. D., A. D., K. M., interview)

The actions of the 'wild group' of guerrillas were not held retrospectively as typical of the behaviour of all guerrillas. One elder explained: 'they were like children. The first born is good and obedient. The next is a delinquent' (Lusulu group, interview). Both civilians and guerrillas commonly blamed the 'youth' running amuck, becoming 'criminals', even 'animals'. The fear of this last group of guerrillas did not colour interpretations of the actions of earlier groups, but was remembered as being in stark contrast to them:

First we were delighted when they came, we'd run up to them. But at the end, they became our enemies . . . We were so happy at first, we'd hear reports of contacts, capturing of weapons and the taking of everything from the dead soldiers.

(S. M., interview)

In fact, before the witch-killings Dandanda had been sought out by numbers of refugees from the neighbouring district of Gokwe because, being under ZIPRA/ZAPU control, it was perceived as a desirable place of order and safety away from the violence of Rhodesian forces and particularly Muzorewa's auxiliaries (Chitete elders, interview).

Memories of the ZIPRA command are also very favourable. A former policeman and ZAPU official, for example, recalled:

How to stop it? We couldn't do that. There was no way to stop it. But the commanders were the ones who really helped. They talked to the people strongly, threatened, 'Look, we'll have war against each other .What evidence do you have?' It was those commanders who managed to calm it down.

(M. D., A. D., K. M., interview)

Some blamed the killings not on guerrillas but on civilians. A senior ZAPU leader explained, 'all this witch-killing was led by peasants trying to bring their misunderstandings against themselves to the guerrillas which was wrong . . . people were selling their neighbours . . . the guerrillas were being misled by local people' (N. K., interview).

Retrospective evaluations of the *inyanga* and *sangoma* mediums who identified witches at the meetings were not wholly condemnatory, though one person mentioned that an *inyanga* involved would be lynched if he ever set foot there again and local kraalheads recalled: 'that *sangoma* was just telling lies, making up any story, that one is guilty, that one must die, that one is clean' (H. K., H. M., interview). However, many recollections were not so critical. Some saw the *inyanga* simply as 'instruments' of the guerrillas, being drawn by what was expected of them (T. S. M., interview). In the individual killings outside the meetings, too, they could be seen as instruments of local hatreds. Other *inyanga* and prophets not directly involved sometimes said that put in such a position themselves, they too would have identified people, and even turned on each other. A prophet from the Apostolic Faith Mission Church in Zion recalled:

One Friday I came home and heard everyone was wanted at Gabela. They wanted *inyanga* and prophets to identify witches and sell-outs. . . . The plan was to start with the *inyanga*. Then we were to be called to confirm the results of the *inyanga*. We were fifteen or twenty prophets called to that meeting. *Inyanga* were told to bring their bones. . . . Had it continued there would have been chaos. It would have been like gambling. We'd have identified people and then turned on each other and some of the *inyanga* and prophets would also have died.

(Mapanawomvu, interview)[19]

The *inyanga* and prophets retained a legitimacy amongst the guerrillas. One of the prominent *inyanga* of the war years who was involved in the Dandanda witch-hunts was given a special space in the guerrilla assembly point after the ceasefire to continue his healing. After leaving the assembly point, he continued to have a successful *inyanga's* business and also claimed to have played a prominent role in post-war community cleansing (though not in the same community as his wartime activities) (C. N., interview).

Accounts agree that the havoc caused by the witch-killings allowed Rhodesian penetration of an otherwise secure area. 'Guerrillas had been very effective . . . but that was all in ruins', the Zionist prophet explained (T. S. M., interview). Many locals were rounded up and interrogated by government forces. A Rhodesian army convoy penetrated the area for the first time since the start of the war. This violence helped the Rhodesians and left a painful legacy, but it did not break the legitimacy of the nationalist cause, nor did it break the legitimacy of ZIPRA as a whole, as people differentiated between the groups of guerrillas they had seen.

Dandanda contextualized

Dandanda violence was not only atypical, it was the worst for guerrilla and civilians deaths in the entire Northern Front. So why was it that violence was more successfully contained elsewhere?

Certain aspects of Dandanda's history militated against strong civilian control even without the problem of guerrilla deaths. Dandanda was Lupane's most recent frontier of settlement, with large-scale immigration of Ndebele-speaking people (into an area of sparse Tonga settlement) occurring only in the late 1960s and 1970s, very shortly before the war. There was little time for new communities to have cohered. The woman whose vengeful spirit was seen as the source of so many problems had arrived in the area with her family only in 1976, the very same year the guerrillas began to arrive. Partly because settlement was so recent, it was one of the places where ZIPRA had to create local party branch structures. These communities lacked trusted veteran nationalists with long-standing followings who could organize civilians in dialogue with guerrillas or effectively exert authority over the guerrillas.

In areas with a longer history of settlement and stronger ZAPU structures, party officials' accounts are often tales of successfully exerting authority over wayward youths and guerrillas before violence escalated out of control. They would liaise with senior commanders in trying to do so, and put themselves at considerable risk. Some senior politicians went to the top party leadership to get advice on this issue and civilians recalled them saying on their return, 'No, we want to take the land, with or without witches. We'll investigate about witches later' (Lupaka elders, interview). In Singwangombe, witch-killings also followed guerrilla deaths, but they were more rapidly controlled. The local provincial party member recalled:

> Four witches were killed here . . . [out of] hatred. People just went to *inyanga* and they'd throw bones. So-and-so would be identified as a witch and they'd be killed. Most . . . were sold by locals and killed by guerrillas. The party intervened, I as provincial member intervened . . . I said, 'Now, can you produce your constitution to show me you have been assigned to kill witches. Where is the document that gives you the power to kill witches? We are the leaders of ZAPU and you are our soldiers. We don't know that constitution. After this talk, the killings stopped . . . I was very strong on that issue.
>
> (S. N., interview)

Dandanda was also far from the base of the ZIPRA NF2 Command.[20] In other areas, the senior commanders could be brought in more quickly and the authority of the ZIPRA High Command could be asserted over guerrillas and junior commanders before violence escalated to such a degree.

In other places Zionists recalled taking a stand against the killing of witches: one such argued that only God had the right to take life. *Inyanga* are also sometimes held to have prevented killings by saying that guerrillas had been poisoned somewhere else, and in some places there was popular objection from ZAPU and elders. Elders (including veteran nationalists) from St Paul's for example, retold the following story:

> Six guerrillas died at one time This is why people were gathered to find out who it was . . . ZIPRA suspected poisoning and *sangoma* were called to smell the witches – these were the local *sangoma* who people knew. The *sangoma* did not identify the people as the killers of the guerrillas. Their verdict was that the guerrillas died here but the poisoning was not done in the area. The *sangoma* were then asked to identify witches . . . but the people objected. They said, 'No, we're not interested in finding witches, we want the ones who killed those guerrillas.' So later a committee was set up to get *sangoma* from far away. . . . In fact Lancaster House saved us, otherwise the issue was going to be resumed and someone would have died for it.
>
> (St Paul's elders, interview).

The most important contributions to containing violence were probably efforts by ZAPU and ZIPRA to alter supply routes and hence prevent guerrillas dying. In some areas, the guerrilla command or party leaders responsible for guerrilla supplies became suspicious about Rhodesian poisoning and their investigations and subsequent actions stopped further deaths from poisoning. Some changed the source of their supplies and outlawed the use of suspect stores. Others decided to get goods straight from the city. A ban on all gifts of supplies and supplies that did not come through the party structures was put in place in some areas. Stories circulated of mysterious gifts of clothing from white people intended for guerrillas. Sometimes particular events caused suspicion to focus on particular items of clothing: as for example, when a guerrilla and a civilian both got sick or died from using the same item. Others spoke of clothes with a strange smell. A ZAPU provincial officer based in Bulawayo during the war recalled:

> some guerrillas got out of hand, started killing innocent individuals
> . . . we discussed that issue [and] . . . influenced our districts and
> branches not to receive clothing from rural stores because you never
> know who is who. This [issue of poisoned clothes and food] did a lot
> of damage in a short period. The local leadership went to the local
> store people to investigate because they were suspicious.
>
> (Y. D., interview)

Conclusion

In the months following the ceasefire, the legacies of wartime witch-hunts were apparent. Some wartime witch-killing cases were retrospectively brought to the courts, and there was one incident in which guerrillas left the assembly point and killed a witch (*Chronicle*, 24 February and 29 May 1991).[21] ZAPU's leader, Joshua Nkomo, addressing a rally in Lupane in August 1980 announced 'I don't want to hear that any member of our party, the Patriotic Front, has held any trial in this part of the country' (*Chronicle*, 22 August 1980). However, the problem of 'kangaroo courts' after independence, so much reported in the press and parliament seems to have been predominantly in the ZANU areas in the East of the country. In Matabeleland, violence associated with wartime witchcraft accusations was quickly contained.

Debates over post-war cleansing did not emerge in Matabeleland after the ceasefire, partly because of the political and military repression which followed independence.[22] It was not until the ZANU government and ZAPU opposition signed the Unity agreement of 1987 that debates over cleansing really came to the fore, encouraged by a political climate of more open criticism of the government and heightened by the suffering provoked by severe drought and the emergence of incurable disease. Since the Unity agreement, itinerant witch-eradicators have been active in rural Matabeleland and have staged community events very similar to those of Chikanga and the other pre-war witch-cleansers. The most influential among these, known as Gawula, was discredited as rapidly as he came to fame. His cleansing was not directed specifically to wartime legacies though arguably the amount of witchcraft was related to ongoing social tensions produced by war.

To conclude this discussion of wartime witch-killings, it is important briefly to state what the events described in this paper are not. Events in Dandanda cannot be reduced to a case of soldiers being drawn into entirely local struggles unrelated to the war. They were not primarily about ongoing struggles over generation, gender and stratification. These were wartime events about power and vulnerability in the relationship between guerrillas and the civilians who supported them.

Guerrillas were, of course, drawn into local disputes and jealousies, but in efforts to prevent this happening, party officials and other civilians were also drawn into wider debates over military strategy and the goals of nationalism. The solution to violence against civilians involved dialogue with civilians and assertions of authority through the structures of the ZIPRA command and the institutions of the party. The most important pre-war social divide in Dandanda and much of Lupane was that between the most recent waves of Ndebele-speaking immigrants and the earlier settlers of Tonga origin. However, wartime violence was not interpreted in terms of this social cleavage, and its salience seems to have been reduced rather than widened in the course of the war.

This paper has tried to provide a new dimension to the literature on the liberation war. Recent analyses of wartime violence have often emphasized the pain of innocent lives lost, its senselessness or arbitrariness. This is certainly an important part of memories of the war, which continues to be troubling and which people cannot forget. But in focusing on retrospective accounts of the causes of guerrilla deaths, attempts to understand them and efforts to contain violence against civilians, I have tried to add other strands of wartime memories in which local communities were more than just passive victims of uncontrolled youth with guns. They were responsible, reflective agents in a moral debate. Guerrillas, likewise, were struggling to understand and control life-threatening situations. Tales of the suffering and ordeals of the war years are often in large part tales of heroism and bravery in taking a stand to contain violence.[23]

It would have been interesting to compare the wartime memories on which I have based my discussion with earlier accounts, and so put them in historical context. However, academic studies of the war conducted shortly after the cessation of hostilities are based in different parts of the country and are influenced by the outlook of their authors. David Lan, for example, who conducted fieldwork in 1980 and whose influential book *Guns and Rain* was discussed earlier, believed in political struggle as good in itself. He was concerned to illustrate that suffering was purposeful and led to goodness and healing.[24] He does not dwell on the pain of living through guerrilla war and treats violence – even that associated with witch-hunting – as the unproblematic removal of evil, as a release from suffering. Lan himself, reflecting on criticism from later scholars notes that his concern to show the relationship between guerrillas and peasants as mutually beneficial 'blinded' him to the pain of the war. Violence and efforts at its containment, like its traumatic memory, could scarcely fit with such an outlook.

In the course of my interviews, people reacted to the information that poisoning was a deliberate Rhodesian tactic to break the relationship between guerrillas and civilians in various ways. For many it merely confirmed previous suspicions. Guerrillas in particular, were often aware of the investigations of the ZIPRA command. But for those civilians to whom the information was new, it was also inconclusive. It certainly could not resolve many of the moral and political questions raised by the witch-hunts, including the sense of collective involvement, nor could it ease the painful memory of lives needlessly lost during the war years. In providing information on the 'hows' of guerrilla deaths, knowledge about Rhodesian use of poisons also does not answer the preoccupying 'whys' of those deaths: why one victim and not another, why one village and not its neighbour.[25] The knowledge that the Rhodesians used poisons also leaves open the question of whether local poisoning agents knew they were being used in this role.[26] And it certainly does not preclude witches' involvement.

The violence I have described illustrates the fragility of the relationship between guerrillas and civilians in the liberated areas and how vulnerable it was to Rhodesian poisoning. However, wartime efforts at containment are remarkable for the scope of individuals they involved. They are memorable not only for the instances where they failed, but also for the many instances where they succeeded.

Notes

This research forms part of a broader collaborative project between JoAnn McGregor, funded by the Economic and Social Research Council, Grant No. R00023 527601, and Jocelyn Alexander and Terence Ranger, funded by the Leverhulme Trust. I am most grateful to my research assistants Callistus Mkwananzi and Nicholas Nkomo, and to the University of Zimbabwe and the Ministry of Local Government for their support. Grateful thanks also to Wendy James, Mark Leopold, Richard Werbner and the editors of this volume for their comments on earlier drafts of the paper.

1   A fuller account of the war, including a broader discussion of guerrilla and civilian narratives, and further detail on military strategy and history is provided in our jointly written forthcoming book J. Alexander, J. McGregor and T. Ranger, *Violence*

and Memory: One Hundred Years in the 'Dark' Forests of Matabeleland, 1896–1996.

2   ZANLA lines of command may have been weaker and ZANLA also lacked well developed rural nationalist party structures. The literature on the war has sometimes characterized ZANLA as a 'peasant' army of relatively young, poorly trained and disciplined recruits in comparison to ZIPRA's older, better disciplined and longer trained recruits who often had experience of urban employment. ZIPRA had also developed a capacity for conventional warfare. See Ranger and Bhebe 1995: 6–23.

3   Richard Werbner also found a stress on bravery in accounts of wartime violence, particularly in women's accounts of fierceness (*chibindi*) in defending their homes: see Werbner 1991: 157.

4   ZANLA operational areas were also very severely affected. Indeed, most of documentation on poisoning relates to the ZANLA areas.

5   The most detailed coverage of poisoning and other Selous Scout operations is in the academic studies of Ellert 1980: 124–161; Brickhill 1992–3; Flower 1987; and Stiff's unacademic book (1985).

6   It is possible that some of the violent events described below were perpetrated by such 'turned' guerrillas.

7   Their analyses also reflect the different wartime histories of the districts on which they are based, as discussed by Alexander 1995.

8   I am using the term 'witch' to translate the Ndebele term *umthakathi* (pl. *abathakathi*) and the term 'sell-out' for the Ndebele term *umthengisi* (pl. *Abathengisi*), which in addition to referring to sell-outs is also the common term for vendors or traders, derived from the verb *ukuthengisa*, to sell).

9   T. O. Ranger notes the resurfacing of debates over witchcraft in administrative records in the 1950s for the first time since turn of the century debates over the Witchcraft Suppression Ordinance of 1899. See Ranger unpublished (b): 2.

10 Further detail on naming and notions of difference between evictees and early settlers are discussed in Alexander and McGregor 1997. Most early settlers understood and spoke at least some Ndebele, though they often used Tonga in the home.

11 The reports of M. E. Hayes also document *sangoma* mediums' witch-finding roles, as well as that of other mediums such as *tshomani* spirit mediums, see for example, Hayes, November 1975, CHK 6/LU/Goduka; CHK 6/LU/Mtenjwa and CHK 6/LU/Mabhikwa, documented in Ranger, unpublished (b).

12 Chiefs' statements about the problem of witchcraft and requests for powers to deal with it are documented in the Minutes of the Midlands Provincial Assembly, 28 October 1951 and 27 August 1952, 5 2796/2/1. Evidence for continued hearing of witchcraft cases at chiefs' courts can be found in the reports of M. E. Hayes, for example, November 1975, CHK 6/LU/Mabhikwa, detailed in Ranger, unpublished (b).

13 See for example: Alison Redmayne's description of Chikanga's activity (Redmayne 1970), and Mark Auslander's account of 'Dr Moses' who also operated in Southern Rhodesia (Auslander 1993). The large literature on the Mchape witch-eradication movements is usefully reviewed in Ranger unpublished (a). See also Fields 1985 and Maxwell 1994.

14 Members of the party structures from all over the district and others based in Bulawayo described this ring including: Y. D. Lupanda, 2 Feb. 1996; J. N., E. N. and R. M., Malunku, 6 March 1996. Local ZAPU executive officers also gave

this explanation, interview, M. N., Dandanda, 7 April, 1996. It was also a recurrent explanation in guerrillas' accounts.

15 The plural of *inyanga* is either *zinyanga*, or more commonly simply *inyanga*. I use the latter in the paper.

16 *Ihumba* spirits are not spoken about readily or in the presence of a woman who hosts one because to do so is said to cause the woman to die immediately or in a horrible way, such as by being eaten by termites.

17 Interview, S. M., 30 March 1996. The consequences for the family of the woman accused of being at the head of the poisoning ring were also severe: daughters and other family members were killed.

18 Most accounts of meetings (other than the largest in which fourteen lost their life) put the death toll at between three and five per meeting. There were at least three such meetings.

19 Both interviewees are prophets in the Apostolic Faith Mission Church in Zion.

20 It is approximately 100km from the mobile base established by the NF2 command, located in Southern Lupane, in the Gwaimpa valley.

21 *Chronicle*, May 29 and 29 1981. This case involved three deaths after guerrillas ordered a diviner to name witches at a meeting; the meeting was led by the local ZAPU chair. This and subsequent references to the *Chronicle* can be found in Ranger, unpublished, b.

22 Despite the violence of this war, neither dissidents nor government soldiers killed witches.

23 Accounts of bravery are of course, a theme of other writers, such as Werbner 1991.

24 Lan reflected on his work in a presentation to the Britain Zimbabwe Society on 8 June 1997, discussed in Ranger unpublished (c).

25 Knowledge that poisons were used over a broad area cannot in itself provide confirmation that any particular death, or series of deaths, was related to the poisons. Though witch-killings were undoubtedly worst in areas where many guerrillas died of poisoning, there were also instances of witches being killed which seem to have been unrelated to Rhodesian poisons.

26 This issue is not necessarily important, just as one can perform acts of witchcraft without knowledge or intent.

References

Alexander, J. (1995) 'Things fall apart, the centre can hold: processes of post war political change in Zimbabwe's rural areas' in N. Bhebe and T. Ranger (eds), *Society in Zimbabwe's Liberation War*, London: James Currey, 1995, pp. 175–2.

Alexander, J. and McGregor, J. (1997) 'Modernity and ethnicity in a frontier society. Understanding difference in Northwestern Zimbabwe', *Journal of Southern African Studies*, vol. 23, no. 2, pp. 187–201.

Alexander, J., McGregor, J. and Ranger, T. (forthcoming) *Violence and Memory: One Hundred Years in the 'Dark' Forests of Matabeleland, Zimbabwe*, Oxford: James Currey.

Apter, A. (1993) 'Atinga revisited: Yoruba witchcraft and the cocoa economy, 1950–1951', in J. and J. Comaroff (eds), *Modernity and its Malcontents: Ritual Power in Postcolonial Africa*, London: University of Chicago Press, pp. 111–28.

Auslander, M. (1993) '"Open the wombs!": The symbolic politics of modern Ngoni witch-finding', in J. and J. Comaroff (eds), *Modernity and Its Malcontents: Ritual and Power in Postcolonial Africa*, University of Chicago Press, pp. 167–93.

Bhebe, N. and Ranger, T. (eds.) (1995), *Soldiers in Zimbabwe's Liberation War*, London: James Currey.

Bourdillon, M. (1987) 'Guns and rain: taking structural analysis too far?' *Africa*, vol. 57, no. 2, pp. 263–74.

Brickhill, J. (1992–3) 'Zimbabwe's poisoned legacy: secret war in Southern Africa', *Covert Action*, vol. 43, pp. 4–59.

Brickhill, J. (1995) 'Daring to storm the heavens: the military strategy of ZAPU, 1976–79', in N. Bhebe and T. Ranger (eds) *Soldiers in Zimbabwe's Liberation War*, London: James Currey, pp. 48–72.

Comaroff, J. and J. (eds) (1993) *Modernity and Its Malcontents: Ritual and Power in Postcolonial Africa*, Chicago and London: University of Chicago Press.

Chronicle, 22 August 1980 and 24 February 1981.

Douglas, M. (ed.) (1970) *Witchcraft Confessions and Accusations*, London: Tavistock.

Ellert, H. (1993) *The Rhodesian Front War: Counter-Insurgency and Guerilla Warfare 1962–1980*, 2nd edn., Zimbabwe: Mambo Press.

Fields, K. (1985) *Revival and Rebellion in Colonial Africa*, New York: Princeton University Press.

Flower, K. (1987) *Serving Secretly. An Intelligence Chief on Record. Rhodesia into Zimbabwe 1964–1981*, London: John Murray.

Kriger, N. (1992) *Zimbabwe's Guerilla War. Peasant Voices*, Cambridge : Cambridge University Press.

Lan, D. (1985) *Guns and Rain: Guerillas and Spirit Mediums in Zimbabwe*, London: James Currey.

—— (1997) Presentation at Britain Zimbabwe Society meeting, 7–8 June.

Maxwell, D. (1994) 'A social and conceptual history of North-East Zimbabwe 1890–1990', Oxford, unpublished Ph.D. thesis.

Nkomo, N. (unpublished) *Between the Hammer and the Anvil: The Autobiography of Nicholas Nkomo*.

Ranger, T. (unpublished a) 'Mchape: A study in diffusion and interpretation' (1992).

—— (unpublished b) 'Patterns of witchcraft belief and control in Northern Matabeleland: gleaning the archives' p. 2.

—— (unpublished c) 'Zimbabwe lives. report on the BZS research days June 7 and 8 1997' (1997).

—— (forthcoming) 'Zimbabwe Since 1960', in *History of Central Africa*, London: Longman.

Redmayne, A. (1970) 'Chikanga: an African diviner with an international reputation', in M. Douglas (ed.) *Witchcraft Confessions and Accusations*, London: Tavistock Publications, pp. 103–29.

Stiff, P. (1985) *See You in November. Rhodesia's No-holds Barred Intelligence War*, Alberton, South Africa: Galago.

Werbner, R. (1991) *Tears of the Dead. The Social Biography of an African Family*, Edinburgh University Press.

ᅟ

—— (1995) 'In memory: a heritage of war in Southwestern Zimbabwe' in N. Bhebe and T. Ranger (eds), *Society in Zimbabwe's Liberation War*, London: James Currey, pp. 192–206.

Interviews

Apostolic Faith Mission Church leaders, Mapanawomvu, 28 August 1996.
C. M. and C. N., Mzda, 28 January 1996.
C. N., Mzola, 28 January 1996.
Elders, Chitete village, Dandanda, 10 December 1994.
Elders, Lupaka, 9 February 1996.
Elders, Dandanda, 10 December 1994.
Elders, St Paul's, 13 September 1996.
E. S., 25 September 1996 (interview conducted by J. Alexander).
Group interview, Lusulu, 26 February 1996.
G. S., Chitete, 10 December 1994.
H. K. and H. M., Gegema and Gogo villages, 10 December 1994.

J. N., E. N. and R. M., Malunku, 6 March 1996,
M. D., A. D., K. M., Lake Alice, 19 February 1996.
M. N., Dandanda, 7 April 1996.
N. K., Mzola East, 16 September 1996.
Nkomo, N. and Dube, R., Bulawayo, 4 September 1996 (interview conducted jointly with J. Alexander).
Nkomo, N., Lupane, 19 February 1996.
O. D., 27 September 1996 (interview conducted by J. Alexander).
S. M., Lupane, 30 March 1996.
S. N., Singwangombe, 21 February 1996.
S. T., Chitete, 10 December 1994.
T. S. M., Pupu, 20 February 1996.
Y. D., Lupanda, 22 February 1996.

8

NAMING AND CLAIMING

The integration of traumatic experience and
the reconstruction of self in survivors' stories
of sexual abuse

Susan D. Rose

> Each segment of our conduct and experience bears a twofold
> meaning: it revolves about its own center, contains as much breadth
> and depth, joy and suffering, as the immediate experience [allows],
> and at the same time is a segment of a course of life.
>
> (Simmel 1971: 187)

With this passage, Georg Simmel launches into his exploration of 'The
Adventurer', an essay that profoundly and playfully explores the ways in which the
'adventure' is an integral part of a life, yet marked by its discontinuity with it:

> The most general form of adventure is its dropping out of the continuity
> of life. . . . What we call an adventure stands in contrast to that
> interlocking of life-links, to that feeling that those countercurrents,
> turnings, and knots still, after all, spin forth a continuous tread.
>
> (Ibid.: 187–8)

Strikingly, Simmel's analysis of 'adventure' applies well, if paradoxically,
to the experience of trauma. Traumas, like adventures, are often marked in
parenthetical time.[1] But while Simmel may 'ascribe to an adventure a beginning and an end much sharper than those to be discovered in other forms of
our experiences' (ibid.: 188), the traumatic event often resides in more
ephemeral time, remaining unintegrated or 'frozen' in time. As psychiatrist
Dori Laub, who writes about the experiences, memories, and narratives of
Holocaust survivors, argues:

> The traumatic event, although real, took place outside the
> parameters of 'normal' reality. . . . This absence of categories that

define it lends it a quality of 'otherness,' a salience, a timelessness, and a ubiquity that puts it outside the range of associatively linked experiences. . . . Trauma survivors live not with memories of the past, but with an event that could not and did not proceed through to its completion . . . and therefore . . . continues into the present.

(Laub 1992: 69)

In what ways may trauma be considered the shadow-side of adventure – similar in form though oppositional in meaning – that draws one in rather than out? Trauma, like adventure:

is certainly part of our existence, directly contiguous with other parts which precede and follow it; at the same time, however, in its deeper meaning it occurs outside the usual continuity of this life. Nevertheless, it is distinct from all that is accidental and alien, merely touching one's outer shell. While it falls outside the context of life, it falls, with this same movement, as it were, back into that context again . . . it is a foreign body in our existence which is yet somehow connected with the center; the outside, if only by a long and unfamiliar detour, is formally an aspect of the inside.

(Simmel 1971: 188)

This connection between inner lives and outer manifestations is illustrated well by shirts contributed to the Central Pennsylvania Clothesline Project.[2] (See Figures 8.1 and 8.2.) Organized in conjunction with the national project based in Massachusetts and part of the international movement against violence directed at women, the Project invited women to construct T-shirts that expressed not only the violence they suffered but also the healing and recovery they were experiencing. The exhibit was assembled as part of the 1993 Public Affairs Symposium on 'Violence in America' at Dickinson College. Initially interviews with twenty women were conducted; follow-up interviews were then done at the national exhibit in Washington D.C. where over 5,000 shirts were displayed in April 1995.

The resulting video documentary, *Clothesline,* integrates images of these shirts and interviews with women who speak about the making and meaning of their shirts.[3] The documentary opens with a clothesline of shirts made by women: white shirts (contributed by family or friends) represent women who had been killed; blue or green shirts had been made by victims of childhood sexual abuse or incest; red, pink, or orange shirts had been constructed by victims of rape and sexual assault; and purple shirts by women who had suffered violence because of being targeted as lesbian. The women drew upon different images and materials to portray the abuse and healing they experienced: black felt and burlap hearts, pieces from childhood dresses, broken candles, ripped-out hearts, lace daggers, and photographs of graduation day.

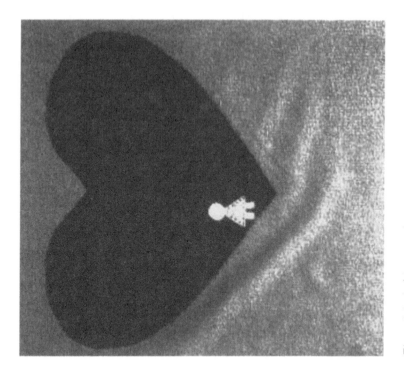

Figure 8.2 A shirt contributed to the Central Pennsylvania Clothesline Project

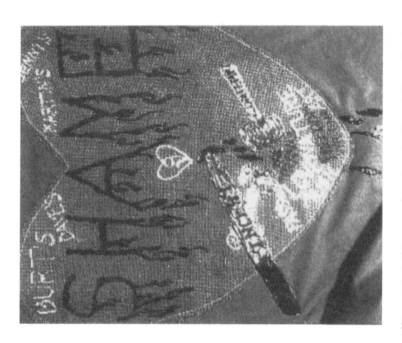

Figure 8.1 A shirt contributed to the Central Pennsylvania Clothesline Project

On one shirt, a burlap heart configuring the experience of pain and healing illustrates the embodiment of that which is both integral and foreign, and presents an outer representation of that which lies within. (See Figure 8.1.)

As Pat describes the making and meaning of her shirt:

> I've always felt that my heart was damaged in some way. And that's why I wanted to start with the heart. I picked burlap because I feel that I'm very rough. I don't feel that I can be caring or compassionate to other people. And I just feel like I have a very rough heart. This is the wound, the incest. It doesn't take like a big part, because I don't feel that it destroyed my whole heart, it's just something that radiated. And the little hammers are what I've used to beat myself into not allowing me to be me, all my life. And these are the things – nature and love and passion and music and things like that – that I consider to be me. And that's what bleeds. The part that's me that isn't allowed to be. The shame which I feel; I carry my father's shame. I am shame. In the middle, the little heart, is God. Because I feel that God is the only one that's brought me through.[4]

Pat simply and exquisitely speaks of the embodied pain and numbness of both *being* and *not being* which is part of the experience of violation, and reveals the layers of meaning that interact with one another, defining and redefining the connections between inner and outer realities. She also speaks of the relationship between violation (the incest) and her father's shame that has bled into her – 'I carry my father's shame. I am shame' – and visually represents it in bleeding red capital letters. She has internalized that sense of shame but in the healing process has begun to unearth it and give it back: 'I decided to name the people that I can remember abusing me. . . . And that's powerful to me because I feel like I need to start giving responsibility to those people. I still carry it as my fault.' And she continues:

> I know there's hope. I know it's out there and I know some day I'm going to get there. It's just, I keep tying to trip myself up on the way. I really have the confidence that I can recover. It [the abuse] will always be there, and it will be a part of me, but it isn't going to define me anymore.

Pat is very articulate about the ways she has embodied and blocked pain. She speaks of wanting to embrace the part of her she left behind as a child, and of reclaiming feeling and compassion for herself and others. In the process, she is both coming to understand and redefine the meaning that sexual abuse has had for her: 'It will always be there . . . but it isn't going to define me anymore.' This is not a matter of 'moving beyond' experience, it is a matter of understanding experience in a new way, one that recognizes both its pervasiveness and its limits. In describing the process, Pat recognizes both the connections and discontinuities between inner and outer selves For Pat and for other survivors of childhood sexual abuse, recovery involves renegotiation of one's identity.

Renegotiation requires dialogue among one's various selves and between those selves and others who can listen. As Laub argues, in order to undo the entrapment of the traumatic reality and its re-enactment, one must engage 'in a process of constructing a narrative, reconstructing a history and essentially, of *re-externalizing* the event (Laub 1992: 69). The act of telling one's story, both through visual and narrative representation, is an important part of the process. Often the narratives of people who have been traumatized reflect what Harvard psychiatrist Judith Herman considers to be the central dialectic of psychological trauma:

> the conflict between the will to deny horrible events and the will to proclaim them aloud. . . . People who have survived atrocities often tell their stories in a highly emotional, contradictory, and fragmented manner which undermines their credibility and thereby serves the twin imperatives of truth-telling and secrecy.
>
> (Herman 1992: 1)

Survivors both seek and fear knowledge. The structure of the narrative reflects this dialectic and the approach-avoidance of the survivor to knowing and feeling that often comes with the experience of trauma. Moreover, the narrative is not static; it continues to develop over time and experience. Within the context of psychotherapy, the telling of a story is often a 'slow, laborious process, a fragmented set of wordless, static images [that are] gradually transformed into a narrative with motion, feeling, and meaning' (Herman 1996). As Laub describes the narrative of a survivor of Auschwitz:

> She was testifying not simply to empirical historical facts, but to the very secret of survival and of resistance to extermination . . . her silence was part of her testimony. It is not merely her speech, but the very boundaries of silence which surround it which attest, today as well as in the past, to this assertion of resistance.
>
> (Laub 1992: 62)

By breaking through the silence, survivors are constructing oppositional narratives that defy the taboo against *talking about* incest and torture, and in the process are re-creating themselves. In resisting traditional narrative forms, survivors often encounter great scepticism and resistance to the telling of their stories. Speaking out is a political as well as a therapeutic act, and as such, is a claim to power. It involves risk as well as promise. And as these women who were ready to speak out remind us, we need to consider what it means *not* to risk. While there are dangers involved in speaking out, there are also dangers in remaining mute. Silence stifles the soul, affects the quality of relationship with others, and accepts an unjust and abusive system of power that renders the victim powerless. It makes abuse possible without holding the abusers accountable. In the process of breaking silence, survivors are not only finding their own voices; they also are collectively creating new narratives that challenge the individual and collective denial of abuse and the reproduction of violence. In dialogue with others who can bear witness, survivors are redefining the experiences that once rendered them powerless.

One contributor to the Clothesline project portrays herself as a little girl without aims situated in the corner of a black heart: (See Figure 8.2.)

> I knew I wanted to have a black heart on it. Maybe it was because I just felt that way about hearts, and about love. That's all very black. That's me – the little purple girl. I cut out little felt arms. And then . . . I left them off.

Liz cannot articulate just why she left off the arms: but she knows it is significant that she cannot attach or position them: 'They didn't fit, I just couldn't get them to fit right.' The absence of arms or hands is commonly found in drawings of traumatized children, and is often interpreted as representing a loss of power and ability to act.[5] Liz, now a successful magazine editor and lay-out designer, has chosen to speak out publicly about her abuse. When asked what she wanted to tell the public, she immediately replied:

> It's important for people to realize that those statistics represent people. Behind every one of those numbers [of abuse] is a person . . . [who is] struggling. . . . It's not just something you get over. And so there's all those hundreds of thousands of walking-wounded women out there. And we're all struggling. I'm trying to find ways to make it less black.

Liz reports that she always remembered the physical abuse inflicted upon her by her father who 'became quite violent after a brain tumor'. She recalls, too, being sent to her aunt's and uncle's for the summers after her mother died. While she talked about 'the vivid memories' she had about the summers there, she also says: 'I just don't remember anything about [the sexual abuse] within that time frame. Although it went on for six summers [from the age of six to twelve], it's like I remember it as one summer.' After graduation from college she experienced a flood of memories.

Liz describes moving in and out of awareness, both at the time the abuse was going on and later, as she recalls the details and remembers more fully the emotional impact it had. As many contemporary feminists and psychotherapists would describe it, recovery actually involves re-membering the connections between body and mind and spirit. It involves picking up the threads of discontinuity and making sense of them; it calls people to reweave the fabric of their being (Davis and Bass 1994). In the process of recovery, the abuse becomes redefined as it becomes more fully understood. For Liz, it became integrated in new ways as the adult-she and the little-girl-she become more aware of one another. The little purple girl with no arms can now be embraced by the adult woman who is re-claiming parts of herself, a process that Liz describes as a journey.

The adventure that leads one into new encounters, stimulates the senses by challenging them with new sounds, smells, sensations.[6] When one leaves behind familiar territory and enters new terrain, adrenalin rushes to prepare one to meet the unknown, the unfamiliar, the stranger who is potentially an enemy but also potentially a friend. The 'alter-adventure' of engaging past trauma may likewise lead one into unexpected, though strangely familiar territory. As one embarks on the interior journey, it may feel as if one is revisiting a minefield. The challenge for the survivor is not only to explore the old terrain but to carve a new landscape out of it. With both the adventure and alter-adventure, the journey invokes risk but also opportunity. By expanding and exploring new boundaries, the adventure/alter-adventure can revitalize. It can also terrify. It can lure us further or paralyse us.

While culture shapes how we interpret experience, what meaning we attach to it, biology puts certain constraints on this. In the case of inescapable trauma, the psychobiological response is more likely to numb than to mobilize one for flight or fight.[7] As psychologist Elizabeth Waites describes it:

> Traumatic experience typically produces an overwhelming need to escape what is, in reality, inescapable. Dissociation is a psychobiological mechanism that allows the mind, in effect, to flee what the body is experiencing. . . . The shock of trauma produces states that are so different from ordinary waking life that they are not easily integrated with more normal experience. As a result of this discontinuity, the traumatic state may be lost to memory or remembered as a dream is sometimes remembered, as something vague and unreal.
>
> (Waites 1993: 14)

Because of its place in our psychic life, remembered trauma, like adventure, tends:

> to take on the quality of dream. It often moves so far away from the center of the ego and course of life which the ego guides and organizes that we may think of it as something experienced by another person [or as something] alien.
>
> (Simmel 1971: 188)

In the case of sexual abuse, this dream-like quality of experience results from the sense of one's self being so assaulted, so bombarded, that one psychologically 'escapes' in order to avoid destruction.

This phenomenon is well described in the narratives of adult survivors of childhood sexual abuse. Dissociation, which gives rise to a form of temporary transcendence, is one of the major defence mechanisms resorted to by traumatized children. The mind or spirit leaves the body and the child may come to feel no pain, may leave the scene entirely, neither experiencing the abuse at the time nor remembering it afterwards. The escape from self – from what is being done to the self – creates a safer space, a retreat. It may be temporary or longer-lasting, depending on the severity and frequency of abuse. The responses of others help shape the meaning of the experience, and the possibilities for either integrating the experience or rejecting it, for either dealing with it in the present or putting it aside to deal with later. Over time, one becomes accustomed, even entrained, to follow certain patterns of response, whether dissociating from or acknowledging pain (Herman 1992; van der Kolk *et al.* 1996).

In the case of adventure, one seeks revitalization through excitement. In the traumatic escape, rather than seeking more stimulation, one seeks less; rather than excitement, one seeks safety.[8] As Liz recalled her escape into the wallpaper:

> I remember being on their bed and he was laying on top of me. And I had my hands stretched out. And I was touching the wallpaper. And it was that flecked wallpaper, you know, the kind with the white stuff with gold specks, and just feeling it. . . . I was trying to focus on it . . . rather than on . . . yeah, I [was] dissociating.

Many survivors of childhood sexual abuse have described the experience of becoming observers of their own abuse, of symbolically leaving their bodies and watching the enactment of abuse from another place, for example, from the ceiling or through a window. This figurative flight may protect them from abuse that might otherwise be impossible to experience and recover from, given the psychological meanings for the self. As Ferenczi, Freud's student, analysand, friend, and colleague wrote in a 1933 paper shunned by his psychoanalytical peers:

> It is difficult to fathom the behavior and the feelings of children following such acts of (specifically sexual) violence. Their first impulse would be: rejection, hatred, disgust, forceful resistance. 'No, no, I don't want this, it is too strong for me, that hurts me. Leave me be.' This . . . would be the immediate reaction, were it not paralysed by tremendous fear. The children feel physically and morally helpless. The overwhelming power and authority of the adults renders them silent.
>
> (In Greven 1990: 158)

The effects of trauma on personality formation and integration vary according to the type and severity of the trauma, and whether or not one is able to speak of and process the trauma (Terr 1990). Both experience and expression are critical here. As Waites argues,

> The integration of identity is closely allied to the development and experience of autobiographical memory, a sense of personal continuity and consistency over historical time that forms the background for the individual's interactions with others and serves as a reference point for self-reflective activities.
>
> (Waites 1993: 14)

For some, experiences of severe abuse have led to dissociative identity disorders (DID), formerly referred to as multiple personality disorder (MPD) Cathy, who identifies herself as having MPD, symbolically portrays the divides within by splitting her shirt in half:

> Well, this is the side that is the part of me that was in bondage. And then over here, this side, is freedom from it. . . . And then I put this name, Audrey here because I have another persona and her name is Audrey Katherine Lovett. And she gets me out of a lot of jams and she's my best friend, but it's really me. I give her a lot of credit when it should be me that takes the credit – because she does all the good. And, so, it's really me. She's gotten me into a couple of jams though too, along the way. And then this represents my arms because I was very, very destructive. I've got scars all over my arms.

Cathy points out quite literally the outer manifestations of her inner pain, and the ways in which her abuse led to internal divisions and multiple personas. She also divides the shirt with the words 'despair' and 'hope'.

> So I put here . . . 'despair'. And then I come over here and I put 'hope'. . . . In some ways I did this the way I thought people would want to see it, and to portray it in a better way than sometimes I feel. . . . Sometimes I feel that to survive is punishment. . . . But I didn't feel it was offering survivors anything. And so I decided to put 'hope' there instead. And for the most part I feel more hopeful than I ever have in my life.

This sense of hopefulness grew out of supportive dialogue with professionals and other survivors, and dialogue between her own split selves:

> There's no reason why I should be breathing, but for some reason I am a survivor. And I need to learn to accept that, and go with it, instead of resisting it. And I know it will take the rest of my life.

After years of severe familial abuse, foster care, and recurrent hospitaliza-
tions, Cathy is for the first time living on her own and employed. She is
grateful to a supportive community of people who can listen to the stories of
abuse she has to tell, help her sort out the meaning of those experiences, and
move on:

> It's great to know that there's people that are there for you, who
> believe you. . . . I might have a long journey ahead of me but I'm
> willing to do it. And I've got the support to do it this time. And
> there ain't no stopping me.

For another contributor, the split is displayed through the images she
drew on the front and back of her shirt. As Marty describes it:

> It's got sort of a healthy family on one side and a very dysfunctional
> family on the other. . . . Actually this is the front. What I always did
> in the past was, I sort of used the good things in my life to sort of
> cover up the bad things and that contaminated the good things,
> because it made them unclean. So, what I did was, I put this on the
> front so I could just . . . be out with this. And just say, this was
> wrong, it was wrong, and it was reality. And then the good things
> won't be contaminated.

Marty then discusses her motivation for working through her childhood
experiences of abuse:

> I live apart from myself. You know, I kind of float around. And I want,
> I'm twenty-six years old, and I want to experience the rest of my life.
> And there's something that follows me around. And it's just terrible.
> And I need to admit that it exists because otherwise, you know, I get
> real crazy inside. And I feel separate from my life. I'm just sort of
> watching it from a distance. And it's not feeling real to me. And I have
> a real sense that I don't want to lose the next twenty-five years of my
> life and wake up and be, you know, have lost all those years.

Some theorists and therapists argue that until the selves are integrated, re-
united, and one is able to tell the story of the abuse as experienced and
witnessed, the self cannot alter the meaning, and therefore the impact of the
abuse. Other therapists and survivors argue that integration does not
necessarily have to take place, that for some survivors, there may be a
conscious choice or subliminal warning not to force integration but to allow
the co-existence of parts of the self. In either case, awareness of one's
experiences and recognition of the complexity of one's self/selves is
fundamental to embracing rather than 'losing oneself'.

To lose oneself is to become so involved in something that one is no longer self-conscious about what one is doing. One is, in a sense, taken away. Whether in the context of work, or making love, or dealing with trauma, being so engaged can be powerful and productive as long as one can return to an awareness of self again. It is not losing one's self per se that is to be avoided, for we may find ourselves anew in the process of being lost and found. The danger is to lose touch for so long that one becomes unaware of some of the most potent sources of action and motivation (Miller 1981: 1990). To be 'lost in the moment', is one thing. To be lost for months, or years, or for a lifetime is quite another; it is to become alienated from one's self, and less responsible *to* and *for* one's self.

In daring to remember and speak about what they remember, survivors encounter both loss and gain. Sylvia Fraser, in *My Father's House: a Memoir of Incest and Healing*, reveals this as she describes her process of recovering and integrating memories of childhood abuse:

> In retrospect, I feel about my life the way some people feel about war. If you survive, then it becomes a good war. Danger makes you active, it makes you alert, it forces you to experience and thus to learn. I know now the cost of my life, the real price that has been paid. Contact with inner pain has immunized me against most petty hurts. Hopes I still have in abundance, but very few needs. My pride of intellect has been shattered. If I didn't know about half my own life, what other knowledge can I trust? Yet even here I see a gift, for in place of my narrow, pragmatic world of cause and effect . . . I have burst into an infinite world full of wonder.
>
> (Fraser 1987: 253)

In order to step back into the fullness of being and embrace the wholeness, in both its good and bad aspects, survivors speak of the need to pick up the strands of their being; to re-member the connections between the body, mind, and spirit and to re-integrate knowing and feeling. This is not a mater of finding the one, authentic or monolithic self, but rather of recognizing the multiplicity and complexity of one's experiences and the continual evolving of identity (Bruner 1990; Lifton 1993; Strozier and Flynn 1996).

The task of re-connecting to oneself and others, however, is not an easy one. There are many reasons why people forget or deny (Freyd 1996), why parts of our being go into hiding to protect, or at times expose, or wage war with other parts. The challenge is to develop not only an awareness of all these parts but also a sense of empathy with that self-as-other which may have been created as a means of enduring trauma. If the trauma is survived and a sense of safety is secured, then a reunion of the split selves may be possible. A recognition of other-as-self may create a sense of identification, of empathic understanding. Rather than an 'other' co-existing as a stranger or

170

foreign body within, it may come to be seen as a friend, even an integral part of one's being. Even though one may experience oneself-as-other as a way of surviving great violation, the selves are materially embodied together, and help to define one another. Not to identify and embrace the other-as-self is to deny the diverse experiences, both connective and discontinuous, that have helped shape who one is.

The consequences of this denial may take many forms: alienation, projection, psychosomatic symptoms, disembodiment. One may come to feel disconnected from self or others; unaware of what one is doing or feeling; unaccepting of responsibility for what one does. The defence mechanisms of denial and dissociation are used by abusers and witnesses of abuse as well as by survivors. This helps explain how ordinarily decent people can also come to torture and abuse others, and how people can witness such atrocities and still deny that such abuse exists.[9]

Judith Herman argues in her study of post-traumatic stress disorder (PTSD) among war veterans and sexual-abuse survivors: 'The ordinary response to atrocities is to banish them from consciousness. Certain violations of the social compact are too terrible to utter aloud: this is the meaning of the word unspeakable'. She goes on to argue that:

> Atrocities, however, refuse to be buried. Equally as powerful as the desire to deny atrocities is the conviction that denial does not work. . . . Remembering and telling the truth about terrible events are prerequisites both for the restoration of the social order and for the healing of individual victims.
>
> (Herman 1992: 1)

In order to gain a greater understanding of the impact and reproduction of violence, we need to examine the interactions of psychological and biological processes with cultural and social forces. We need to ask, under what conditions and through what means victims are likely to be silenced or enabled to speak; likely to forget, recall, or retrieve memories; likely to panic, become numb, or resist; to dissociate or integrate experience; to identify with or challenge the perpetrator? How do various kinds of social support affect the experiences and responses of survivors to violence and resistance? Violence in its various forms and intensities challenges not only theoretical models but also emotional responses. It is therefore critical that 'we', as individuals and the body politic, examine our willingness to explore the sources and consequences of familial, institutional, and cultural violence, and our resistance to doing so. Where do the sources of support and challenge lie? Where does denial cover up violence, and where are violence and denial confronted? Which stories are told, which are buried? What do we believe and what do we refuse to believe? What do we know of violence? What do we not know? And why?

'Knowing', let alone recalling, involves complex processes that are mediated by cultural, social, political, and psychological factors. Being human means having the capacity to reflect upon the past and alter the present in its light, as well as to reinterpret the past in light of the present. As Kenneth Gergen argues, the 'immense repository of our past encounters may come to be salient in different ways as we review them reflexively or come to reconceptualize them' (Gergen 1982: 18). Jerome Bruner further argues in *Acts of Meaning* that, 'Experience in and memory of the social world are powerfully structured not only by deeply internalized and narrativized conceptions of folk psychology but also by the historically rooted institutions that a culture elaborates to support and enforce them (Bruner 1990: 57). Therefore, it should come as no surprise that the processes of knowing, forgetting, and remembering are as complex as human beings themselves, who continually have to negotiate their social worlds, and their understanding of what is true in the present as well as in the past. These are philosophical, political, and sociological issues as well as psychological ones. It is clear that one's position of power in society (marked by 'race', class, gender, age, etc.) influences whether one is seen as credible and authoritative. It is no coincidence that formal resistance to memory recovery is associated not with survivors of car accidents, stroke victims, or even war veterans but with survivors of childhood sexual abuse.[10]

As Milan Kundera writes in *The Book of Laughter and Forgetting* (1994), 'Man's struggle against power is the struggle of memory against forgetting'. The resistance to acknowledging and then acting upon the reality and pervasiveness of child sexual abuse in the United States is well documented. It is difficult to deal with the number of children who are taken to emergency rooms and who die each year as a result of abuse. But denying that that reality exists does not alleviate the suffering of those children nor prevent the reproduction of violence. Neither does denying the experience of adult survivors of child abuse. In order to understand the degree of violence in the United States today, we need to examine the process and function of denial – at individual, institutional, and cultural levels. As Herman reminds us, while atrocities may be repressed, they are not forgotten (Herman 1992: 7).

The consequences for those who are enabled to tell their stories and for those who are silenced are clearly different, as psychologist Lenore Terr shows in her work on childhood trauma. In a systematic, longitudinal research study of children who had experienced a range of traumatic incidents (from kidnapping to car accidents to sexual abuse), Terr found that the psychological and social adjustment of traumatized children depended less on the severity or duration of the trauma and more on whether or not the child was able to speak of the trauma, and if so, how people responded (Terr 1990: 1994). Were they able to listen, and to act as witness in support of the child without blaming or silencing the child?

For those whose speaking meets with denial or derision, the original betrayal is reinforced and the secondary trauma becomes retraumatizing. Pat for example, says that for a long time she was more angry at her mother for not protecting her than at her father who sexually abused her.[11] At the same time, she recognizes that her mother's continuing denial and inability to deal with the incest is rooted in her own abuse history:

> That's how she survived her abuse. . . . My mother is very honest about her denial. She does not want to know. When I told her, she said it didn't surprise her at all. . . . But she also said, 'I don't want to know anything bad about him.' And then she gave me the, 'Oh, you're doing so wonderfully'. . . . She can't handle anything that's negative.

Pat clearly identifies the patterns of denial that enable the perpetuation of abuse:

> What I would say to the public is that I strongly believe you are the problem. The perpetrators are given permission. It's the people like my mother who had to turn their back – and I say that to myself too, because that's how I survived, turning my back on people. . . . Like being at work where people would make abusive comments or make fun of people sexually, I just couldn't deal with it. And it's only going to change if we've got the guts to turn and look at ourselves and ask 'Why? Why are we so afraid to face it?'

There are many reasons why denial is an easier, if less effective, mechanism than acknowledging and dealing with an abusive relationship, especially when it occurs within the context of the family. It is hard to listen to stories of abuse for they threaten our identity as human beings; they challenge our notions of family and our sense of ourselves as belonging to a civilized society. And the strongest resistance, as Alice Miller (1981) argues, stems from self-defensiveness, for listening to such stories may unearth the listener's own repressed experiences of pain. We conveniently find ways to avoid what is hard to believe, to bury and conceal that which is not supposed to be. From time to time we are made aware of the existence and consequences of domestic violence and political torture, and of the coping strategies of victims and witnesses, as earlier writings and studies show, but the opening through which recognition can turn to action is quickly sealed off from collective investigation.[12] Silence protects both perpetrators and the notion (no matter how illusory) of a harmonious community and family; it also retraumatizes and isolates victims.

Ultimately, recovering from trauma is not just an individual act but a collective process: it demands dialogue. While bearing witness to trauma is a process that involves the listener, many people are unable or unwilling to listen, and trauma-survivor narratives often meet with great resistance from the larger society. A backlash against speaking out occurs because it exposes the atrocities in our midst and challenges both those who abuse power and those who stand by as muted witnesses. It is 'easier' to side with abusers than to serve as effective witnesses to the abused, as Herman clearly articulates:

> It is very tempting to take the side of the perpetrator. All the perpetrator asks is that the bystander do nothing. He appeals to the universal desire to see, hear, and speak no evil. The victim, on the contrary, asks the bystander to share the burden of pain. The victim demands action, engagement, and remembering. In order to escape accountability for his crimes, the perpetrator does everything in his power to promote forgetting. Secrecy and silence are the perpetrator's first line of defense. If secrecy fails, the perpetrator attacks the credibility of his victim. If he cannot silence her absolutely, he tries to make sure that no one listens. To this end he marshals an impressive array of arguments, from the most blatant denial to the most sophisticated and elegant rationalization. After every atrocity one can expect to hear the same predictable apologies; it never happened; the victim lies; the victim exaggerates; the victim brought it upon herself, and in any case, it is time to forget the past and move on. The more powerful the perpetrator, the greater is his prerogative to name and define reality, and the more completely his arguments prevail.
>
> (Herman 1992: 7–8)

The organized resistance to survivors speaking out is both predictable and revealing. The False Memory Syndrome Foundation (FMSF), organized by the parents of Jennifer Freyd, a psychology professor at the University of Oregon, is a prime example. Freyd's parents organized FMSF a couple of months after Jennifer entered therapy. Although she had not spoken to the public or her parents about her childhood abuse, they went on the offensive by organizing the FMSF, whose major aim is to repudiate claims of recovered memories. After Jennifer declined their invitation to serve on the Board of Directors, her parents pressed the attack by sending unsolicited materials that questioned their daughter's integrity and character to her colleagues while she was undergoing her tenure review. The invasion of privacy and violation of boundaries in these contemporary and public actions reveal, in and of themselves, the problematic nature of her parents' relationship with her.

Interestingly, Professor Freyd's research focuses on the epistemology of knowing. Her new book, *Betrayal Trauma: the Logic of Forgetting Childhood Abuse*, draws upon current psychological and neurophysiological research to posit a theory of betrayal trauma which explicates why it makes sense for children who have been abused by family members to forget that abuse. As Bickerton points out in his review of *Betrayal Trauma*, 'Freyd marshals the psychological, neurological, and cognitive-science literature with impressive skill' (Bickerton 1997: 20) to suggest that when pain comes from betrayal by someone very close to a child, and the abuser (and everyone else) acts as though nothing is amiss, the child – who is dependent upon those adults – will find ways to minimize, deny, or forget the abuse in order to survive. This is especially true in a culture that tends to believe and support adults, while questioning the credibility and experience of children (see Ceci and Bruck 1995).

Given the social forces that act to preserve patriarchal and parental power, and to protect adult perpetrators, it is no surprise that many survivors of sexual abuse have found it nearly impossible to speak of their abuse. Social, institutional, and cultural forces have often colluded to silence such stories which threaten the ideal of family harmony and community order. To reveal the range and depth of perversion and abuse is to threaten that very order. The irony, of course, is that not to reveal it, is to ensure the reproduction of violence and distortion, and thus ultimately the collapse of the very systems people are trying to protect.

In attempting to speak out, survivors must not only tell their story of abuse but counter the abuser's version that is typically normalized by dominant cultural narratives about victimhood, the family, and relationships between parents and children. The survivor of childhood sexual abuse has to break through the traditional story line that places blame and responsibility on the victim, and calls (in the Fourth Commandment) for children to obey their parents without a reciprocal emphasis on the responsibility of parents to children.[13] The challenge for survivors of childhood sexual abuse is to create a new language by which they can speak of abuse and of parents who violate their responsibility to children. In challenging the old story, survivors are seeking a new positionality *vis-à-vis* the dominant discourse. They are creating alternative narratives that enable them to speak of childhood sexual abuse and to resituate blame and responsibility, to give the shame back to those who abused them rather than accepting it as their own fate. In radically challenging the 'official story' that upholds the status quo, these new stories do not come without struggle (Rose 1993).

In the act of violence, the perpetrator controls the story he enacts. This is seen in such expressions as: 'she asked for it', 'that'll teach her a lesson', 'she made me do it, it was her fault', 'spare the rod, spoil the child'. Within the context of this traditional and patriarchal narrative, the targeted person becomes a victim because she deserves it. 'Our sense of the normative is nourished in narrative, but so', argues Bruner, 'is our sense of breach and exception. Stories make "reality" a mitigated reality' (Bruner 1990: 97). Trauma narratives (whether they recount experiences with sexual abuse, lynching, or political torture) point to the unjustified violence done to people, and hold abusers rather than victims accountable. They expose the illegitimate use of force, power and authority, and in so doing, de-authorize the credibility and legitimacy of the abusers.

By naming and claiming the experience of abuse and survival as their own story, survivors reconstruct the story of abuse rather than accepting it as the shameful bequest of parental violation. The survivor narrative names the violation as an act of cruelty, control, or hubris, not as justified punishment visited upon a recalcitrant inferior or 'sidekick'. This act of naming and narrating seizes the story from the violator and gives witness to the struggle of the survivor and to her multidimensional self. The survivor is no longer objectified, her identity no longer relegated to a unidimensional victimized or stigmatized status; rather she may emerge from the fire as a strong, resourceful, and diversified self.

Although silence may serve as a refuge, it is also a place of bondage. In speaking out, the victim-survivor finds her own voice through which she can tell her story. Instead of living with the split, polarized identities of the good-bad selves projected onto her by the abuser, she can come to appreciate and experiment with both the resistance and the accommodation that was part of her survival strategy. Taking the story away from the abuser, and redefining the experience and oneself in relation to it, is an act of self-determination. As a consequence, resourcefulness and responsibility rather than reaction can come to characterize relationships and life choices. Volition, rather than violation, then becomes the driving force and opens up the possibilities for healing.

Notes

Many thanks to Kim Rogers, Graham Dawson and Linda Crockett for their thorough and thoughtful readings and insightful comments on earlier drafts.

1   Although for those whose abuse begins early and is chronic, trauma may be the consistent and continuing reality.
2   Growing out of a grass-roots group in Cape Cod, the National Network for the Clothesline Project is now located at P.O. Box 727, East Dennis, MA 02641, USA. When the project first started in 1991, there was one clothesline with thirty-one shirts on it. By February 1995, 250 clotheslines representing 35,000 shirts had been assembled around the country. In April 1995, more than 5,000 shirts were exhibited as part of the National Clothesline Project on the mall in Washington, DC.
3   A 53-minute documentary film, *Clothesline*, based on interviews with women who contributed artwork to the Central Pennsylvania Clothesline Project, was co-produced by Lonna Malmsheimer and Susan Rose. It is available through South Mountain Productions, 93 Old Town Rd., Gardners, PA 17324, USA.
4   All excerpts are from transcripts of interviews with women who contributed to the Central Pennsylvania Clothesline Project in February 1993, Carlisle, Pa. Each of the interviewees is referred to by first name.
5   For more detailed discussions of drawings as diagnostic tools and the significance of the omission of hands, arms and feet, as well as the uses of art therapy,

see Peacock 1991, Spigelman *et al.* 1992, Magwaza *et al.* 1993, Burgess and Hartman 1993, Burgess 1981, Di Leo 1973, Kelley 1984 and Lemley 1990.

6   The response to new challenges can be arousing and energizing, and at optimal levels, can facilitate learning, problem solving, and a sense of competence. But trauma, in contrast to interesting challenges, can overtax the mechanisms for responding to new or dangerous situations. Systems regulating arousal may become hypersensitive, too easily switched on or too difficult to moderate or turn off. (Waites 1993: chapter 1).

7   Inescapable shock tends to produce lasting and deleterious psychobiological changes. See Krystal 1990, van der Kolk 1987, van der Kolk *et al.* 1996.

8   The adventure can draw us into an exciting exchange with worlds beyond our ordinary experience. But these times of adventure need to be complemented by periods of reflection. If the adventure is not to become just a frenetic run from self as ordinarily perceived and experienced, then periods of quiet reflection and integration need to follow. If we do not move inward, and contemplate that which we have experienced, then we are forever on the run. Or if the process of reflection is too interrupted, we – and our experiences with adventure (or trauma) – become fragmented, splintered, dismembered. If people are not given the space to reflect, or are warned not to remember, then they are more likely to forget and stay split.

9   See, for example, Kristof 1997. This article focuses on the stories of Second World War Japanese veterans who, more than fifty years later, are still haunted by the memories of crimes they committed against other men, women, and children during the war.

10 For current brain and memory research exploring the ways in which experience is recorded, and how the processing and storage of traumatic memories may be quite different from the processing of more ordinary experiences, see van der Kolk *et al.* 1996. As we gain better data about how bio-chemical and neurological processes interact with trauma, we will be better able to assess the processing, storage, and retrieval of a range of events along the spectrum from ordinary to traumatic. See Herman 1992 and 1996 for a review of studies which indicate that traumatic memories from childhood have been retrieved after a period of dense amnesia and later confirmed beyond a reasonable doubt. See also Terr 1994.

11 This is a common response of incest survivors who feel betrayed by their mothers who failed to protect them then; they are often more angry at them than at their abusers. This holds true, conversely, for fathers who stood by while their wives abused their children. One explanation is that the ineffective witness who did not protect the victim is a less threatening object of anger.

12 See Herman 1992, Greven 1990, Gordon 1988, Pleck 1987, Rose 1993.

13 For a more detailed discussion see Rose 1993, Greven 1990, Brown and Bohn 1989, Poling 1991 and Jay 1992.

References

Bickerton, D. (1997) review of Freyd, *Betrayal Trauma*, in *New York Times Book Review*, 26 Jan., p. 20.

Brown, J., and Bohn, C. R. (eds) (1989) *Christianity, Patriarchy and Abuse: a Feminist Critique*, New York.

Bruner, J. (1990) *Acts of Meaning*, Cambridge.

Burgess, A. (1981) 'Children's drawings as indicators of sexual trauma', *Perspectives in Psychiatric Care*, vol. 19, pp. 50–8.

Burgess, A. and Hartman, C. (1993) 'Children's drawings', in *Child Abuse and Neglect*, vol. 17, pp. 161–8.

Ceci, S. and Bruck, M. (1995) *Jeopardy in the Courtroom: a Scientific Analysis of Children's Testimony*, Washington, DC.

Davis, L. and Bass, E. (1994) *The Courage to Heal*, New York.

Di Leo, J. (1973) *Children's Drawings as Diagnostic Aids*, New York.

Ferenczi, S. (1933) 'Confusion of tongues', quoted in Greven 1990: 158.

Fraser, S. (1987) *My Father's House: a Memoir of Incest and Healing*, New York.

Freyd, J. (1996) *Betrayal Trauma: the Logic of Forgetting Childhood Abuse*, Cambridge.

Gergen, K. (1982) *Towards Transformation in Social Knowledge*, New York.

Gordon, L. (1988) *Heroes in Their Own Lives: the Politics and History of Family Violence*, New York.

Greven, P. (1990) *Spare the Child: Religious Roots of Punishment and the Psychological Impact of Physical Abuse*, New York.

Herman, J. (1992) *Trauma and Recovery*, New York.

—— (1996) 'Crime and memory', in C. Strozier and M. Flynn (eds), *Trauma and Self*, Boston pp. 3–18.

Jay, N. (1992) *Throughout Your Generations Forever: Sacrifice, Religion, and Paternity*, Chicago.

Kelley, S. (1984) 'The use of art therapy with sexually abused children', *Journal of Psychosocial Nursing*, vol. 22, pp. 12–18.

Kristof, N. (1997) 'A Japanese generation haunted by its past', *New York Times* 22 Jan. A1, p. 8.

Krystal, J. H. (1990) 'Animal models for posttraumatic stress disorder', in E. L. Gillen (ed.), *Biological Assessment and Treatment of Posttraumatic Stress Disorder*, Washington.

Kundera, M. (1994) *The Book of Laughter and Forgetting*, New York.

Laub, D. (1992) 'Bearing witness', in S. Felman and D. Laub, *Testimony: Crises of Witnessing in Literature, Psychoanalysis and History*, New York.

Lemley, B. (1990) 'Pictures of the pain', *Social Issues Resources Series – Mental Health* vol. 4, p. 14.

Lifton, R. J. (1993) *The Protean Self: Human Resilience in an Age of Fragmentation*, New York.

Magwaza, A., Killian, B., Petersen, I. and Pillay, Y. (1993) 'The effects of chronic violence on preschool children living in South African townships', *Child Abuse and Neglect*, vol. 17, pp. 795–803.

Miller, A. (1981) *Prisoners of Childhood*, New York; also published in paperback as *The Drama of the Gifted Child* (1983).

—— (1990) *For Your Own Good: Hidden Cruelty in Child-rearing and the Roots of Violence*, New York.

Peacock, M. E. (1991) 'A personal construct approach to art therapy in the treatment of post sexual abuse trauma', *American Journal of Art Therapy*, vol. 29, pp. 100–9.

Pleck, E. (1987) *Domestic Tyranny: the Making of American Social Policy against Family Violence from Colonial Times to the Present*, New York.

Poling, J. N. (1991) *Abuse of Power: A Theological Problem*, Nashville.

Rose, S. (1993) 'Child sacrifice: projective Christianity', *Anima* vol. 20, pp. 1–18.

Simmel, G. (1971) 'The adventurer', in *On Individuality and Social Forms*, Chicago.

Spigelman, G., Spigelman, A. and Engelsson, I. (1992) 'An analysis of family drawings', *Journal of Divorce and Remarriage*, vol. 18, pp. 31–53.

Strozier and Flynn (eds) (1996) *Trauma and Self*, Boston.

Terr, L. (1990) *Too Scared to Cry*, New York.

—— (1994) *Unchained Memories: True Stories of Traumatic Memories, Lost and Found*, New York.

van der Kolk, B. (1987) *Psychological Trauma*, Washington, DC.

van der Kolk, B., McFarlane, A. and Weisaeth, L. (eds) (1996) *Traumatic Stress: the Effects of Overwhelming Experience on Mind, Body, and Society*, New York.

Waites, E. (1993) *Trauma and Survival*, New York.

9

TRAUMA, MEMORY, POLITICS

The Irish Troubles

Graham Dawson

Trauma, reconciliation and the Irish past

The Irish historical past is often described as 'traumatic'. The sixteenth-century plantations, the 1641 Rebellion, the Union with Britain, the Famine, the Great War, the War of Independence, the Civil War – and, of course, the Troubles of the past thirty years – have all been referred to as traumas.[1] Above all, in nationalist history-writing and popular memory from the nineteenth century down to the present, the experience of trauma has defined the very essence of the story of Ireland (Brady 1994; Bradshaw 1994); as a narrative of oppression and suffering inflicted upon the Irish people by English (and later, British) colonialism over eight centuries; of Irish endurance and resistance throughout this time; and of the achievement of a partial and incomplete independence from tyranny in 1922, qualified by the continuance of traumatic colonial dominance in the British statelet of Northern Ireland.

This interpretation of Ireland's past is less often recognized in England, nor is it common to see its account of a traumatic history as one that embraces Britain too (but see Boyce 1972: 185).[2] The possibility of recognizing a traumatic element in the imperial mission was largely precluded by British colonial discourse which construed the narrative of Empire as a heroic adventure to civilize the world (Dawson 1994). The imperial narrative denied the validity of the nationalist historical perspective, in Ireland as elsewhere: palpable suffering – during the Famine, for example – was held to be the responsibility of the colonized people themselves rather than of those who governed them. Where incontestable evidence of the brutality of British rule did surface, condemnation of state actions tended to start from (rather than call into question) 'traditional assumptions that Britain stood for justice, righteousness and good laws' (Boyce 1972: 99).

This tradition of British liberalism nevertheless provided a basis for naming the traumas inflicted on others to secure the British Empire. During the Irish War of Independence (1919–21), anti-republican reprisals directed against Irish homesteads and communities by the Black and Tans and Auxiliaries provoked a broadly constituted and vociferous public campaign of protest in England. A Labour Party Commission sent to investigate the condition of Ireland in November 1920 reported that 'things are being done in the name of Britain which must make her name stink in the nostrils of the whole world' (ibid.); while in the Peace With Ireland Council, Conservatives and socialists joined with Liberals to publicize and condemn the British 'terror', and to call for an end to the conflict (ibid.: 61–102, 229 n. 119). Among its supporters, the radical liberal historian and journalist, J. L. Hammond, demanded a public enquiry into the reprisals 'on the grounds of justice to the British people' as well as to the Irish. Attempting to convey, in his reports from Ireland, his sense of the reciprocal damage caused to English civil and political culture by this war waged by the imperial state, Hammond endorsed the truth of a comment made to him by an Irishman: 'This is a tragedy . . . but it is your tragedy, not ours' (ibid.: 100).

However, this has never been a popular perception of 'Irish history' in England. When in June 1921 the Dublin Castle official, Sir John Anderson, wrote to the Chief Secretary for Ireland, Sir Hamar Greenwood, advocating treaty negotiations to resolve the conflict, his assessment of the public mood in England was that 'their one instinctive desire in relation to Ireland is to forget' (ibid.: 134). The political settlement of 1922, granting an independent Free State in twenty-six counties whilst maintaining a unionist-dominated 'Home Rule' parliament for the six counties of Northern Ireland, created the conditions for precisely such a historical forgetting. In the post-1945 period, this tendency to forget significant dimensions of Britain's own imperial history has been exacerbated by the problematical impact of decolonization (begun in Ireland) and the loss of empire upon British national culture and identity. Metaphors of an English cultural 'amnesia' regarding the causes and development of the current Troubles are indeed widespread among Irish commentators (e.g. Kiberd 1985: 93, Kirkaldy 1992: 40). Small wonder, in such a cultural context, that the reciprocal impact of 'Ireland's traumatic past' upon England is barely considered or understood.

On the surface the Downing Street Declaration of December 1993, signed by the British Prime Minister, John Major, and the Irish Taoiseach, Albert Reynolds, appeared to buck this historic trend. The Declaration stated that:

The most urgent and important issue facing the people of Ireland, North and South, and the British and Irish governments together, is to remove the causes of conflict, to overcome the legacy of history and to heal the divisions which have resulted, recognizing that the absence of a lasting and satisfactory settlement of relationships between the peoples of both islands has contributed to continuing tragedy and suffering.

The text expressed 'the inestimable value, to both their peoples . . . of healing the divisions in Ireland', which can come about 'only through the agreement and co-operation of the people, North and South, representing both traditions in Ireland'. New arrangements would be sought 'to lay the foundations for a more peaceful and harmonious future devoid of the violence and bitter divisions which have scarred the past generation' (Downing Street Declaration).

Incorporating the principles outlined in the unpublished Hume-Adams agreement, the Declaration created the political basis for the ceasefire of the Irish Republican Army (IRA) on 31 August 1994, for the ensuing ceasefire declared by the Combined Loyalist Military Command several weeks later, and for the two governments' Framework Document of 22 February 1995 setting out the conditions for inclusive, all-party talks on the future of Northern Ireland. The Declaration tapped into a deep desire for peace in Northern Ireland and (albeit less urgently experienced) in the Irish Republic and in Britain too. It appeared to recognize the full complexity of relations involved in the conflict. And it spoke the language of healing: the bitter divisions, the scars of violence, the tragedy and suffering, would be ended by a process of reconciliation and agreement that would 'remove the causes of conflict' and 'overcome the legacy of history'.

This latter phrase, however, must give pause for thought. How was this 'legacy of history' to be understood, and how did the two governments envisage its 'overcoming'? Closer scrutiny of statements made by the Irish and British leaders in the months leading up to and immediately following the Declaration suggests that the proposed settlement took little account of the magnitude and character of that historical 'tragedy and suffering'. What was being advocated was, rather, a wholesale abandonment of Irish nationalist popular memory.

The Irish Foreign Minister, Dick Spring, speaking at the Irish Labour Party conference in April 1993, argued: 'Let us be prepared to cast off the chains of history, to stop being prisoners of our upbringing' (Walker 1996: 65). A few weeks after this, Taoiseach Albert Reynolds suggested: 'We are not tied up in our past. We want to move forward, to look at the changes required to ensure that both communities can live together'. In November, Reynolds echoed Spring even more closely: 'We must not be the prisoners of history' (ibid.: 66). Here, the dynamic metaphor of liberation (of casting off chains, of breaking free) is detached from its traditional reference – to Irish national liberation from the historic shackles of British imperialism – and turned against that very aspiration. The nationalist narrative of liberation itself becomes the chain of bondage, while reconciliation is offered as the key to freedom.

The strategic utility of 'overcoming the legacy of history' in this way was revealed by John Major – writing in, of all places, the Belfast-based nationalist newspaper, the *Irish News* – in February 1994: 'We cannot live in the past. Dreadful deeds have been done by all sides in past centuries. We should all regret that, but those of us alive today are not responsible for them. Our generation must look to the future' (*Irish News* 1994). If this rhetorical appeal invites us to consign 'dreadful deeds' firmly to the distant past, the reality is that some 3,500 people have died during the last thirty years as a direct result of the Troubles (Sutton 1994). Their families and friends continue to bear the psychic scars of these deaths. Many of those responsible are not only alive today but are serving sentences for terrorist offences in British and Irish gaols. (These prisoners, both republican and loyalist, were instrumental in securing political agreement to the ceasefires within their communities.) Others – like the British soldiers and their military and political superiors, responsible for shooting dead fourteen unarmed civilians in Derry in January 1972 – have never been called to account.

The politics of reconciliation promoted by the two governments is designed primarily to take the IRA out of Irish politics and to stabilize the Northern Ireland state, laying the basis for a permanent political settlement in the mutual interests of capital and state security in both the Irish Republic and Britain. In furthering this they have developed what, to borrow Heather Goodall's terms, I shall call an 'institutional amnesia': a practice of 'state-organized forgetting' concerning the causes and consequences of the conflict (Goodall 1994: 58–9).

If this strategy has a long history in Britain, its deployment in the Irish Republic coincides with the backlash against militant republicanism during 1972, the most violent year of the conflict, as the death toll in the North escalated and refugees poured south (Coogan 1996: 182–9). An assault on nationalist popular memory was launched in the public media, promoted by 'powerfully organized cadres within the Irish intelligentsia' and underpinned by the work of 'revisionist' historians (Kiberd 1991: 5, Brady 1994, Boyce and O'Day 1996). This 'anti-nationalist revisionism' (Kiberd 1991: 8) laid the ideological foundations for a political rapprochement between the British and Irish governments, eventually formalized in the Anglo-Irish Agreement of 1985, which has sought to bring official Irish and British narratives concerning the past, the present, and the future into a common alignment. Reconciliation between the conflicting communities in Northern Ireland is to be established on this basis.

Where the language of reconciliation speaks of forgetting the past, however, this amounts to a denial of the psychic and political realities of those communities. In such a situation – where violent conflict has only recently ended, remains fresh in living memory, and is liable to break out again (as happened with the ending of the IRA ceasefire in February 1996) – the psychic and political legacies of history are not 'overcome' quite so readily: they remain a source of profound tension within and between the warring communities. That which the language of reconciliation would smooth over and erase, the language of trauma insists upon: it names the realities of Northern Ireland as traumatic, and points to the necessity of remembering in order to go forward to any viable alternative future. Nevertheless, traumas are remembered only in the face of powerful pressures to forget, and it is to these that I turn next.

Trauma, memory, and forgetting in the Irish Troubles

As a popular expression in everyday use, trauma refers to the psychological impact of some violent or otherwise shocking event, producing deep-rooted effects which are difficult to come to terms with. Etymology reminds us that this popular usage rests upon a more specific psychoanalytic concept that in turn draws from and redefines a term in pathology derived from the Greek. Since at least the mid-seventeenth century, the meaning of trauma was 'a wound, or external bodily injury; also, the condition [of shock] caused by this'. Psychoanalysis extended this to psychopathology, redefining trauma as 'a disturbing experience which affects the mind or nerves of a person so as to induce hysteria or "psychic" conditions'; and, after 1916, as 'a mental shock'.[3]

In the development of Freud's thinking, the concept appears initially in his work on female hysteria, with the discovery that '[h]ysterics suffer mainly from reminiscences' of traumatic events in childhood, repressed into the unconscious (Freud and Breuer 1895: 58). During the First World War, Freud developed the concept to explain the phenomenon of 'shell shock' or 'war neurosis', and proposed the idea of a 'repetition compulsion' operating as a means of psychic defence against the traumatic memory (Freud 1920; see also Ferenczi *et al.* 1921). For Freud, although the psychic trace of the determining event and the emotional charge provoked by it resist symbolization, assimilation and integration within the psyche, they nevertheless persist in a state of disconnection producing intense, unconscious emotional energy. This finds displaced and often delayed expression in a range of symbolic effects: hysterical symptoms, speech disturbances, hallucinations, dreams, forms of compulsive behaviour – and amnesias.

As the language of psychoanalysis has permeated the vocabularies of political discourse, journalism, and history-writing, the term 'trauma' has been extended to encompass psychic processes that impact upon whole communities and cultures. This poses the theoretical problem of how a concept developed to explain the effects of corporeal and psychic shock upon the individual might be applied to a social group whilst avoiding the danger of ascribing to that group a collective psyche (as if it were 'like' an individual) (Ignatieff 1996).

For my purposes here, I suggest that the term 'trauma' – while retaining its power to identify psychic effects at the level of the individual – also provides a useful metaphor enabling the identification of collective processes for which no other language exists. Typically, the metaphor entails three proposals about the past. First, it indicates a psychic dimension to the conflicts of history; a sense that profound suffering has been inflicted upon and endured by a people, a community, or a nation, and that both the suffering and the response to it are integral to the historical record. Second, the term connotes the persistence into the present of a harmful past whose scars have not healed, but whose disturbing effects might remain difficult to grasp or acknowledge. Third, 'trauma' involves a relation of memory, whereby the suffering of the past is remembered, often incompletely, by a community in forms of cultural representation and commemoration. Alternatively, it may be forgotten, rendered invisible or unspeakable by a process of cultural (as well as individual) amnesia.

If we are to understand why traumatic memories are forgotten, it is first necessary to remind ourselves of their disturbing content. In what follows, Mary Holland describes two examples from the war in the North of Ireland of survivors' efforts to remember and to tell a story about their trauma.

> A woman writes many years after her father's death: 'You lived for 11 days after the bomb. They say your arms and legs fell off when you died. I was 12 years old and very frightened. Frightened to look at your charred face, your badly swollen lips and eyes, the tubes in your throat. Amazingly, I remember a few jokes you tried to tell me before the end. I think you must have known how scared I was. The smell of burning flesh never really goes away. God, what you must have felt, knowing that your own child, the little girl you used to hold in your arms, was afraid to hug you, even to be left alone with you'. Only now, with children of her own, can she tell her father how angry she felt that his death left her mother and family on their own.
>
> A father whose son was killed in an explosion describes the pieces of human remains in gardens and on rooftops, with steam rising from them. He sees a young soldier crying, being comforted by one of his mates. Later he is called to the morgue to identify his son's body, but it is impossible. There are only pieces of flesh and limbs with a tongue placed on the top. 'Why were we summoned by the police to view these remains? I do not know'.
>
> (Holland 1997)

There are immense difficulties in speaking and writing about such memories. Remembering a traumatic event is a process riven with ambivalence. Is it good to remember? Does the attempt to represent the traumatic past help a survivor to come to terms with it, perhaps to bear the pain? Or is it risking too much, ploughing up things too painful or disturbing to remember, things that are best buried, consigned to silence, forgotten? Those who do attempt it are struggling to shape the traumatic event into narrative form, to integrate it into their world of meaning, to fashion words that are in some sense adequate to the dislocation and the horror. But they are also seeking recognition of that pain, disturbance, dislocation, and horror, from others. The remembering and forgetting of trauma is necessarily a communal process centred upon a struggle for social recognition.[4]

These particular stories are among thousands of others collected from all over Northern Ireland since early 1996 by a Belfast-based project called *An Crann* (The Tree), as the core of a new 'storytelling museum' about the Troubles ('Voices of the victims' 1996). According to the writer, Damian Gorman, who launched the project in December 1994 'when both ceasefires were in operation', the primary aim of the project is to ' recover the story of what happened to us' during the war: 'everybody's personal history is part of a shared history. . . . Obviously there are very many people who have suffered. And the idea is to piece all those testimonies together as parts of a mosaic' (ibid.: 40). The psychic struggle waged by the individual survivor to integrate traumatic memory within viable maps of meaning is given a social correlate in this effort to read and understand personal testimonies as elements in a larger, collective history. Responding to the point that 'some might say the project is opening old wounds that maybe would be better healed over', Gorman replies:

> Some people do . . . say to me that the best thing to do is to bury it as deeply as possible. . . . In a lot of people's lives things come up and they fold them away as if there is some reinforced concrete chamber of the human heart into which these things can be put, and there isn't. These things pulse away, and they distort, and they do harm. They can seep out into the rest of your life. And just as I believe that is the case for an individual, so it is the case for a community and there are an awful lot of things that we need to hear.
> ('Voices of the Victims' 1996: 40)

A second aim quickly emerged from the process of meeting and talking with people: to cultivate 'the practice of listening . . . to just make a space into which people can say their piece, [because] it's in spaces like that where important things can take root, like tolerance and forgiveness' (ibid.). With this, *An Crann* has become an endeavour not only to record but to heal the traumatic past, working on the connections between the psychic and the social, the individual and the communal, telling and listening. Contrary to the practice of 'state-organized forgetting', with its impulsion to 'overthrow' and 'cast off' the past, *An Crann* calls for more remembering. This is a necessary condition of authentic reconciliation, since the buried past will otherwise continue to exert a malign influence in a range of morbid symptoms, silences and emotional reactions.

However, this necessary process confronts the profound difficulties involved not only in telling, but also in reading, listening and bearing witness to traumatic memories. We struggle to relate ourselves, imaginatively and emotionally, to the traumas of others. Antjie Krog, a South African poet covering for radio news the investigations of the Truth and Reconciliation Commission into human rights violations committed during the apartheid era, has written very powerfully about the harrowing process of listening, day after day, to testimonies of trauma. By the second week of the hearings, whilst answering questions on an actuality broadcast, 'I stammer. I freeze. I am without language'. A counsellor from the Commission tells the journalists, 'You will experience the same symptoms as the victims. You will find yourself powerless, without help, without words'.

> [R]eporting on the truth commission has indeed left most of us physically exhausted and mentally frayed. . . . Water covers the cheeks and we cannot type. Or think. And this was how we often ended up at the daily press conference – bewildered and close to tears at the feet of Archbishop Tutu. By the end of the four weeks they were no longer press conferences – he was comforting us. . . . Every week we are stretched thinner and thinner over different pitches of grief . . . [H]ow many people can one see crying, how much torn-loose sorrow can one accommodate?
>
> (Krog 1997: 6)

Accounts like this support the psychoanalytic theory of transference which suggests that traumatic events are transmitted from one psyche to another. Disturbance, pain and horror, remembered and represented to another, enter the listener by 'introjection' and may reproduce themselves there – as embodiments or evocations, perhaps, of psychic scenarios buried deeply within the internal world of each of us. There they encounter (or, better, call into being) the many forms of a necessary psychic defence – whether resistance, denial and disavowal, or the anaesthetic of emotional exhaustion – mobilized to 'split off' these painful and destructive feelings from the self. This expulsion of unwanted elements from the self tends to be accomplished by their imaginative 'projection' into people, places and objects in the social world, which thereby become the 'bearers' of violence, of death and of loss, that return to haunt the self from the outside, as a threatening external Other.[5] Memories of trauma are produced through this encounter with psychic defence and denial. If those remembering must exert their telling to push through their own resistances, often they confront those of their listeners as well. To relate to the trauma of another is to risk undoing the work of psychic defence upon which the ordinary world of the self appears to be based, and admitting the traumatic. Helping a survivor bear and detoxify the effects of traumatic experience involves a psychic openness to, and an ability

187

to tolerate, one's own pain, fear and disturbance. Defensive disavowal, on the other hand, offers a means to seal the traumatic into the zone of the Other, safely split off – both psychically and socially – behind a secure border of demarcation.

This psychoanalytic account of psychic defence against trauma, as a means to preserve a less painful normality, may illuminate certain cultural responses in Britain and the Republic to the conflict 'in' Northern Ireland. Its hostile representation as an atavistic tribal war between primitives, each side being 'as bad as the other' and beyond the pale of civilized concern; the contemptuous and dismissive wish to 'leave them to it'; the fear that poisonous influences from 'up there' might pervade and contaminate normal life 'here': these can be understood as so many cultural manifestations of psychic denial and disavowal. Damian Gorman, speaking during the temporary peace of the first IRA ceasefire (31 August 1994 – 9 February 1996), identifies this process at work within Northern Ireland itself when he remarks that:

> With the *Crann* I have been aware of the fear in people whose relatives have been killed that they will be left behind, because there is such a yearning among society at large to get away from that time. They feel they will inevitably be sidelined, because they are living, pulsing reminders of that time of death and sectarian murder. The view is that we cannot take those people with us, for if we do we can never forget all of that.
>
> ('Voices of the victims' 1996: 43)

'State-organized forgetting', with its seductive offer to cast off the chains of history, appeals to precisely this yearning, whilst actively exacerbating the difficulties of social recognition and the fears of abandonment – of being left to deal with the past alone – experienced by the bereaved.

A comparable 'leaving behind' has affected those bereaved and injured by the IRA's bombing campaign in England. In a BBC documentary investigating the long-term psychological after-effects of the Birmingham pub bombings – which killed twenty-one people and injured 162, many seriously, on 21 November 1974 – a number of the survivors spoke publicly for the first time to explain that 'they feel their story has been forgotten' (*Aftershock* 1994).[6] Although the atrocity had 'shattered' their lives and frequently their 'peace of mind', and continues to 'cast a shadow over us' twenty years later, there had been no civic commemoration, and the official attitude appeared to be that 'its an embarrassment': 'they don't want to remember' (ibid.). Similarly, Sharon Smith, a resident of the Barkantine Housing Estate devastated by the Docklands bomb ending the IRA ceasefire, has condemned governmental neglect of its psychological impact: 'No-one seems to care, they've just left us here to cope with it' (*Guardian* 1997a: 2). Gorman sees *An Crann* as a challenge to this tendency of the wider public, particularly those in Northern Ireland intent on embracing the promise of a peaceful future, 'to detach from the whole process'. The voices of the survivors constitute, for Gorman, a communal resource for confronting a shared history in which all are 'implicated' ('Voices of the victims': 43).

There is, of course, more than one way of construing that shared history. Gorman rightly emphasizes the broader collective value and significance of survivors' stories. However, the difficulties inherent in remembering and witnessing trauma are compounded in the context of a war, where political antagonism is continually fuelled by – and in turn helps to reproduce – the bitternesses and hatreds of violent conflict. In August 1995 a documentary entitled *Trouble With Peace*, broadcast to mark the first anniversary of the IRA ceasefire, included an interview with a loyalist woman, Sandra Rock, whose brother Sammy – a member of a loyalist paramilitary group – had been killed by the Irish National Liberation Army in 1993. She said:

> Why the peace made me angry was because I don't want the ones who murdered my brother to get off scot-free. I really wanted the ones that murdered my brother murdered. I want thems to be dead. And I want their families to go through what I've been going through. . . . A lot of these people are saying, 'I forgive them, I forgive them'. I can't find it in my heart to forgive the ones that murdered my brother and I never will. And I hate those people. Hate them. And I do wish them dead. That's why I hate peace.
>
> (*Trouble With Peace* 1995)[7]

This is a chilling repudiation of the language of reconciliation, and provides a powerful illustration of the inadequacy of 'state-organized forgetting' as a response to the realities of the war. Sandra Rock and others like her – in Ireland and Britain – cannot simply 'shake off' the loss, anger and hatred generated by bereavement, nor the impulse to mitigate the psychic distress and alleviate the pressure of suffering through revenge: the wish to push back onto the Other the suffering that the Other has placed onto you, in a further cycle of politically motivated violence – as if the loved brother could thereby be made to live on.[8]

Social recognition of these realities is available in Northern Ireland, however, within those local, mainly working-class communities – whether loyalist or republican, unionist or nationalist – which are most deeply and routinely enmeshed in the war. The language of trauma is deployed in the public commemoration of the war dead that occurs regularly in these communities. Relating to and representing communal memories of past traumas, this establishes a politics of suffering. Political identity is strengthened through communal bonding and aligned with the psychic needs of the survivors of violence. In this process, the personal suffering and mourning of the survivors is publicly recognized, affirmed, and given dignity and meaning through its incorporation into a unionist/loyalist – or nationalist/republican – political narrative about past, present, and future.

Placed within this broader narrative framework, the particular event achieves a more general significance as an event in a communal history. This can be seen, for example, in the commemoration of the IRA bomb atrocity of 23 October 1993, when nine members of the loyalist community (including two children) were killed in a no-warning attack on Frizzell's Fish Shop on the Shankill Road. Under the headline, 'We will remember them', an editorial in the *Shankill People* newspaper praised 'the bravery and humanity' of 'those who dived into the blasted ruins . . . to search for the victims, oblivious to their own safety', as 'worthy of their forefathers on the Somme' (*Shankhill People* 1993: 4). Here, the spirit of self-sacrifice manifest in today's embattled community is both measured and ennobled by association with the loyalist volunteers of the Ulster Division during the Great War, some 5,000 of whom were killed serving their country on the first day of the Battle of the Somme, 1 July 1916.

The same process is evident in the commemoration of Bloody Sunday, the name given by the nationalist community to the events of 30 January 1972 in Derry, when a battalion of the 1st Parachute Regiment sealed some 10,000 civil rights demonstrators into the nationalist ghetto of the Bogside, attacked with rubber bullets and water cannon those who tried to climb a street barrier, and then began shooting with high-velocity rifles. 'They fired repeatedly into the crowd, and then at people fleeing and at others trying to reach the wounded' (Farrell 1980: 289). Fourteen unarmed civilians were shot dead, seven of whom were under nineteen years old, and seventeen others received wounds, some serious. John Hume, the leader of the 'constitutional nationalist' Social Democratic and Labour Party and a Derry MP at Westminster and Strasbourg, speaking at the twenty-fifth anniversary commemorative demonstration in Derry on 2 February 1997, recalled Bloody Sunday as 'the most traumatic day in the lifetime of every citizen of this city and certainly of mine as their representative'. The pain, he said, went very deep (cited in Sharrock 1997a: 7). Among those able to corroborate this was Kay Duddy, whose seventeen-year-old brother Jackie was one of those shot dead: she was reported as saying that the anniversary had brought back 'terrible, terrible memories' (ibid.). In naming the event, the nationalist community was both recalling and drawing a direct parallel with a previous 'Bloody Sunday'. This took place in Dublin on 21 November 1920, during the Independence War of 1919–21, when twelve civilians were killed after British forces fired into an Irish football match in reprisal for a series of IRA assassinations. The very naming locates the significance of the Derry atrocity within the longer history of the Irish struggle for national liberation from British imperial rule.

These politicized narratives of memory offer immense psychic resources of strength, hope, and resilience to the members of the embattled communities.

They provide collective, cultural means to combat the disintegration and withdrawal of the self that so often marks the presence of the traumatic. By empowering the survivors, who thereby cease to be passive 'victims', they energize the political will. They promise that redemption of suffering is possible and that it will be made ultimately meaningful through the achievement of the political demands of the community. And they ensure that the dead 'have not died in vain', that they live on as a touchstone and inspiration for those who have survived them and who continue their struggle.

However, in thus underpinning and mobilizing psychic energy on behalf of the communities locked in antagonism, this politicization of memory simultaneously generates paradox. Public commemoration itself is turned into a battlefield where selective, discrepant and antagonistic narratives of the past clash and compete. When, for example, republicans remember that crucial year, 1916, they commemorate the heroic martyrs of the Easter Rising who gave their lives in a doomed revolt which nevertheless began the revolution leading to an independent Irish state. In so doing, they forget the Irish dead of the Great War – seen as Britain's imperialist war – which is the exclusive focus of loyalist remembering of 1916 (Walker 1996: 87–91, 99–104). The commemoration of one traumatic event is precisely the amnesia of the other.

While remembering and offering public recognition for the traumas of 'our' community, politicized communal memories thus tend to withhold recognition, to forget, and to deny the traumas of the Other: recognition of the trauma is felt to imply recognition of the political narrative that articulates its significance. To deny social recognition to trauma, however, is not to ignore but to entrench it. The hostilities of armed conflict thus tend to impact back upon mourning and commemoration, a process made most explicit in the common phenomenon in Northern Ireland of actual violent attacks upon commemorative events, funerals, gravestones, and memorials.[9]

The politics of memory: Bloody Sunday

The paradoxes of political commemoration are especially clear in the case of Derry's Bloody Sunday. The traumatic impact of this event upon nationalists and republicans derived primarily from its stark exposure of the fundamental injustice and violence inherent in the maintenance of 'the Protestant supremacist state' (Foster 1989: 592) of Northern Ireland. But this was compounded by vigorous efforts at a public cover-up made on behalf of the British state, to clear its name and erase its responsibility for the massacre from the historical record. The Army's press statement claimed that the Paras had returned fire after coming under attack from 'seen gunmen and nailbombers', and that 'fire continued to be returned only at identified targets' (cited in Coogan 1996: 160). The implication, that those killed had been gunmen or nailbombers, was refuted by the Widgery Tribunal's official report on the events. Nevertheless, the report declined to condemn the killings, allowing the British press to claim that 'Widgery clears paratroops for Bloody Sunday' (*Daily Telegraph*), and even that 'Widgery blames IRA' (*Daily Express*) (cited in Curtis 1984: 50).[10]

After the Tribunal, the Army's official fiction was reproduced rather than questioned in Britain for many years, through censorship and denial of alternative perspectives. In 1978, for example, a BBC film about Derry called *A City on the Border* 'showed a mother putting flowers on her son's grave, which bore the words, "Murdered by British Paratroopers on Bloody Sunday"'. The woman laying her bunch of flowers on the grave stayed in: but the shot of the tombstone was cut on the instruction of the Controller of BBC1. The British public was not to know the significance of her action' (Curtis 1984: 51). An orchestrated public amnesia enveloped the political significance of the trauma, bereavement, and commemoration for nationalists in the North of Ireland, that was not dispelled for twenty years.[11]

Under these circumstances, the commemoration of the dead of Bloody Sunday is necessarily a political act, an instance of what the Palestinian-American writer and activist, Edward Said (1997), has called 'speaking truth to power'. The connections between past and present were pointed up by Sinn Féin President, Gerry Adams, in his speech at the twenty-fifth anniversary demonstration: 'Widgery was a lie, and Bloody Sunday remains pertinent today because it is an open wound. Bloody Sunday is the Sunday which has never ended' (cited in Sharrock 1997a). Trauma persists because of continuing injustice, not least in the implication that the dead were somehow not innocent. Hence speaker after speaker at this commemoration, as every year since 1972, echoed demands that 'the whole incident be reinvestigated', and that 'the British Government accepts full responsibility for the events' with a public apology (Mullen, in Chaudhary 1997a). These demands are currently supported by 'the Taoiseach . . . the leader of the opposition in the Republic, and the leaders of the two main nationalist parties in the North . . . [and] clearly the majority opinion in Ireland' (Rolston 1996: 8–9). Kay Duddy hoped that, 'Perhaps when we have had their names cleared we can come to terms with it and finally lay them to rest' (Sharrock 1997a). Yet while efforts to secure this necessary recognition are channelled through an inescapably political campaign, tensions and contradictions inevitably exist within the community between the requirements of public commemoration and the personal needs of mourning relatives and survivors. One, Mickey Bradley, who was shot whilst going to the aid of a wounded friend near the Rossville Flats, has objected to the event having 'become political' – 'we are here to commemorate our loved ones'(ibid.) – but calls nevertheless for 'the officers who gave the orders to open fire on us [to be] prosecuted. They are the real criminals' (Chaudhary 1997b: 4).

Bloody Sunday is a particularly illuminating case in two further respects. It exemplifies how the politicization of commemoration produced by the

Troubles is related both to inter-communal antagonism within Northern Ireland, and to the widespread cultural forgetting of the Irish conflict in England. Besides challenging the 'official amnesia' of the British state, the Bloody Sunday commemoration has also had to negotiate a current of triumphalism within loyalist memory. As the lyrics of one song in the Ulster Defence Association's *Detainee Song Book* (1974) go: 'Went to Derry not on a hunch/Knew I'd get a taig [Catholic] before lunch/Bang, Bang, Bang, Bloody Sunday/This is my, my, my beautiful day' (Bell 1976: 2). Recognition of the atrocity by unionists has been at best grudging. Their difficulty in 'sympathis[ing] with the relatives of the victims seeking an official government apology', stems from a perception that the killings had 'become so bound up in republican propaganda' (*Belfast News Letter* 1997). This position was reiterated by the Ulster Unionist security spokesperson, Ken Maginnis, who again dismissed calls for a new inquiry in his response to the twenty-fifth anniversary events (Sharrock 1997b), and by the leader of the Democratic Unionists in Derry, Gregory Campbell. The latter was reported as saying: 'Quite obviously the paratroopers took action that they ought not to have taken and innocent people died, but every year since that Sinn Féin and the IRA manipulate this event' (Sharrock 1997a). In 1997 – twenty-five years after the event – there has been a sign of a more generous spirit of recognition among unionists. An editorial statement by the staunchly unionist newspaper, the *Belfast News Letter*, condemned the shootings as 'unforgivable' and an 'appalling over-reaction' by the paratroopers, who 'opened fire indiscriminately with scant regard for the lives of others who were guilty of nothing': 'those who lost innocent loved ones deserve nothing less than a heartfelt, unambiguous apology from the highest possible source' (*Belfast News Letter* 1997).

English cultural amnesia about the event is more than a matter of traditional ignorance about the historical suffering of Northern Irish nationalist and republican communities (though it certainly does demonstrate this). Bloody Sunday is 'our tragedy' too, because it was an atrocity perpetrated 'in our name', and because it provided the catalyst for the start of the republican bombing campaign in England (Dillon 1996: 146–52). The psychoanalyst Rob Weatherill has argued that when we allow no 'place for death in our own lives', when we respond to it by 'the denial of death, [by] our refusal to take it on board'; then it returns in our lives as 'a trauma that comes from the *outside* . . . [a] radically excluded Other, which arises as if from another universe' (Weatherill 1994: 80–1, 83). When, on 22 February 1972, the Official IRA planted a bomb in a revenge attack on the Parachute Regiment's HQ in Aldershot, killing six civilian workers and a Catholic chaplain, the traumas of the Irish war indeed 'returned' – were 'brought home' – to England.

The English people have no equivalent to the politicized communal narratives of Northern Ireland as resources for making sense of the traumas of the war. Survivors often speak of a bombing as 'senseless' (see, e.g. *Aftershock* 1994). A counsellor, Jo Robertshaw, has suggested that, for the children of Warrington – traumatized by the town-centre bomb of 20 March 1993 that killed three-year-old Johnathan Ball and twelve-year-old Tim Parry – 'the overwhelming difficulty was the question why' (Jury 1994). Barry Chambers, a deputy-head teacher, noticed that: 'In the weeks following the bomb, the kids were saying "what is it about?" We realized there was a gap' (ibid.). Significantly, one year after the bomb, many children now wanted (in the words of sixteen-year-old Stephen Anderson) 'to find out why it happened and why it has been happening for so long' (ibid.). Steps had been taken to introduce Irish history into the curriculum of Warrington's St Thomas Boteler School, and the Warrington Project had been formed to establish contacts and exchanges with schools and communities in Ireland (ibid.). Here, the perception of a link between 'our suffering' and 'their suffering', together with a need to recover and make sense of a lost past, generates an alternative response to trauma. A strategy of remembering for reparation replaces denial, disavowal, and amnesia.

Remembering, recognition, and reparation: the cultural politics of peace

To speak of 'overcom[ing] the legacy of the past' in the Irish conflict, in an attempt to make peace by drawing a line under the past and 'moving on', is problematic for at least two reasons. It colludes with, and reproduces, the historic British denial of responsibility for the traumas of colonialism in Ireland; and it leaves intact deep sources of grief, grievance, and antagonism that are rooted in the recent history of the Troubles. An alternative perspective has been articulated by Martin Finucane of the Irish Campaign for Truth (launched in January 1995): 'If we are to overcome our past, we must come to terms with it and we can only do that if we know the truth about it' (Rolston 1996: 10).

Coming to terms with the past has, I have argued, a psychic as well as a political dimension, both of which need to be addressed and understood in their complex interaction. Real tensions and difficulties, both theoretical and practical in kind, are involved in holding together these two dimensions and integrating them into a coherent analysis. The relations between trauma and cultural processes of remembering and forgetting are characterized by an inherent ambivalence even without the further complications, contradictions, and paradoxes that accrue through the politics of an armed conflict. If the difficulties of 'coming to terms with' a traumatic past in the face of psychic defence and resistance are profound in whatever circumstance, they are greatly aggravated by the intense pressures of a war zone. Conceptual difficulties in making sense of the inter-relations between the psychic and the political are compounded by the danger of reductionism, whereby the importance of one dimension is asserted either without reference to, or in explicit negation of, the other. Thus, in gatherings of the politically minded, talk of 'the psyche' – of mourning, distress, emotional realities – can be dismissed as an irrelevant distraction from the serious political issues. In contrast, among those concerned with the psychic dimension, there is a tendency to define and explore these issues in terms of the personal, the private, the individual, the human. This is in contradistinction to social and political processes, which are reduced, oversimplified, and allowed no constitutive role in bringing about the many different kinds of traumatic experience.[12]

Despite these difficulties, the language of trauma nevertheless brings into focus the realities of psychic damage within the cultural, historical, and political relations in which the Irish and British peoples are mutually entwined and implicated. It challenges the strategies of containment, the amnesias, operating in much of the dominant cultural and political discourse on 'the national past' – and the current conflict – in both Britain and Ireland. It insists that there is a psychic as well as a cultural dynamic to remembering and forgetting, threaded through efforts at a political settlement capable of realigning past, present, and future. And it confronts the problem of whether, and how, it is possible to further the difficult process of psychic reparation necessary to any genuine reconciliation of deep-rooted and violent conflict; of whether, and how, it is possible to undo the plethora of psychic defences erected, like so many internal 'peace-lines', in defence against the traumas of the war.

There is no easy solution to these problems – no magic remedy to heal the traumatic past. However, at the core of any valid project of reparation must be initiatives that extend social – and public – recognition of trauma. I have argued throughout this essay that securing social recognition is a necessary part of the psychic process undergone by the bereaved and the traumatized as they struggle to come to terms with horror and loss. At the most fundamental level, the public acknowledgement of a violent death or injury, and the naming and calling-to-account of those responsible, establishes an objective foundation without which it may be impossible (in Kay Duddy's words) to 'finally lay [the dead] to rest'. Public recognition of the individuality of the dead and the particular circumstances of their death also supports the emotional work of mourning, which mobilizes profound desires to keep alive the name and value of the deceased in memory, thereby 'repairing' the damage wreaked within the 'inner world' of the psyche (Dawson 1994: 40–3, 117–20). Evidence of the desire for some form of public recognition is afforded by the unexpected success of a recent publication, *Bear in Mind These Dead* (1994), which simply recorded chronologically the names of all who have died in the current Troubles, with their age, the place and manner of death, and those responsible. The publisher was astonished when the entire print-run of 1,200 copies sold out with demand still high, and likened the function served by the booklet to that of the Vietnam memorial wall in Washington D.C. (Sutton 1994).[13]

The social recognition of trauma may be particularly valuable when it is extended to others across the communal and national divides, in a symbolic attempt to undo or reverse the reproduction of antagonism and hatred. One striking, recent instance of this was the attendance of leading loyalist, Gusty Spence, at the funeral in November 1996 of his friend, Kevin Lynch, a former IRA commander. Spence, now co-ordinator for the Progressive Unionist Party which represents the political views of the Ulster Volunteer Force, was himself a UVF paramilitary imprisoned for murder (Sharrock 1996).

Another recent example stemmed from the assassination by an IRA sniper of Lance-Bombardier Stephen Restorick at an Army checkpoint in South Armagh on 12 February 1997. A witness to the killing, local resident, Lorraine McElroy, who was wounded by the same bullet and accepted the family's invitation to the funeral in Peterborough, told the press that: 'People ask me if I'm nervous, as a[n Irish] Catholic, of going to a British soldier's funeral. But I'm not going to a British soldier's funeral. I'm going to the funeral of a young man who died in front of me' (*Guardian* 1997b). In the event, Mrs McElroy was prevented from attending due to the onset of symptoms believed to be those of post-traumatic stress disorder (Linton 1997). Hopes were expressed at the service 'that [Stephen Restorick's] death will be a catalyst to restart the peace process and bring both sides together to talk' (*Guardian* 1997c). His mother, Rita Restorick, 'out of a need to make some sense of her son's death', wrote to Gerry Adams appealing for the IRA ceasefire to be restored, and to other political leaders in Northern Ireland urging them to negotiate with Sinn Féin (Sharrock 1997c).[14]

As the Warrington Project demonstrates, such initiatives may be broadened into a genuinely communal practice of reparative remembering. Other opportunities are afforded by public commemorations, as in the belated recognition by unionists of Bloody Sunday, and in the proliferating forms of what Jane Leonard has termed 'inclusive commemoration', involving joint, cross-communal and inter-national participation particularly in events to mark the two world wars, the Irish Famine and the 1798 Rebellion (Leonard 1996a: 21–2). Like any challenge to dominant constructions of public memory, such initiatives may entail considerable difficulties and risks.

The most potent form in which social recognition may be extended across the frontiers of conflict is that of an acknowledgement and apology to the victims of a particular traumatic event by those responsible for it, either directly as perpetrators or indirectly as political representatives. When the Combined Loyalist Military Command announced its ceasefire on 13 October 1994, its statement (read by Gusty Spence) continued: 'In all sincerity we offer the loved ones of all innocent victims over the past twenty-five years abject and true remorse. No words of ours will compensate for the intolerable suffering they have undergone during the conflict' (Coogan 1996:

452). Sinn Féin leaders have made repeated apologies for IRA actions in recent years: Gerry Adams, for example, described the Frizzell's Fish Shop bombing as 'wrong' and a 'great tragedy, a devastating tragedy', offering 'my complete and absolute sympathy' (Boycott 1993), and in response to Rita Restorick's letter, 'generally gave his condolences and apologized for the grief that has been caused' (Sharrock 1997c).

Statements of this kind are often maligned as hypocritical and self-serving, especially whilst the violence continues. Yet these expressions of recognition, remorse and apology from both sides of the political divide represent serious attempts to undo the workings of defensive disavowal, hatred, and revenge, and to grapple with the contradictions of embroilment within an armed conflict. Besides their immediate value for survivors (Rita Restorick expressed herself 'pleased' at the Adams letter) the effectiveness of such gestures lies in their potential to elicit mutual recognition across the political divide. Ultimately, the quality of such exchanges will be judged by their contribution to ending hostilities and facilitating negotiations towards a just and lasting political settlement. The latter, in turn, is a condition of any thorough-going process of reconciliation. However, there is no guarantee that the social recognition of trauma will be placed at the centre of a political settlement. Here, the power of the state to help or hinder reparative remembering is decisive.

Fundamental to the project of reparation, therefore, are efforts to push 'truth and justice' onto the political agenda in a manner that involves the British state. The Sinn Féin leadership has consistently argued against the 'selective condemnation' of violence, whereby the IRA is demonized as solely responsible for causing death and suffering, whilst any action by the British military and the RUC is justified as a legitimate response to terrorism by the forces of 'law and order', and their collusion with the sectarian loyalist paramilitary groups (throughout the era of the unionist state ruled from Stormont, and continuing under direct rule from London) is denied and covered-up. Speaking at the 1995 Bloody Sunday commemoration, Adams argued that:

> There cannot be a healing process, a process of reconciliation unless all of us address honestly and openly the hurts we have caused. But everyone must do this – republicans and unionists and loyalists, and especially the British government. If John Major is genuinely committed to peace in this country, he should make a start by apologising to the people of Derry for the atrocity of Bloody Sunday.
>
> (Adams, quoted in Rolston 1996: 7)

The calls from throughout Ireland for an official apology for Bloody Sunday, and for a calling-to-account of the British soldiers and politicians responsible, have wider implications in that they demand 'acknowledgement of the truth that the British state has committed human rights violations' (ibid.: 38). This would involve a major shift in stance, away from the state's ideological self-representation as the honest broker towards an admission of its role as an active party to the conflict.

As Bill Rolston points out in his survey of the literature of human rights, the state 'has every reason to deny its extra-judicial violence' (unlike 'insurgent or counter-state groups' which tend 'to claim their operations as proof of their own strength and ability'):

> There is something particularly offensive about the human rights violations of the state. The state, after all, claims a monopoly on the legitimate use of force, the right to establish and oversee mechanisms of justice, and the key role in guaranteeing the life, happiness and security of its citizens. . . . An inability to have any influence over the state's behaviour makes for intense vulnerability on the part of victims of state abuses of power. One can always hope that the state can identify and bring to trial or detention someone from a non-state organisation who has abused one's human rights. But who guards the guards?
>
> (Ibid.: 20)

For these reasons, there is a particular desire for, and onus upon, public recognition by the state of traumas inflicted on its behalf.

Notwithstanding the talk of 'reconciliation' and 'healing' in the Downing Street Declaration, the Conservative Government proved unresponsive to the calls for justice and redress emanating from Ireland. This prompted the formation of the Irish Campaign for Truth and its call (following some fifteen international precedents between 1974 and 1994) for the establishment of a truth commission (ibid.: 17): that is, an official, state-sponsored investigative body set up to advance an inclusive process of truth-telling and public acknowledgement of human rights violations in a society emerging from a period of violent conflict and state repression. Rolston acknowledges both 'the dilemma . . . in seeking justice while the offending regime is still in power', and the current lack of popular support in Ireland for the truth commission proposal: 'even during the eighteen-month cease-fire [the question of human rights abuses] was not a central element in political debate' (ibid.: 21, 48). He concedes, too, the unlikelihood of willing collaboration by the British state – whether to make apology, to release information on security force activities, or to facilitate 'the prosecution of state personnel for past human rights abuses' – under any new political arrangements that might be achieved in Ireland as a result of the peace process (ibid.: 50).[15] Nevertheless, Rolston is right in his insistence that 'the right to truth [is] a crucial political demand', fundamental to 'the attempt to construct a just peace'; and that, even without state endorsement, a broadly-based truth commission enjoying legitimacy both within Ireland and internationally could make a valuable contribution in promoting social recognition of the traumatic past, 'in the interests of reconciliation and healing' (ibid.: 48–9, 51).

A truth commission would be of value not only in Ireland but in Britain too, where a veil of official secrecy continues to obscure the past, and to impede a necessary reassessment of the state's role in, and the social and cultural impact of, the conflict. There are encouraging signs that a process of reparative remembering is currently underway, with 'the stories we need to hear' increasingly being aired on television and film, in fictional writing and other cultural forms. For example, investigative documentaries – on Bloody Sunday, the Birmingham pub-bombings, and the miscarriages of justice in the cases of the Birmingham Six and Guildford Four – have done much to promote recognition by the British people of what has been done in their name, and of the costs of war that they have borne. A number of high-profile feature films have introduced British audiences to Irish nationalist and republican perspectives (on anti-Irish racism, the Famine, the republican prisoners' hunger strikes of 1980-1, and the struggle for Irish independence) which, only a few years ago, would have been anathema.[16] Receptivity to initiatives that aim to unlock the fixities of the remembered past has been boosted by the political peace process, and especially by the joint ceasefires, during which the anti-terrorist broadcasting ban was lifted and new cultural spaces opened up in both Ireland and Britain.[17] A truth commission would help to deepen and extend the process that is currently underway, investigating the damage, psychic and social, wreaked by the war. It would clarify its origins in the intertwined histories of the two islands, recover this as indeed a part of 'British history', and thus begin to undo the work of colonial disavowal.

Kay Duddy's hopes are that, 'Perhaps when we have had their names cleared we can come to terms with it and finally lay them to rest' (Sharrock 1997a). Perhaps. But there are limits to any 'healing' of psychic damage. The psychotherapist, Susie Orbach, reflecting on the South African process of 'truth and reconciliation', points out:

> [A]s the Truth Commission openly acknowledges, it would be naive to think that it can wipe away the emotional pain of the individuals whose lives have been marked by acts perpetrated under apartheid. Those wounds never completely heal. . . . The trauma is never fully in the past, but lives on in the present. Perhaps the most we can hope for is that if the wrongdoing and trauma are recognised in the present, future generations will experience the repercussions as their history rather than as their present.

> (Orbach 1996: 6)

Reparation may not always be possible for the generations marked by communal trauma, and this can also be reproduced through family relationships into the following generation.[18] Trauma persists – but reparation is about mobilizing the resources of hope, so that living can go on in its wake. In time a new society may be created, where the hard work of reparation can be undertaken in freedom from violence and fear.

Postscript

Since this essay was completed in July 1997, multi-party talks on the future of Northern Ireland have taken place under the aegis of the new Labour Government in Britain and the new Fianna Fail-led Coalition Government in the Republic of Ireland. In the context of these ongoing political negotiations, the British Government announced a new public, judicial inquiry into the events of Bloody Sunday (MacAskill 1998, Walsh 1998). On 10 April 1998 the talks concluded with an Agreement between the parties and the two governments (NIO 1998). This was prefaced by a six-point Declaration of Support, the second point affirming that: 'The tragedies of the past have left a deep and profoundly regrettable legacy of suffering. We must never forget those who have died or been injured, and their families. But we can best honour them through a fresh start, in which we firmly dedicate ourselves to the achievement of reconciliation, tolerance, and mutual trust, and to the vindication of the human rights of all (ibid.: 1). Provision is made in the Agreement for new Human Rights Commissions to be established north and south of the border and for their representatives to meet in a joint committee (ibid.: 16–18). In a section explicitly concerned with 'Reconciliation and Victims of Violence', the Agreement affirms that 'it is essential to acknowledge and address the suffering of the victims of violence as a necessary element of reconciliation'; and it recognizes that 'victims have a right to remember as well as to contribute to a changed society'. A Northern Ireland Victims Commission will investigate these issues, and the Agreement includes a commitment to allocate resources in support of community-based initiatives . . . that are supportive and sensitive to the needs of victims' (ibid.: 18).

Notes

This essay was written and revised between January and July 1997. Earlier versions were presented as papers at the Critical Dialogues Seminar, Dept. of Sociology, University of Essex, 27 February 1997; the Faculty of Art, Design, and Humanities Open Seminar, University of Brighton, 3 March 1997; and the London History Workshop, 2 June 1997. I am grateful to all who contributed to those discussions; and to Sue Dare, Susannah Radstone, and Alistair Thomson for their critical reading of drafts. Developments in the Irish peace process, which have occurred since the completion of the essay and which bear directly upon its themes, are noted in a brief postscript.

1   See, respectively, Walker (1996: 61); Leonard (1996a: 5); Boyce and O'Day

(1996, 63, 90 and 97); Bourke (1996: 145 and 231); Boyce and O'Day (1996: 54); Longley (1991: 43).

2 I use 'Britain' and 'British' when referring to the state, to Empire, and in a general sense to the culture of England, Scotland, and Wales; and 'England' and 'English' when a more specific focus is intended.

3 Chambers Twentieth Century Dictionary.

4 For my concept of 'social recognition', see Dawson (1994: 22–6, 205–6, 259–77, passim).

5 The psychoanalytic concepts used here are those developed in the Kleinian tradition. See Dawson (1994: 27–52) and Frosh (1987: 242–8).

6 For this phenomenon in the Irish Republic, see Sharrock (1994).

7 Cf. the response of some loyalist mourners after the IRA's Shankill Road bomb, 23 October 1993: 'I just think they are IRA scum. . . . I just hope the UVF and the UFF go in and get them sorted. If I had a gun myself I would go out and shoot them.' Margeret Martin, cited in Weale (1993: 3).

8 For the psychic significance of revenge, see Dawson (1994: 93–9, 112–3, 119).

9 Examples include the IRA's bombing of the Remembrance Day ceremony at Enniskillen, 8 November 1987, and the fatal attack by loyalist Michael Stone on the funeral at Milltown Cemetery, Belfast, 16 March 1988, of the three IRA Volunteers killed in Gibraltar; both described in Bew and Gillespie (1993). See also Leonard (1996a: 20) and Leonard (1996b).

10 According to Don Mullen (1997), the report 'failed to take proper account of all the available evidence.'

11 Significant interventions were made by two TV films, Remember Bloody Sunday, broadcast BBC2, 30 January 1992; and Sunday, Bloody Sunday, broadcast Channel 4, 30 January 1997.

12 On the difficulties of integrating psychic and socio-political analyses, see Dawson (1996: 75–102).

13 Representative of Beyond the Pale Publications, in conversation with the author, 19 November 1996, Belfast.

14 Sharrock suggests that this is 'the first time the parents of a soldier murdererd by the IRA has (sic) written in such terms to the leader of its political wing'.

15 For early signs that this might change under the 'New Labour' Government elected on 1 May 1997, see Sharrock (1997c: 3).

16 For documentaries see, for example, Who Bombed Birmingham? (1990), Remember Bloody Sunday (1992), Aftershock (1994) and Sunday, Bloody Sunday (1997). Features include In the Name of the Father (1993), The Hanging Gale (1995), Some Mother's Son (1996), and Michael Collins (1996). A recent high-profile novel, exploring the repercussions of political violence with origins in the armed conflict of the early 1920s, is Seamus Deane, Reading in the Dark (1996), shortlisted for the Booker Prize.

17 For example Michael Collins, produced during this period, survived calls from the British right for it to be banned as an IRA propaganda film. It provoked a far-reaching debate about the history of the Anglo-Irish and Civil Wars and their relationship to the ongoing national question, confronting both British amnesia and what Edna Longley (1991: 43) has described as the 'traumatized silence' about the Civil War in Irish popular memory. See Jordan (1996); Lee (1996a); Lee (1996b).

18 See, for example, the accounts now emerging from children of Holocaust survivors (Karpf 1996).

References

Aftershock: the Untold Story of the Birmingham Pub Bombings, broadcast on BBC2, 9 November 1994.

Belfast News Letter (3 Feb. 1997), Editorial, cited in D. Sharrock, 'Bloody Sunday inquiry calls grow', *Guardian*, 4 Feb. 1997: 5.

Bell, G. (1976) *The Protestants of Ulster*, London.

Bew, P. and Gillespie, G. (1993) *Northern Ireland: A Chronology of the Troubles*, Dublin.

Bourke, J. (1996) *Dismembering the Male: Men's Bodies, Britain and the Great War*, London.

Boyce, D. G. (1972) *Englishmen and Irish Troubles: British Public Opinion and the Making of Irish Policy 1918–1922*, London.

Boyce, D. G. and O'Day, A. (eds) (1996) *The Making of Modern Irish History: Revisionism and the Revisionist Controversy*, London and New York.

Boycott, O. (1993) 'Adams denies tactics split', *Guardian,* 26 Oct. 1993: 3.

Bradshaw, B. (1994) 'Nationalism and historical scholarship', in C. Brady (ed.), *Interpreting Irish History: The Debate on Historical Revisionism*, Dublin and Portland, : 191–216.

Brady, C. (ed.) (1994) *Interpreting Irish History: The Debate on Historical Revisionism*, Dublin and Portland.

Chaudhary, V. (1997a) 'Killings doubts will not go away', *Guardian*, 18 Jan. 1997: 4.

—— (1997b) 'My whole world was turned upside down', *Guardian*, 18 Jan. 1997: 4.

Coogan, T. P. (1996) *The Troubles: Ireland's Ordeal 1966–1996 and the Search for Peace*, London.

Curtis, L. (1984) *Ireland: The Propaganda War. The British Media and the 'Battle for Hearts and Minds'*, London.

Dawson, G. (1994) *Soldier Heroes: British Adventure, Empire and the Imagining of Masculinities*, London and New York.

—— (1996) 'The paradox of authority: psychoanalysis, history and cultural criticism', *Angelaki*, vol. 2: 75–102.

Deane, S. (1996) *Reading in the Dark*, London.

Dillon, M. (1996) *Twenty-five Years of Terror: The IRA's War Against the British*, London.

Downing Street Declaration, reproduced in full in *Guardian*, 16 Dec. 1993: 2.

Farrell, M. (1980) *Northern Ireland: The Orange State*, London.

Ferenczi, S. *et al.* (eds) (1921) *Psycho-Analysis and the War Neuroses*, London.

Foster, R. (1989) *Modern Ireland 1600–1972*, London.

Freud, S. (1920) 'Beyond the pleasure principle', in *On Metapsychology*, ed. A. Richards (1984), London.

Freud, S. and Breuer, J. (1895) *Studies on Hysteria*, ed. A. Richards (1974), London.

Frosh, S. (1987) *The Politics of Psychoanalysis*, London.

Goodall, H. (1994) 'Colonialism and catastrophe: contested memories of nuclear testing and measles epidemics at Ernabella', in K. Darian-Smith and P. Hamilton (eds), *Memory and History in Twentieth-Century Australia,* Melbourne.

Guardian (1997a) 'The blast that shattered the Docklands', 'The Week' supplement, 15 Feb.: 15.

—— (1997b) 'Ulster woman to attend funeral of British soldier shot in front of her', 15 Feb. 1997: 4.

—— (1997c) 'Murder of soldier should act as catalyst to restart peace process, funeral told', 25 Feb. 1997: 4.

Holland, M. (1997) 'The secrets of troubled minds', *Observer,* 19 Jan. 1997.

Ignatieff, M. (1996) 'Articles of faith', in 'Wounded nations, broken lives', *Index on Censorship, Irish News,* vol. 25, no. 5.

Irish News, 25 February 1994

Jordan, N. (1996) 'Truths we must tell', *Guardian Friday Review,* 25 Oct. 1996: 2–3, 19.

Jury, L. (1994) 'Pupils who escaped IRA bombs seek answer to a very tough question', *Guardian,* 19 March 1994: 5.

Karpf, A. (1996) *The War After: Living With the Holocaust,* London.

Kiberd, D. (1985) 'Anglo-Irish attitudes', in Field Day Company, *Ireland's Field Day,* Derry.

—— (1991) 'The elephant of revolutionary forgetfulness', in M. Ní Dhonnchada and T. Dorgan (eds) *Revising the Rising,* Derry.

Kirkaldy, J. (1992) 'Anglo-Irish relations: things have changed', *Irish Studies Review,* vol. 1: 40.

Krog, A. (1997) 'Cry, beloved country', *Guardian,* 18 Jan. 1997.

Lee, J. (1996a) 'Reeling back the years', *Sunday Tribune,* 3 Nov. 1996: 14–15.

—— (1996b) '*Michael Collins* and the teaching of Irish history', *Sunday Tribune,* 17 Nov. 1996: 16.

Leonard, J. (1996a) *The Culture of Commemoration: The Culture of War Commemoration,* Dublin.

—— (1996b) 'The twinge of memory: Armistice Day and Remembrance Sunday in Dublin since 1919', in R. English and G. Walker (eds), *Unionism in Modern Ireland,* Dublin: 99–114.

Linton, M. (1977) 'Shooting witness has breakdown', *Guardian,* 17 Feb. 1977: 5.

Longley, E. (1991) 'The Rising, the Somme and Irish memory', in M. Ní Dhonnchadha and T. Dorgan (eds), *Revising the Rising,* Derry.

MacAskill, E. (1998) 'Bloody Sunday inquiry', *Guardian,* 29 Jan. 1998: 1.

Mullen, D. (ed.) (1997) *Eyewitness: Bloody Sunday,* Dublin.

Ní Dhonnchadha, M. and Dorgan, T. (eds) (1991) *Revising the Rising,* Derry.

NIO (1998) *The Agreement: Agreement Reached in the Multi-Party Negotiations* (Northern Ireland Office).

Orbach, S. (1996) 'When truth is not enough', *Guardian Weekend,* 26 Oct. 1996: 6.

Remember Bloody Sunday, broadcast BBC2, 30 January 1992.

Rolston, B. (1996) *Turning the Page Without Closing the Book: the Right to Truth in the Irish Context,* Dublin.

Said, E. (1997) 'The pen and the sword': in discussion with Jacqueline Rose at the Brighton Festival, Brighton, England, 14 May 1997.

Shankill People, 'We will remember them', Memorial Issue, November 1993.

Sharrock, D. (1994) 'Families remember forgotten massacre', *Guardian*, 16 May 1994.

—— (1996) 'Gusty wind of change', *Guardian*, 16 Dec. 1996: 6–7.

—— (1997a) 'New Bloody Sunday inquiry plea rebuffed as up to 20,000 join march', *Guardian*, 3 Feb. 1997: 7.

—— (1997b) 'Bloody Sunday inquiry calls grow', *Guardian*, 4 Feb. 1997: 5.

—— (1997c) 'IRA victim's kin hail letter', *Guardian*, 12 March 1997: 6.

—— (1997d) 'Blair says sorry for Britain's "failure" in the Irish famine', *Guardian*, 2 June 1997: 3.

Sunday, Bloody Sunday, broadcast Channel 4, 30 January 1997.

Sutton, M. (1994) *Bear in Mind These Dead: An Index of Deaths from the Conflict in Ireland, 1969–1993*, Belfast.

Trouble With Peace, broadcast Channel 4, 30 August 1995.

'Voices of the victims' (1996) interview with Damian Gorman, *Causeway*, vol. 3, no. 3: 39–43.

Walker, B. (1996) *Dancing to History's Tune: History, Myth and Politics in Ireland*, Belfast.

Walsh, D. (1998) 'Inquiry to shed light on shadows of Widgery', *Irish Times*, 30 Jan. 1998, http://www.irish-times.com.

Weale, S. (1993) 'Peace and revenge vie as Belfast mourns', *Guardian*, 26 Oct. 1993: 3.

Weatherill, R. (1994) *Cultural Collapse*, London.

Who Bombed Birmingham? (Granada), broadcast on ITV, 28 March 1990.

Part 2

DEBATES AND REVIEWS

10

REALITY OR NOTHING!

False and repressed memories and autobiography

J. P. Roos

Dennis Potter's last TV-series, *Cold Lazarus*, tells how the deep-frozen brain of a TV-writer – a thinly veiled Potter himself – is reactivated after 300 years. His brain begins to produce visual memories, which are the object of both scientific and commercial interest: a group of scientists debates them and a ruthless TV mogul plans to broadcast them as the ultimate 'reality TV'. In the memories, the subject is alternately a little boy or the man at the age of his death, sometimes in the clothes of the boy. At one point the little boy is sexually abused by a village marginal, a memory which is unclear and dim at places. Later memories, in contrast, are shown very graphically and narratively and in utmost detail.

The point of the series is that the activating of memories demands conscious participation from the brain, although the scientists presume that it has no will of its own. In fact, the memory work recreates the personality of the writer. The brain becomes more and more distressed, sending messages of wanting to be free from the memory work (to the astonishment of the scientists who did not believe that the brain could regain consciousness). The happy end is brought about by a member of the team, posing as (or actually being, I don't remember!) a 'ronnie': a Reality or Nothing terrorist who tries to free the world from the clutches of global entertainment monopolies that separate the people from reality. The 'ronnie' destroys the machine to which the brain is connected, thus liberating the brain from its memories, and simultaneously killing it.

In this story, producing memories is seen as a painful, difficult but very precise process. The brain, free from all kinds of mental or bodily hindrances, remembers everything, exactly.

This also seems to be the view of the so-called recovered-memory therapy movement, which believes that there are events which are so difficult and horrible (and sexual) that they are totally repressed, to emerge at some later date, prompted by some association or similarity. The problem with this assumption is that it is extremely difficult to verify such memory recovery, either because there is no independent confirmation of the event or because we can never know whether it really was forgotten at all.[1]

This said, I don't wish to deny the possibility of re-remembering forgotten events stored in the unconscious parts of the brain. The well-known Proustian Madeleine remembrance is an innocuous case of the same phenomenon, except that there is no repression behind the forgotten event. In fact, madeleine-type associative long-forgotten memories are extremely common, almost daily occurrences. Another type of real memory recovery happens when somebody starts writing autobiographical reminiscences; working at one's past is sure to bring about fresh memories (how reliable they are is another question).

The problems I want to address are first, whether it is possible to repress completely from one's memory important events in one's life, and second, what implications this has for autobiographies (that is, whether one might write entirely different life stories depending on one's memories). This is a question which actually underlies most of the history of psychoanalysis from its beginning, as Freud himself can be described as the first repressed memory therapist.[2]

An instance of recovered memory which is important because it has affirmed the reality of recovered memories in court and as a consequence sent a person in jail for murder and rape, is the case of Eileen Lipsker (Terr 1994).

Eileen Lipsker had a highly troubled childhood and youth (alcohol, a violent father, a mother with mental problems, divorce, sexual promiscuity, drug use etc.). She later married and had two children, the older an eight-year-old daughter. One day she happened to look at her daughter in a position which brought back a similar position of her best friend, who had been eight years old when she was raped and killed. The following days and weeks brought back previously repressed memories of having seen her father – an occasionally violent man and heavy drinker – kill her friend during an outing. After these first memories Eileen also recovered memories of being sexually abused by the father. The memory of the murder as described by Eileen was very vivid and detailed.

Eileen was already in therapy because of marital difficulties and probably also problems related to her past. After discussions with her therapist, she came forward with her accusations. The father was brought to justice and condemned in the end, even though there was no other evidence connecting him to the murder. The father denied the murder but did not deny the allegations of incest, which certainly increased the reliability of Eileen's testimony. (The defence chose a strategy intended to show that Eileen had reason to hate her father so much that she could even invent a murder accusation.) It was later revealed that all details described by Eileen Lipsker had been published previously and that the possibility of the father's guilt was already entertained by Eileen's estranged mother and sister, while at the time Eileen was completely silent about her presence in the scene of murder.

In all, Terr's version of the case of Eileen Lipsker did not sound very plausible. There were several reasons to suspect her testimony and the role of her therapist was central. In fact, the wave of recovered memory cases may have given Eileen Lipsker the idea of coming forward with her accusations in a new form. Even if they were true, we can not know whether she had remembered the event all the time, but had been ashamed to come forward after her initial silence. In fact, the conviction of Eileen's father has since been overturned and he has been released (Pendergrast 1996, Showalter 1997). I don't know whether he is now, in turn, suing his daughter and her therapist, or maybe even the expert witness Terr.

This debate over the truth or falsity of repressed memories has been raging for several years, mainly in the USA.[3] On the one hand, many psychotherapists believe that children and young adults can repress difficult and traumatic memories, and then recover them.[4] This has led to several court cases and other situations where children have made serious accusations against their parents, other relatives or friends of the family. The opposite point of view is that such fatal memories as rape, sexual abuse, violence, cannot be repressed and that their 'recovery' is always spurious. Either the memory has always existed or it is pure fantasy (or a mixture of fantasy and real events, as is any product of the unconscious). In the famous Chris 'experiment' a young boy was told a completely false story about his having lost his way in a shopping centre, when he was very small. Some years later, when he was told that this had never happened, he refused to believe it, because the memory had become completely real for him (Loftus and Ketcham 1994). This proves at least that memories, whether real or unreal, have the same reality for those who have them. When they exist, it is impossible to distinguish them from real events. And when the memories don't exist, it doesn't help much if we are told that we should remember them (how many times have we been told that such and such thing has happened but we have no memory of it?).

This problem has not been discussed in relation to autobiography, but it is important from a theoretical point of view. Is the writing or telling of an autobiography in any way related to the process of memory recovery? If so, what about false memory? What implications does this discussion have for the realist approach to life stories?

The recovered-or-false memory debate has until now mainly taken place in the USA (and the UK). This debate is in many ways typically American: naive exaggerations, extreme positions on both sides, dramatic court cases, monetary considerations.[5] In Europe, the situation is much more subdued: discussions inside professions, confrontation between therapy-oriented social workers, doctors and families. In Europe there is also much more often a situation where there is conflict between families and the state itself; in extreme cases social welfare administrations have taken custody of children against the will of the parents. The well-known Swedish child 'Gulags' have stigmatized the European welfare state as a leviathan-like system which crushes the individual, beginning with the child (Aminoff 1996).[6] In European cases also, it is not so much false memory that is at issue as the trustworthiness of children and the interpretations of therapists.[7]

The false memory debate is an extreme example of the problem of the trustworthiness and reality of life stories as a whole. Even more generally, it fuels the debate between realistic and textual positions in the analysis of life stories. This problem has been a classic question in philosophy. Bertrand Russell described memorably in his autobiography how happy he was when he finally could believe that tables or houses really existed and were not just imaginary constructs (Monk 1997). It was declared a non-question by Wittgenstein for whom there were only things to be discussed with language and images which could not be expressed with words at all. This debate of external vs. linguistic reality was introduced into the social sciences gradually via linguistics, psychoanalysis, literary studies and post-modern theory. In brief, it is a question of whether there is an external reality ('real life') of which the life story is a more or less faithful rendering or if we should rather see life as being a narrative, a social or language construct, ever changing and always newly constructed so that all the different versions are equally true.

Ian Hacking (1997) has given an interesting example of social construction: the 'construction' of child abuse. Child abuse was 'discovered' in the 1960s when doctors noticed that children's fractures were the result of severe beatings. By 1975 child abuse had become sexual, so that the actual mistreatment and violence had been practically forgotten. Mistreatment of children has always existed and has always been considered wrong even though the tolerance of corporal punishment has somewhat diminished. The social construction, then, is relatively independent of the phenomenon itself, precisely as a realist (like myself) would say. It would be absurd to say that child abuse (in its sexual meaning) is a pure social construction of the 1970s. But as Hacking notes, it has now become an absolute Evil, so that discussion of sexuality of children has become extremely difficult (think also of the difficulties of remaking and distributing Lolita).

I have participated elsewhere (1994, 1997) in this debate (see also Bertaux 1996, 1997). My own position is that people may have somewhat different versions of their life stories during different periods of their lives and that contextual effects are very important (for instance depending on whether the story is written for their children or if its context is work). Nevertheless, the basic story is very much the same and, more importantly, the individual always strives to render the version that most adequately represents his or her life, as presently understood by the writer. The changes introduced in the life story are more often than not results of an improved understanding or knowledge bringing the story closer to the 'real life', not new arbitrary versions attempting to create a new identity.

Bertrand Russell reports from a privately conducted experiment with one of his women friends: 'If you try to persuade an ordinary uneducated person that she cannot call up a visual picture of a friend sitting in a chair, but can only use words describing what such an occurrence would be like, she will conclude that you are mad' (Monk 1997). My own favourite example is the quite ordinary distinction between external reality and its linguistic expression which we experience when we try to find a word for a thing which we have in mind, but cannot express it in words: an extremely frustrating experience. You know perfectly what it is you want to express, but you cannot do it in words.

The false memory debate is precisely about this: are the 'new' memories which completely change a person's view of his or her previous life (memories of being sexually abused by close relatives, or other equally traumatic and terrible events which suddenly emerge from the subconscious and can become extremely concrete and realistic) really true or are they just imaginary products? Are they created in cooperation with a professional therapist who specializes in such memories, or after reading books on the subject etc., or can they even be caused by the general atmosphere, media publicity and so on? Are they real or just constructs? This is an extreme case of the more ordinary question of how a life story is connected to the real life. Or, in other words, it is an extreme case of the thesis of social or narrative constructionism.

For a realistically-oriented life-story researcher, this question is a very tricky one: we usually assume that people's stories are mainly true and that they usually fail by omission, not by fabrication or pure invention. And we (the realists) are unwilling to admit that there is a strong tendency to construct different versions depending on the social situations in which they are told. Therefore, if there is a possibility that people can produce whole episodes (and very central ones) of their lives out of thin air (even though they believe these episodes are true), the realist position seems very weak indeed. On the other hand, false memories are a very strong argument for the postmodern view of social reality: people may construct whatever stories they wish and these need not have any connection with real events. Incidentally, note that the therapists producing these memories are ambivalent realists: their livelihood depends on the belief of the reality of the recovered memories (and they criticise Freudian psycho-analysis for having denied this reality), but they are not so keen on the necessity of proof (Pendergrast 1996).

Of course a realist may choose to believe in the recovered memories which usually give a very dramatic picture of a previously rather dull or 'normal' reality. But in this case he or she will also have to deal with extremely conflicting descriptions of the same reality: the stories before and after the 'recovery', and the versions of other relatives who are usually quite unaware of what has been (supposedly) happening. The best solution for the realist would be to require proof, corroboration of the memories, and a healthy suspicion of the more dramatic and unbelievable versions (such as satanic rituals, extreme forms of sexual abuse and fantastic children's stories).

I shall not discuss here the problem of individual or family secrets, those situations where some event has been kept a secret for a long time and then suddenly revealed. Secrets are another very interesting, related question. It can be said that most families and individuals have their intimate secrets, in many cases quite dramatic ones (Vigouroux 1993). Some of these secrets may be precisely the kind revealed through 'recovered' memories. In the Eileen Lipsker case, discussed above, one plausible explanation is that Eileen reveals a family secret in a 'socially acceptable' way (this is my own explanation for it, assuming that her father was guilty). Here I explicitly discuss cases where it is claimed that something has happened to the person, that he or she has completely forgotten the event (repressed it) and that at some later stage he or, more often, she suddenly remembers it, recovers it, usually with the help of a psychotherapist who specializes in recovered memories. I am not interested in the more extreme (and patently false) cases of satanic rituals, UFOs, snowballing stories of whole communities involved and the like (Ofshe and Watters 1994, Showalter 1997), which are forms of mass or collective hysteria. My concern is with those cases where there is a memory which the person genuinely believes and where it is really possible that the event has taken place.

A related question is what the children remember and can tell about sexual abuse, violence and other traumatic events. They are usually quite unreliable as witnesses, not because they want to invent things or make them up, but rather because they can be easily influenced and are very difficult as interview subjects. This is a problem when therapists or the police come up with questions that lead the child into specific conclusions. In Finland, there is one very famous case which showed how difficult it is to stop the process once the witch hunt has been started (Ristoja, Aulikki and Thomas 1996).

I have not personally encountered cases of life stories where people have recovered previously forgotten memories. In their life stories they may use previous diaries which describe events of which they have no direct memories, but otherwise they tell what they remember and have remembered. They may attempt to go back as far in the childhood as possible and also attempt to distinguish those memories told by others and those remembered authentically (this is also possible to deduce on the basis of the remembered episode; a child cannot usually know complicated terms or places and the memory is always somewhat unclear). But I have *not* encountered spontaneous autobiographies with recovered memories. If there is incest or violence, this maybe something that the author has kept a secret but now revealed in the autobiography (the cases of incest related in the stories are relatively innocuous, with some notable exceptions).

According to Frederic Crews (1997) there are no cases in which repression has been 'proved' to exist during the past sixty years. Whenever Mark Pendergrast (1996) tried to get corroboration for cases cited by defenders of recovered memory, he found no solid evidence. There are, however some cases where we have independent evidence of traumatic events in childhood such as accidents, kidnapping and revealed cases of child abuse (and of course one could think of other such events, for example, children taken from their parents when extremely young). In these cases it is possible to ask the now-adult persons what they remember of the event. In all cases they must now be aware of the facts; it would be unethical to remind them. Some of them admit to remembering the events all the time, some don't remember what happened to them, but none report a spontaneous recovery of the memory.

What is most astonishing is that there is so little research which seeks corroborative evidence for repression. In an article devoted to this question there are only two references of this kind among literally hundreds discussing the phenomenon of repressed memory (Conway 1997, Pendergrast 1996). In the case of recovered sexual abuse memories, it is obvious that the other witness(es) of the event will have a strong incentive to deny it, but one should still expect that during the period in which 'recovered' memories have been known, there should be some actually proven cases, not only claims and counter-claims. Frederic Crews (1997: 165) mentions one case where it has been proven that a recovered memory of sexual molestation was real. Even here, the question about its repression is not clear: the incident was not very traumatic and it may simply have been forgotten.

In other words, the recovered-memory discussion throws more light on the debate concerning reality and construction of life stories than on the actual question of repression of memories. Here I think that the main problem lies in the risks brought about by accepting the idea that life stories are just constructs which should not be taken as representations of reality.

The main risk here is that the analysis of life stories becomes in a sense independent of the actual story. We become free to give any interpretations we wish, even ones absolutely contrary to the claims of the narrators. We lose all (or most) sense of reality. It is in my view much better to err on the side of mistaken belief in the reality of the story than mistakenly believe that the story is completely malleable.

A Finnish colleague, Matti Hyvärinen, has on several occasions discussed the life story of a Finnish leftist student activist 'Anu Rantanen', whom he interviewed several years ago. The story itself is not very complicated. As a young student, Anu Rantanen becomes involved in the communist student movement, is very active and for a time even becomes chairperson of a local group. All the time, however, she describes herself as unsure of herself and feeling completely alienated from her true self, who is not at all the outward oriented, politically dogmatic activist everybody else perceives. What is most intriguing in her story is that while she herself says that she gave up on the ideology quite early, immediately after the peak period of the movement (in the mid-1970s), she actually resigned from the Communist Party only in the mid-1980s, hanging around as a passive but paying member for a long time.

Since Hyvärinen presented this case for the first time (1994), he has changed his position completely ('this is my sixth version' he says in 1997!) The first version described Anu Rantanen as an apolitical person who just happened to be politically active and was somewhat mystified about the long process of separation. The most recent version shows Anu Rantanen as a person true to herself and politically very conscious, so that her story becomes a coherent and very political story rather than the earlier incoherent, conflicting and very unpolitical one. In the last version, the slow process of separation follows logically from her identity as a withdrawn, self-effacing woman. Her self-rhetoric is no longer seen as conflicting with her actual life, but is perceived as actually very coherent: being a dogmatic and leading activist in conflict with her own feelings was only logical for a quiet and self-effacing person (who does not wish to show off by coming clean).

For me, Hyvärinen is a good example of the extreme fictive-story approach. Anything is possible. The rhetoric is everything; the 'simple' question of what kind of life do the stories describe is much less interesting than questions about production of gender and identity in the life stories, both narratively and textually.

Why should one have to suppose that people are producing gender in their stories, independently of their 'real' gender produced by social and biological facts or that their future lives would be influenced by their way of telling about their past lives. If I could paraphrase Bertrand Russell, we could find hypothetical 'ordinary' people and ask them how they are producing their genders, or how they are influencing their lives by their stories, or even to whom they are telling their life stories? As Russell says, they would consider the person asking such questions to be quite mad (or at least incomprehensible). Or take another example: in most European languages, there is the cumbersome division between he and she (not to speak of gendered nouns!), so that a gender-conscious author must either avoid the third person or use he/she (or she/he). Miraculously, in Finnish such a distinction does not exist: there is only one third person pronoun which refers to both genders, and there are no gendered articles as in French or German. Does this mean that we Finns have a different conception of gender than other people? The textualists should certainly think so. The only consequence I am aware of, is that we have great difficulties in distinguishing between gendered words in other languages, but certainly not between 'real' gender (or not less or more than anybody else).

Hyvärinen in turn criticizes my position, in which I have claimed that ordinary people write their stories better when they are free from literary conventions and that all kinds of obvious literary means function more or less as a veil between the 'real thing' and the story. Against that, Hyvärinen posits the linguistic turn, in which the feeling of reality and authenticity is created only by the different literary or stylistic genres, or vocabulary, not by any relation to the life itself, of which it is impossible to know anything. In addition, in Hyvärinen's view, all stories are directed to a public, and thus are strictly contextual. He gives as an example a reading of Augustine's *Confessions*, which lends itself readily to a rhetorical interpretation, being simultaneously a 'true confession' and a document whose objective is to convert people and convince those already converted.

Augustine is a good counter-example of what ordinary life stories usually attempt to do, but its 'rhetoric' of truth, and especially the idea that God sees everything, has strongly affected the idea of autobiography. Without Rousseau and Augustine, we would not have the idea of the truth as a basic requirement of autobiography. This is also a good instance of the influence of great literary autobiographies in ordinary life stories, in which it is not so much the model or style that is important but a principle (often misunderstood), the origin of which is usually unknown to the author. Even though Hyvärinen comes round to the view that the realistic starting point is also important (referentiality and reality are essential parts of the life story for him, unlike many constructivists), he tries, it seems to me, to reconcile things which cannot be reconciled. Either there is an attempt to approximate reality through narrative or else there is a rhetorical construction of one's past and future life.

The problem with constructivism is its elusiveness. A good example of this is Dausien's 1996 analysis of differences between women's and men's autobiographical interviews. The analysis shows that men differ from women in telling stories where they are single heroes and other personages (such as wives or children) don't exist. Women, on the other hand, describe interaction, the complexity of life where they have to be responsible for the family as well as a career, caring for the home and so forth. Dausien presents this as social construction of gender. To the question whether this distinction could simply be the result of social reality, where men are not responsible for family, where their life is centred around work, and similar factors, the answer is that this is also social construction. In my sense it is not: social construction is construction only if from same materials we can construct really different alternatives, as in the case of Lego pieces. If the social 'construction' is determined by social reality, there is no quarrel. The problem is that you get often both kinds of messages (see Sokal 1997).[8]

One excellent way to demonstrate the impossibility of the fictive autobiography position is if we introduce this same discussion in the field of biography. Biography and autobiography are in some ways very different and biographers usually see it as an important endeavour to show how false and misleading a person's autobiography is, as the literary autobiographies often seem to be.[9] My point is simply that if a biographer would by way of introduction tell that he or she is a textualist/narrativist/postmodernist for whom the actual reality of the events related in the biography are irrelevant or simply a textual construction, we should also be prepared to judge the biography only by its literary and textual merits.[10] My question is: why should we treat autobiographies differently from biographies, even if the author is simultaneously the subject of the life story?[11]

Daniel Bertaux's recent contributions against the narrativist turn (1996, 1997a, 1997b) err in the other direction. He is an empirically oriented but theoretically informed researcher, who is singularly well placed to discuss the rise of life story approach in the 1970s and 1980s, having been one of the main movers and participant observers. Bertaux has chosen to lump together narrativists, constructivists and textualists, as well as those who work with single biographies, as enemies of realism and of the sociological point of view. For me, the unique quality of Daniel Bertaux has always been his ability to combine a fine sociological imagination with an excellent story-telling and analysing ability. For him to fulminate against narrativists is truly a *contradictio in adjecto*, whereas both constructivism and textualism are certainly enemies of realism. The idea that historical reality presents itself in the form of a narrative is quite plausible, as well as the idea that the narrative already implies an interpretation of reality. What makes this standpoint realist is simply the idea that the story is a function of the real events and that the story-teller tries to come close to these events.

Bertaux gives an interesting example of both the stability of one's story and of how the story changes when the positions change (Bertaux 1996). In his still unpublished but already classic baker study, the bakery workers were unanimous in telling how difficult and terrible their period as apprentices was, whereas the bakers were reluctant to discuss this period and only when questioned admitted that it was difficult, emphasizing much more what they learned. Note that here we may, in a sense, speak of repressed memory! The constructivist point of view is of course that the past is constructed in a way that depends on the present. The realist response is that we can, with the help of these different perspectives, reconstruct the social reality and the opposing social positions of the storytellers, but that the perspective of the workers is certainly more true and complete, as far as the apprentice experience is concerned. It is simply necessary to collect stories from different positions, in order to get at the reality (which is not denied by the bakers themselves). If we want to get a complete story of the bakers' lives, we must include their experience as apprentices.

In other words, the 'repressed' sections in the life story should be discovered, rather than invented or interpreted freely by a textualist analyzer. From a postmodernist point of view, life stories have been compared to an onion. You can peel the onion endlessly and never get at the truth, but it is possible to go further and compare the analysis of the life story to adding new layers, richer and more complex, to the lived life. The more we analyse, we get farther from the truth! For me, a life is much more like an artichoke, where the best part comes when you have 'peeled' the whole fruit off (and tasted every separate leaf!).

To come back to the repressed memory discussion, it is important from a realist point of view to get at the truth behind all kinds of hidden and falsified versions of life stories and family stories (Golofast 1997). But this truth cannot be gleaned from the processes of the unconscious but rather from tri-angulated stories, where different members of the same social or family group discuss the same events. Here, Daniel Bertaux's realistic sociological approach is a much better guide than his different, actually very vague, exhortations about social constructivism, narrativity and textuality.

Notes

This paper was originally presented at the European Sociological Association Conference, University of Essex 27–30 August 1997, Research Network 1, Biographical Perspectives on European Societies. I thank Selma Leydesdorff and Paul Thompson for their comments.

1 Crews *et al.* (1997) offers one of the best statements against repressed memories. See also Pendergrast (1996).
2 There is a myth that seduction theory was something else, but actually it was not (see Webster 1996).
3 For aspects of the debate see Crews *et al.* (1997), Blume (1991), Conway (1997), Loftus and Ketcham (1994), Pendergrast (1996) and Showalter (1997).
4 Repression is closely related to disassociation. For a classic dissociative identity, previous multiple personality case, see Spiegel (1997).
5 Lawyers and therapists have vested interests on either side: one theory argues that when many therapies were replaced by medication and insurance companies tightened their compensation for therapy, the now unemployed therapists had to find a new source of income from the police. See Money (1997).
6 They still exist.
7 The therapists use the same doubtful techniques to get children to remember events and eventually produce them (see Olsson 1994).
8 Sokal complains about this but has been able to find quotations where the causality relationship is explicitly from conscious construction to social reality.
9 A notable exception is Monk (1997). His biography of Bertrand Russell relates only one actual error in Russell's autobiography as well as one serious omission (Russell's affair with Vivien Eliot).
10 As in some cases we must, when the author has given free reins to his imagination as in Samuel (1996), who opens his devastating critique of a biography of Raymond Williams with the funeral scene, written convincingly from a first person perspective, but patently false because the author was not there and did not talk to persons present.
11 As the textualists anyway separate the author, the 'I' of the story and the 'I' constructed by the reader, there should be no difference in principle between autobiography and biography. See also Stanley (1992).

References

Aminoff, E. (1996) *Lapsen Parhaaksi. Viisi Vuotta Ruotsin Lapsivainojen Uhrina (In the Best Interest of the Child. Five Years as a Victim of the Swedish Child Round-ups)*, Porvoo.

Bertaux, D. (1996) 'A response to Thierry Kochyut's "Biographical and empiricist illusions"', *Biography and Society Newsletter,* December, corrected version.

—— (1997a) 'The usefulness of life stories for a realist and meaningful sociology', in V. Voronkov and E. Zdravomyslova (eds), *Biografitsheskii Metod v Isutsenii Postsotsialistitshekih Obsestv,* Sankt Peterburg.

—— (1997b) *Les Récits de Vie. Perspective Ethnosociologicque,* Paris.

Blume, S. (1991) *Secret Survivors. Uncovering Incest and Its Aftereffects in Women,* New York.

Conway, M. (ed.) (1997) *Recovered Memories and False Memories,* Oxford.

Crews, F. *et al.* (eds) (1997) *The Memory Wars. Freud's Legacy in Dispute,* London.

Dausien, B. (1996) *Biographie und Geschlecht. Zur Biographischen Konstrucktion Sozialer Wirklichkeit in Frauenlebensgeschichten,* Bremen.

Golofast, V. (1997) 'Three levels of biographical narratives', in V. Voronkov and E. Zdravomyslova (eds), *Biografitsheskii Metod v Isutsenii Postsotsialistitshekih Obsestv,* Sankt Peterburg.

Hacking, I. (1997) 'Taking bad arguments seriously', *London Review of Books,* vol. 19, no. 16.

Hyvärinen, M. (1994) *Viimeiset Taistot (The Last Battles),* Tampere.

—— (1997) 'Rhetoric and conversion in student politics: looking backward', in T. Carver and M. Hyvärinen (eds), *Interpreting the Political. New Methodologies,* London.

Loftus, E. and Ketcham, K. *The Myth of Repressed Memory: False Memories and Allegations of Sexual Abuse,* New York.

Monk, R. (1997) *Russell. The Spirit of Solitude,* London.

Money, J. (1997) 'Sexology: Good, bad and human rights', Inaugural Speech, 13 World Congress of Sexology, Valencia 25–29 June.

Ofshe, R. and Watters, E. (1994) *Making Monsters. False Memories, Psychotherapy and Sexual Hysteria,* New York.

Olsson H. (1994) *Catrine och Räittvisan (Catrine and the justice),* Stockholm.

Pendergrast, M. (1996) *Victims of Memory: Incest Accusations and Shattered Lives,* London.

Ristoja, A. and Ristoja, T. (1996) 'The Niko story: Can there be a happy end to abuse accusation cases', *Issues in Child Abuse Accusations,* vol. 8, no. 1:. 34–44.

Roos, J. P. (1994) 'The true life revisited. Autobiography and referentiality after the posts', *Autobiography,* vol. 3, 1 Feb.: 1–16.

—— (1997) 'Context, authenticity, referentiality, reflexivity: Back to basics in autobiography', in V. Voronkov and E. Zdravomyslova (eds), *Biografitsheskii Metod v Isutsenii Postsotsialistitshekih Obsestv,* Sankt Peterburg.

Samuel, R. (1996) 'Making it Up', *London Review of Books,* 4 July: 8–12.

Showalter, E. (1997) *Hystories. Hysterical Epidemics and Modern Culture,* London.

Sokal, A. (1997) 'What the social text affair does and does not prove' in N. Koertge (ed.), *A House Built on Sand: Exposing Postmodernist Myths About Science,* Oxford.

Spiegel, H. (1997) 'Sybil: the making of a disease. An interview with Dr. Herbert Spiegel', *New York Review of Books,* 24 April.

Stanley, L. (1992) *The Autobiographical I*, Manchester.

Terr, L. (1994) *Unchained Memories. The True Stories of Traumatic Memories Lost and Found*, New York.

Vigouroux, F. (1993) *Le Secret de Famille*, Paris.

Webster, R. (1996) *Why Freud Was Wrong. Sin, Science and Psychoanalysis*, London.

11

HUMAN DISASTER, SOCIAL TRAUMA AND COMMUNITY MEMORY

Arthur A. Hansen

Linda Tamura, *The Hood River Issei: An Oral History of Japanese Settlers in Oregon's Hood River Valley* (Urbana, Ill.: University of Illinois Press, 1993)

Sucheng Chan (ed.), *Hmong Means Free: Life in Laos and America* (Philadelphia: Temple University Press, 1994)

When pondering these two excellent books focused, respectively, on an 'old' and a 'new' Asian American population, I encountered an intriguing volume by the sociologist Kai Erikson (1994) that persuaded me to construe them in terms of 'human disaster research'. The volume by Tamura, a third-generation Japanese American (*Sansei*) born and raised in the small Oregon community in which her study is set, centres upon the 'disaster' of the Second World War eviction and detention experience of, primarily, her *Nisei* parents' and *Issei* grandparents' generations (as represented in taped interviews by the author with fourteen surviving Hood River *Issei*).[1] Similarly, Chan's edited anthology of 'interviews' (more accurately, life stories) transacted by her Hmong students at the University of California, Santa Barbara, concentrates on the linked 'disaster' of war, flight, and resettlement endured by their parents and grandparents in Southeast Asia and the United States over the last four decades. At the heart of both of these books is the problematic relationship between traumatized communities and the intergenerational transmission of the remembered past.

Erikson's concern is not with natural disasters but ones caused by human beings. Victims of such disasters commonly testify to feeling fear, self-doubt, helplessness, numbness, estrangement, vulnerability, and the erosion of a sense of security, resulting in a form of trauma. Erikson believes that trauma can serve as a broad social concept as well as a more narrowly clinical one, and that trauma extends not just to individuals but to whole communities. Moreover, trauma can not merely be the consequence of a discrete happening or acute event but can derive from a persisting condition based upon accumulated life experiences.

While shared trauma can function as a source both for creating and impairing community, Erikson stresses its damaging capacity. The experience of human-caused communal trauma:

> can mean not only a loss of confidence in the self but a loss of confidence in the scaffolding of family and community, in the structures of human government, in the larger logic by which humankind lives, and in the ways of nature itself.

As for communalized traumas engendered by human disasters involving toxic contamination, Erikson maintains that they represent 'a new species of trouble' wherein those so victimized are unnerved to the point where they feel that 'something dark and baneful has worked its way into the grain of everyday social life' and that this condition is likely to obtain forever.[2]

Although not plagued by toxic contamination *per se,* people of Japanese ancestry in the United States have been poisoned by unremitting and periodically virulent racial prejudice since the restructuring of the global economy in the late nineteenth century propelled them as a labouring class across the Pacific, particularly to the farms and cities of West Coast states. The constructed narrative voices of Tamura's *Issei* neighbours in Hood River (eleven women and three men), distributed throughout the text within ten chronological-cum-topical sections, vouch for the legal and extralegal actions levelled against *Nikkei* (Japanese Americans). These culminated (but did not cease) with that ethnic community's exiling and incarceration by the US government during the Second World War.

Perhaps to avoid exacerbating the inherited trauma of their *Sansei* interviewer, however, the *Issei* narrators muffled both the traumatizing impact on them and their community of any single event (for example, the unconstitutional wartime imprisonment in desolate interior concentration camps) and the historic skein of racist measures directed at *Nikkei*. These included First World War-era laws in western states forbidding land ownership by immigrant Japanese, a 1924 act by Congress prohibiting Asian immigration, the 1944 removal by the Hood River American Legion post of *Nisei* servicemen's names from the town's memorial plaque, and organized resistance by chauvinistic groups to the return of Japanese Americans to their pre-war West Coast homes.

To better comprehend how Japanese Americans in Hood River Valley (and, by implication, in all of Japanese America) came to feel contaminated by flagrant racism, one should supplement Tamura's book with Lauren Kessler's recent study (1993) of Hood River's most well-known *Nikkei* family, the Yasuis. Based on but not communicated through oral history interviews, Kessler's powerful book relates in throbbing detail how traumatizing racism and attendant feelings of shame and betrayal triggered both the 1957 suicide of the Yasui family's highly successful and once proud *Issei* patriarch and the 1945 decision by about half of his pre-war co-ethnics in Hood River Valley to establish their post-war homes elsewhere.

A 1991 article by sociologist Wendy Ng is useful in clarifying both the temper of the interviews that Tamura conducted with her *Issei* informants and the dynamics of what Ng depicts as 'community memory'.[3] Communities, Ng argues, are 'created by individuals through their interactions with one another, based upon a common history, [and] a part of this creation of community is the . . . memory of the past which individuals bring to the community: a community memory'. Prior to 1981, *Issei* and *Nisei* were reluctant to talk about their past, especially their Second World War expulsion and confinement behind barbed wire.[4] This historical silence was upheld more obdurately within the community and its constituent families than in interactions with outsiders.[5] Although *Sansei* identity politics in the 1960s and 1970s had stimulated *Nikkei* elders into confronting their history, however disturbing, it was the twenty days of hearings by the Commission on Wartime Relocation and Internment of Civilians (CWRIC) that transformed the social discourse about the past within the Japanese American community.[6]

The commission was established by the US Congress to review the facts and circumstances of the Japanese-American evacuation and to recommend appropriate remedies. Between July and December of 1981, hearings were held in Washington D.C., New York, Chicago, Los Angeles, San Francisco and Seattle. Of the 750 who testified before the Commission, the great majority were *Nikkei*.[7] Roger Daniels, the Evacuation's leading student, has characterized their testimony as 'the most impressive aspect' of the CWRIC hearings. After forty years of denying their emotions, writes Daniels,

> The dam burst and the denial ended during the hearings as the detainees one after the other testified with great passion about what they had endured. Many wept openly, some broke down, and, when at the Los Angeles hearings Senator [Samuel I.] Hayakawa testified against monetary redress, the audience, largely Japanese American, disrupted the hearing with shouts, boos, and hisses.
>
> (Daniels 1993: 96–7)[8]

Clearly, the CWRIC hearings catalysed the profusion of Japanese American community and family studies produced in the 1980s by *Nikkei* scholars attuned to oral historiography and/or life history methodology.[9]

Notwithstanding the unclogging of the collective memory channels of the Japanese-American community achieved through the CWRIC hearings, Ng informs us that *Issei* and *Nisei* continued 'to remember the camp experience in selective ways to avoid reliving the trauma of the past'. In all communities, of course, the past is remembered subjectively. What concerns Ng, however, is how the selective interpretation of past events in *Nikkei* history, particularly the Evacuation, is transmitted by those in the Japanese American community who directly experienced it to those who *did* not. Consequently, in 1987–8, she conducted in-depth interviews with *Sansei* who, like Linda Tamura, were born and raised in Hood River, Oregon, after the Second World War. In these semi-structured, open-ended interviews focusing on family, work, and community life, Ng discovered that her *Sansei* informants had learned about their community's past in a patterned way. With respect to their grandparents' and, especially, their parents' detention in camp, information was communicated to the third generation by a combination of 'scattered stories and peculiar behaviour', though the *Sansei* were 'fully aware that the experience had been traumatic as well as dislocating'. Many *Sansei* told Ng that their *Nisei* parents privatised their time in camp by not discussing it openly, treated it casually as though it had lacked significant meaning for them, or presented either a positive or a neutral picture of that part of their past.

Another major theme to emerge from Ng's interviews was that the grandparental and parental transmission of the past was invariably accompanied by admonitions to the *Sansei* generation that they were Americans and should not 'make a big deal out of being Japanese'. For example, even though many *Sansei* had been raised in extended households with exclusively Japanese-speaking grandparents and bilingual parents, they were enjoined not to speak Japanese. (This situation helps to explain why Tamura required the translation assistance of a *Nisei* uncle to transact interviews with Hood River *Issei*, including her own grandmother.) At the same time, *Sansei* were to excel in school because they were Japanese. The contradiction here is apparent, not real, since the intent of this advice was for *Sansei* to become model American citizens ('all American') as a way of coping with the racism that still ran deeply within the social institutions and cultural practices of the Hood River community. 'The collective memory of the community,' concludes Ng, 'transmits, not intentionally, but on a subverted level, a less-than positive attitude about Japanese ethnicity'.

Though the themes articulated by Ng are apparent in the interviews in *The Hood River Issei*, Tamura mitigates their power in two important ways. First, she contextualizes her interviews within a historical narrative that is supported by relevant primary and secondary sources and approached from a comparative perspective. Consequently, community memory and the Hood River situation are placed in a dialectical relationship with history and the Japanese American experience. Second, Tamura imposes a *Sansei* perspective which, though never strident or distended from her sources, emphasizes a community legacy of resistance to oppression, ethnic pride, and the belief, to quote Ng, that 'individuals are responsible for creating their sense of the past and are active participants in creating their own history'.

Accountability for historical representation and agency is palpable within

223

the other book under review here, *Hmong Means Free,* which editor Sucheng Chan labels the first work consisting exclusively of first-person Hmong narratives.[10] Chan, who along with Ronald Takaki spearheaded the rapid intellectual and institutional maturity of Asian American studies in recent years, had increasingly turned her scholarly attention away from older Asian immigrant communities in the United States, such as Japanese Americans, and toward the refugee communities of Southeast Asian people who fled to the US following the Communists' coming to power in 1975.[11]

In her preface Chan explains:

> As their numbers increased, I realized it was important to document their traumatic experiences during the war, during their flight, and after their arrival in the United States. But since I do not know the Vietnamese, Cambodian, Lao, or Hmong languages, I had to find indirect ways to record their stories.
>
> (Chan 1994a)

Prior to her 1989 appointment at the Santa Barbara campus of the University of California, Chan had taught a course on 'The Vietnamese Experience in America' at three sister University of California campuses (Berkeley, Los Angeles, and San Diego) and concentrated on getting her Vietnamese students to write autobiographical essays chronicling their ordeal. At Santa Barbara, for the first time, she found Hmong students enrolled in her Asian American history classes. These students were part of the more than 100,000 Hmong who had fled to the United States, 40,000 to California alone. A few of them so valued Chan's curricular inclusion of their community's history that they volunteered to assist her in interviewing older Hmong about their plight. Ultimately, four students – Thek Moua, Lee Fang, Vu Pao Tcha, and Maijue Xiong – became Chan's 'collaborators'.

Working with these collaborators in collecting Hmong life histories posed a series of difficulties for Chan *vis-à-vis* canonical oral history practice in the United States. Originally intending to have her student interviewers use a schedule of questions, she abandoned this plan upon discovering that in Hmong culture younger people are expected to be deferential to their elders and thus are regarded as rude when interrupting their conversational discourse with formal interrogation. She also scrapped any design for a positivistic representative sample of interviewees. Instead, she asked her students to concentrate upon gathering the life stories of selected members of their own families (and those of two local community leaders), reasoning that they, more than 'outsiders', would be motivated to transmit their heritage in a free and open manner. Students were advised simply to ask their kin to talk about their lives and to discuss anything they regarded as meaningful.

'With this change in approach,' explains Chan, 'the potential *interviewees* became *narrators*'. Indeed, their narrator status was amplified by a combination of circumstances and collaborators' resourcefulness. Between visits to their family homes in central and southern California, the students left behind a tape recorder and requested that a designated narrator talk into it when time permitted. This unorthodox arrangement often led to intensely personal accounts, as when women expressed bitterness about their mistreatment within Hmong society and the family circle: 'Your grandpa never loved me. . . . He was always unjust to me. If this is the life that every woman in this world has to live, then it's not worth it to be a wife'.[12]

Chan further deviated from standard oral history operating procedure during the processing of the project's 'interviews'. In translating the Hmong tapes into English-language transcripts, the four student collaborators (whose written autobiographies also appear in *Hmong Means Free*) sometimes employed colloquial expressions or technical terms that they had acquired in the United States. Another layer of mediation was added through Chan editing of the interview transcripts for publication. Authenticity was sacrificed on the altar of sensitivity when Chan, herself an immigrant from China as a teenager, capitulated to the collaborators' request that she 'clean up' their translations (and thereby spare them from gratuitous humiliation). 'They know, and I know', reasons Chan, 'that one distinct form that racism in America has taken is the singsong pidgin English that many writers have used to depict the speech of Asian immigrants.' While sympathetic to the new ethnography's concern with unequal power relations between indigenous informants and scholars in the interview situation, Chan justifies her 'twice-mediated tales' because they make it 'possible for the narrators to share the stories of their lives with non-Hmong readers'.

Since the end of the war in Southeast Asia, the Hmong have attracted more attention from writers and scholars than any other refugee group to migrate from that area to the United States except the Vietnamese. This point is conveyed by Chan's selected bibliography of English-language sources, but is exemplified by her lengthy and luminous introductory essay, 'The Hmong Experience in Asia and the United States'.[13] Nonetheless, a work highlighting oral narratives like *Hmong Means Free* is consonant with traditional Hmong culture. Until several decades ago the Hmong lacked a written language, and even today few Hmong adults can read and write. Hmong, therefore, depend on oral communication and base their history chiefly on oral traditions (Ng 1993: 51).

What those traditions have transmitted through successive generations is a legacy primarily of persecution. In the eighteenth and nineteenth centuries, while the Hmong lived in south-western China, their Manchu overlords had labelled them 'Miao' ('barbarian' or 'savage') and targeted them for genocide when they defied being humiliated, oppressed, and enslaved. After some Hmong migrated southward to the mountainous regions of Southeast Asia, including Laos, French imperial administrators imposed great hardship on them through taxation, fines, corrupt practices and forced labour. Following the French expulsion from Laos in 1954 and the US government enlistment of the Hmong in the 1960s and early 1970s to 'contain' the spread of Communism in Southeast Asia, thousands of soldiers were wounded and killed, whole villages were wiped out and extreme suffering was endemic. Once the Communist Pathet Lao came to power in 1975, former Hmong fighters were treated as traitors and consigned to re-education camps, where they were tortured, starved and worked to death. Those Hmong who during the late 1970s resisted the Lao People's Democratic Republic (LPDR) were crushed by a combination of napalm, defoliants, and biological and chemical poisons. As for the thousands of Hmong who, under harrowing circumstances, escaped through the jungles to Thailand during the interval between 1975 and 1985, they endured months, sometimes years, of very taxing conditions in refugee camps before being resettled in the United States and other countries.

The life stories in *Hmong Means Free* are generally consistent with this tale of community tragedy. Whereas the *Issei* narratives in the Tamura volume tend to understate the degree of trauma experienced, the narratives told by Hmong elders seemingly hyperbolize it. For example, in discussing the alleged use by Communists of biological and chemical poisons against Hmong resisters, editor Chan (an antiwar activist in the 1960s and 1970s) writes: 'Many observers do not believe the refugees' tales and insist that no evidence of any poisons has been found.'

Also implicitly sceptical about 'the unmediated "real" Hmong history based primarily on their culture as lived and as transmitted in their oral traditions' is anthropologist Franklin Ng (1993: 63) who co-ordinates the Asian American Studies program at the California State University campus at Fresno (the centre of the US Hmong community). In the term papers of his refugee Hmong students, Ng has noticed that they have selectively utilized printed English-language sources about Hmong history to complement their internal, community-based folklore and oral traditions. To sustain the melodramatic past endorsed by their elders, however, the students have had to screen out the written sources' unpalatable details and problematic dimensions. What must be arrayed, say, against the claim that the Laotian Communist government singled out the Hmong for persecution or extinction, writes Ng, is how some Hmong co-operated with the Communists and even meted out many of the harsher reprisals to Hmong resisters (ibid.: 54-63).

What apart from differing cultural styles can be adduced to support the contrasting mode of historical representation between *Nikkei* and Hmong narrators? One could argue that the answer to this question is bound up in the maxim that 'History is a dialogue in the present with the past, about the future'. If Hmong 'historians' telescope and magnify the traumatic character of their community's past to their progeny, perhaps it is partly because these new Asian Americans are deeply alienated from American culture and society and perfervidly hope to return someday to Laos with their families, reclaim their slash-and-burn agricultural economy, reconstitute their traditional lifestyle, and regain their primordial identity.[14] However ironic it seems, the Hmong may invoke a heritage of calamity and a sense of difference to strengthen the attenuated bonds of a community and culture undergoing speedy transformation from the Hmong way to the American way.

A more convincing explanation for the Hmong's stylized portrayal of their cataclysmic past, though, works in the opposite direction. Hmong elders are often wistfully nostalgic about the land they left behind: 'I am sad not knowing whether I will ever see the flowers and bamboo groves in Laos again'.[15] However, they are well aware that their future, and more particularly that of their descendants, is likely to be in the United States: 'This country has become ours and we will live the rest of our lives as good citizens. . . . Our children are assimilating into American life . . . they are growing up to be part of the American melting pot'.[16] They are acutely aware, too, that to be accepted as Americans their offspring will be required to pay a steep price in racial prejudice:

> I see some black [African American] people hating us. I do not understand why they do. I do not hate them; why do they hate me and my family so much? They throw rocks and rotten eggs at my house. They call my children names.[17]

Such a scenario, however, pitiful, becomes more bearable when projected upon an ancestral background of perpetual disaster and unrelieved trauma.

In transmitting, for whatever reason, a community memory of trauma to the younger generation in America, refugee Hmong elders (as epitomized by the narrators in *Hmong Means Free*) have elided from their testimonies any mention of the possible culpability of their leaders and the United States government in constructing a heritage of horror. There is, on the one hand, no recognition that Hmong collaboration as anti-Communist mercenary soldiers on the Central Intelligence Agency's payroll during the 'secret war' in Laos might in some instances have been motivated by 'venality and corruption' (Chan 1994a: XIV). Nor, on the other hand, is reference made to the US's ostensible abandonment of the Hmong after 1975, which a well-documented study by Jane Hamilton-Merritt (1993) reveals to have been manifested in official indifference to the LPDR's efforts to exterminate the Hmong with chemical-biological toxins and, thereafter (continuing to the present), 'acquiescence in the policy of forced repatriation of Hmong from Thai refugee camps to the LPDR, where, unprotected by the United Nations, they face certain torture and death' (Reckner 1994). Surely, what this double silence in the community memory is fostering in Hmong Americans is an individual and group identity rooted in an externalisation of evil and an uncritical affirmation of Americanism.

In recent years scholars have presented the Japanese-American community with overwhelming evidence that the Second World War disaster they suffered was caused not just by war hysteria and racism but also a failure of political leadership in both mainstream and *Nikkei* society.[18] This 'truth' has gone a long way toward liberating *Nikkei* from their collective trauma. When Hmong Americans will have their communal rendezvous with history is an open question, but until that time they will remain prisoners of their traumatic and truncated oral tradition. Hopefully the day is not too distant when Hmong may truly begin to mean free.

Notes

1   Unlike virtually every other US ethnic group, Japanese Americans assign names to their generations and perceive them as occupying autonomous social situations and having distinctive historical experiences and cultural outlooks. The *Issei* or immigrant generation, which settled in the United States mainly in the interval between 1885 and 1924, were ineligible for US citizenship until 1952. Their *Nisei* children, most of whom were born between 1915 and 1935, achieved American citizenship by being born in the United States and earned a reputation within the mainstream population for being a highly 'Americanized' and 'silent' generation. The third-generation *Sansei*, born largely between 1945 and 1965, came of age during the 1960s and 1970s and are identified within, if not outside, the Japanese-American community as social activists concerned with civil rights, social justice, and ethnic consciousness. During the Second World War Japanese-American evacuation, roughly one-third of the more than 120,000 imprisoned in concentration camps by the US government were alien *Issei*, with the remaining two-thirds being citizen *Nisei* and *Sansei*.

2   See Erikson (1994 especially 'Epilogue: on trauma': 226–42). These points represent a refinement, enlargement, and extension of Erikson's 1976 argument.

3   All quoted passages attributed to Wendy Ng found in the present review essay are drawn from 'The Collective Memories of Communities' (1991). For a fuller exploration of Ng's ideas on this topic, see her unpublished University of Oregon doctoral dissertation, 'Collective Memory, Social Networks and Generations: The Japanese American Community in Hood River, Oregon' (1989).

4   When Betty E. Mitson and I edited a volume featuring interviews with Japanese Americans about their World War II experiences two decades ago, we chose a title that reflected this situation: *Voices Long Silent: An Oral inquiry into the Japanese American Evacuation* (1974). This title, moreover, resonated with those of two other volumes produced by *Nisei* historians during that period: Bill Hosokawa's *Nisei: The Quiet Americans* (1969) and Yuji Ichioka *et al.*'s *A Buried Past* (1974).

5   To my knowledge, the first oral history of the Japanese American evacuation by a Japanese American was Sansei John Tateishi's edited anthology of interviews (1984).

6   A striking example of developments prior to the Commission was the publication of Michi Nishiura Weglyn's inspired and deeply critical book, *Years of Infamy* (1976). Incarcerated as a *Nisei* teenager in an Arizona camp, this highly

acclaimed theatrical costume designer broke with her comparatively unpolitical and not ethnically focused past to research and write the first historical study of the Japanese American Evacuation by a former internee.

7 For the Commission's findings and recommendations, see *Personal Justice Denied: Report of the Commission on Wartime Relocation of Civilians* (1982). The Civil Rights Act of 1988 enacted into law all five of the Commission's recommendations, including a formal apology by Congress and a one-time, tax-free payment of $20,000 to each surviving internee.

8 One apparent impact of these hearings on Daniels was to render him more favourably disposed to oral history as both a source of documentation and a research method in historical inquiry. Significantly, *The Hood River Issei* is the first title in the Asian American Experience series edited by Daniels (who also contributed the Foreword to Tamura's book) for the University of Illinois Press. Daniels, furthermore, has figured prominently in the concurrent publication of two other Japanese-American community studies grounded in oral history: Taylor (1993) and Matsumoto (1993). Hayakawa (1906–1992), a noted semanticist, achieved celebrity status as a flamboyant conservative in 1968 when, as the newly appointed president of San Francisco State University during the student strike demanding a curriculum that acknowledged the US's multicultural origins, he ripped out the wires from campus protesters' loudspeakers. After switching from the Democratic to the Republican Party, Hayakawa was elected to the US Senate in 1976. During his tenure of office, he was not only an active opponent of redress and reparations for Japanese Americans but also, in 1979, 'advocated putting Iranians in concentration camps during the hostage crisis the way we did with the Japanese in World War II'. See Niiya (1993).

9 See, for example, the following: Akemi Kikumura (1981); Gary Y. Okihiro and Timothy I. Lukes (1985); and David Mas Masumoto (1987). Both Kikumura, an anthropologist, and Okihiro, a historian trained in African studies, have contributed relevant methodological pieces: Kikumura (1986), Okihiro (1984). Redress leader John Tateishi's 1984 study is arguably the quintessential text. In his preface, Tateishi states that those in his community had been traumatized by their forced exclusion and false imprisonment. 'Up to now', he concludes his commentary, 'painful memories have kept Japanese Americans unwilling and unable to talk. But they are silent no more.'

10 For an abbreviated version of this study, see Chan (1994b).

11 See Takaki (1989) and Chan (1990). Takaki and Chan and their respective supporters have clashed in print over the protocol of Takaki's scholarship. See the forum on *Strangers from a Different Shore* in the *Amerasia Journal* 16 (1990), 61–154.

12 Life story of Zr Lo, in ibid., 172.

13 The comparative richness of scholarship on the Hmong community as against other Southeast Asian groups can be readily appreciated by consulting a recent bibliographical essay prepared by Chan for the Asian American Studies Association. See Chan (1994c).

14 I have appropriated the term and concept of primordial identity from Franklin Ng (1993: 61)

15 Quoted from the life story of Xang Mao Xiong in Chan (1994a: 102).

16 Quoted from the life story of Ka Pao Xiong in Chan (1994a: 85).
17 Life story of Boua Neng Moua in Chan (1994a: 214–15).
18 The reference here is to the collaborationist role in the Japanese American evacuation played by the national leadership of the Japanese Americans Citizens League.

References

Chan, S. (1990) *Asian Americans. An Interpretive History,* Boston.

Chan, S. (ed.) (1994a) *Hmong Means Free: Life in Laos and America,* Philadelphia: Temple University Press.

—— (1994b) 'Hmong Life Stories', in F. Ng (ed.), *New Visions in Asian American Studies: Diversity, Community, Power,* Pullman, Washington: 43–62.

—— (1994c) 'A selected bibliography and list of films on the Vietnamese, Cambodian, and Laotian experience in Southeast Asia and the United States', in F. Ng (ed.), *New Visions in Asian American Studies: Diversity, Community, Power,* Pullman, Washington: 63–110.

Commission on Wartime Relocation of Civilians (1982) *Personal Justice Denied: Report of the Commission on Wartime Relocation of Civilians,* Washington D.C.

Daniels, R. (1993) *Prisoners Without Trial: Japanese Americans in World War II,* New York.

Erikson, K. (1976) *Everything in Its Path: Destruction of Community in the Buffalo Creek Flood,* New York.

—— (1994) *A New Species of Trouble: Explorations in Disaster, Trauma, and Community,* New York.

Hamilton-Merritt, J. (1993) *Tragic Mountains: The Hmong, the Americans, and the Secret Wars for Laos, 1942–1992,* Bloomington, Indiana.

Hosokawa, W. (1969) *Nisei: The Quiet Americans,* New York.

Ichioka, Y. *et al.* (eds) *A Buried Past: An Annotated Bibliography of the Japanese American Research Project Collection,* Berkeley, California.

Kessler, L. (1993) *Stubborn Twig: Three Generations in the Life of Japanese American Family,* New York.

Kikumura, A. (1981) *Through Harsh Winters: The Life of A Japanese Immigrant Woman,* Novato, California.

—— (1986) 'Family Life Histories: A Collaborative Venture', *Oral History Review,* vol. 14.

Masumoto, D. M. (1987) *Country Voices. The Oral History of a Japanese American Family Farm Community* , Del Rey, California.

Matsumoto, V. J. (1993) *Farming the Home Place: A Japanese American Community in California, 1919–1982,* Ithaca, N.Y.

Mitson, B. E. and Hansen, A. A. (eds) (1974) *Long Silent: An Oral inquiry into the Japanese American Evacuation,* Fullerton, California.

Ng, F. (1993) 'Towards a second generation Hmong history', *Amerasia Journal* vol. 19.

Ng, W. L. (1991) 'The Collective Memories of Communities', in S. Hune *et al.*, Asian *Americans: Comparative and Global Perspectives,* Washington: Pullman:103–12.

Niiya, B. (ed.) (1993) *Japanese American History: An A-to-Z Reference from 1868 to the Present,* New York.

Okihiro, G. Y. (1984) 'Oral history and the writing of ethnic history,' in D. K. Dunaway and W. K. Baum (eds), *Oral History. An Interdisciplinary Anthology,* Nashville, Tennessee.

Okihiro, G. Y. and Lukes, T. L. (1985) *Japanese Legacy: Farming and Community Life in California's Santa Clara Valley,* Cupertino, California.

Reckner, J. R. (1994) 'Review of Tragic Mountains', *Journal of American History* vol. 81, June: 334–5.

Takaki, R. (1989) *Strangers from a Different Shore: A History of Asian Americans,* Boston.

Tamura, L. (1993) *The Hood River Issei: An Oral History of Japanese Settlers in Oregon's Hood River Valley,* Urbana, Illinois: University of Illinois Press.

Tateishi, J. (ed.) (1984) *And Justice For All: An Oral History of the Japanese American Detention Camps,* New York.

Taylor, S. C. (1993) *Jewel of the Desert. Japanese American Internment at Topaz,* Berkeley, California.

Weglyn, M. N. (1976) *Years of Infamy: The Untold Story of America's Concentration Camps,* New York.

12

TRAUMA AND THE LONG-TERM LIFE STORY

Paul Thompson

Is it possible through the life story approach to gain a really significant understanding of how traumas and setbacks affect people in the long term? Is there any way in which we can tease out the really significant differences which explain why one person can rise above an apparently devastating difficulty, and soar on beyond it, while another may collapse indefinitely in crumpled paralysis?

I have been thinking about this especially in recent years because of my own work for a book on *Growing Up in Stepfamilies,* which I have carried out along with three co-authors, a child psychiatrist and two family therapists. Our intention was to combine the strengths of quantitative and qualitative methods, so we deliberately chose fifty men and women, now in their thirties, but in childhood stepchildren, who had been followed since birth by a longitudinal statistical research programme, the National Child Development Study (NCDS). This programme had taken every child born in Britain in one week in March 1958 and followed them and their parents with interviews – almost wholly structured and statistical – at first frequently, and more recently at intervals of around five years. Using NCDS made our stepfamily research unique in Britain in its basis on a reliable sample, and we hoped to compare the fifty retrospective life story interviews which we carried out with the earlier statistical data and thus strengthen our interpretations of what mattered most for these children in the long run.

The in-depth stories which we recorded are very powerful and worth hearing in themselves. The research has reached some important conclusions. For example, our evidence shows powerfully how crucial grandparents are for most children who have lost a parent through separation or death. We were able to understand in a new way how gender roles make it so much harder for a stepmother to succeed than for a stepfather. A man, of whom less is expected, is therefore best advised not to try to become a full substitute parent, and is more likely to cause trouble if he does. We could show how children suffer unnecessarily from the failure of most parents to explain to them what is happening at a separation or a death, and how especially disastrous it is likely to be in the long run when an infant child is told that a stepfather is a natural father. We could see how very rare it is for a lost parent to cease to be significant in a child's consciousness, and how some adults continue to be haunted by their loss, longing just to find a photograph of their parents or to hear the sound of their voice.

On the other hand, as the work of interpreting the research went on we realised more and more that there were fundamental difficulties in reaching any conclusions on many of the issues which interested us.

One immediate difficulty was an increasing doubt as to whether the sample, although certainly the soundest that any British research on stepfamilies has used, was as impeccable as we had originally thought. It has become increasingly clear to us that the fact that our interviewees stayed in a longitudinal study indicates a relative stability in their lives. This was brought home on the one hand by some of the trails which we followed seeking informants lost to the sample, which might end unsuccessfully, for example, in a rehabilitation centre for drug and alcohol addicts. On the other hand, informants who remained in the study, while certainly including several still suffering deeply damaging after-effects of childhood trauma, and a few pushed into mental illness or criminality, were as a whole relatively successful at work and stable in their emotional lives.

We had no way of knowing whether the large number of 1958 children who are now lost to the whole sample, nearly a third, and still more of the missing former stepchildren, might not be radically more disadvantaged, and indeed precisely the population who swell the clinic lists in need of help. The same problem certainly applies to the Berkeley cohorts (of which more in a moment): for example, more of those who divorced have dropped out than those who have remained married.

This is not an insoluble difficulty. Because those who remain in the study range from the socially stably rooted to those who are unemployed, mentally ill or convicted deviants, it would in principle be possible to redress the balance in the sample by allowing for the bias in those who fall out, provided that the issue was more seriously addressed by the researchers who run longitudinal studies. Unfortunately, perhaps to protect their credibility, they have not given it much attention, and in public concentrate on demonstrating the undoubted thoroughness with which they continue to pursue all members of their cohort. In our case we were not able to discover any clues – apart from simple demographic matchings – as to how far our own fifty informants differed either from the larger group of stepchildren still in the study, or from those who had dropped out earlier.

A second and more intractable problem is the sheer passage of time. Let us consider education. We found that as a whole the children underperformed significantly at school, and they got little special help or understanding from their teachers. Indeed only one child could describe any kind of close relationship with a teacher. Ironically that was an adolescent boy who had an affair with his sports teacher. This finding seems irrelevant today, however, when schools are made to be so much more conscious of the large numbers of pupils from broken and reconstituted families. Again, our stepchildren, who entered the labour market at a time of full employment, did not in fact suffer much from their lower educational achievement; indeed they appeared to have done impressively well and to have risen instead through the workplace. In the present-day period of much higher unemployment, it seems highly unlikely that stepchildren could follow the same path. In other words, there were crucial ways in which our findings might be accurate descriptions of the past, but social and economic change have made them irrelevant in terms of contemporary policy issues.

The passing of time also made our projected comparison between the interviews and the earlier data very meagre. The original interview schedules had already been destroyed, and since most of the questions which we were asking had not occurred to the earlier researchers, there was simply no data for comparison. The advantages of a relatively sound sample remained; but even that was slightly undermined by the in-depth interviews. These revealed that one fifth of our informants had been mis-classified by the original interviews, principally because of deliberate deceptions by parents who wanted to conceal illegitimate births. We longed to read notes of what had actually been said by parents at the time of the interviews, and how the interviewer had interpreted the situation; but none survived.

It was thus with considerable excitement that I learnt of the extraordinarily rich resources of research on human lives over time in the San Francisco Bay area kept at the Institute of Human Development at Berkeley. These had been collected by a team of psychologists there since the late 1920s. They are described in *American Lives: Looking Back at the Children of the Great Depression* by John Clausen, who died in 1995, who had worked for decades at the Institute, and knew better than anyone else the potential of the material held in its archive.

The Oakland longitudinal cohort studies are among the earliest anywhere. Because all the children studied grew up through the depth of the Great Depression, which hit the majority of their families badly, this can effectively be seen as a longitudinal study whose members all began with a traumatic setback. Originally there were three cohorts, begun in 1927, 1928 and 1931, together comprising 517 children all born between 1921 and 1929. They were consolidated in the 1960s, and contact has been maintained until the present, not only locally but with those who have migrated elsewhere in the United States. Researchers have kept in close personal contact with the informants and their families, and staff continue to attend weddings, funerals, sports days, and so on.

The Oakland studies were both medical and social longitudinal studies from the start. They used a wide range of methods, ranging from photographs and X-rays and IQ and other statistical tests, to in-depth interviews, which in some cases were carried out on a monthly basis, and interviewer's notes when called in for help or advice. There are interviews not only with the principal informant, including retrospective life story interviews, but with also in-depth information from parents, siblings and spouses. The records include hundreds of pages of discussion of family relationships and problems as observed by the researchers: I do not know anything of such detail which has survived from the interwar years in Britain, and I would be surprised if anywhere in the world there are people whose lives have been more deeply studied for so long than the 253 who were still in the project in 1982.

Sadly, John Clausen was the last remaining champion of the longitudinal studies. The last new interviews with the whole cohort were carried out in the early 1980s, and its whole future is now in doubt. Current researchers at the Institute are only concerned with human development in infancy. The archivist whom I met in 1996 had been given notice.

One of the immediate attractions of *American Lives* is that it gives a very good idea of the richness of the research material, which has been re-used by many well-known scholars including Erik Erikson, Tamara Hareven, Arlene Skolnick, and by Glen Elder Jnr. for his classic *Children of the Depression.*

Clausen's intention in *American Lives* is to use the cohort material to explain why some of these children suffered from their earlier setbacks right through their lives, while others did well enough. Not only did all of them grow up in the depression decades, so that many had unemployed fathers, but a third of them lost a parent, either through death or desertion. Clausen interweaves his analysis with presentations of fascinating case studies, which he partly checked with the subjects.

Unfortunately the long passage of time between the planning of the research and the eventual emergence of this book tells against it. Clausen's basic interpretative idea, that those who succeed had acquired 'planful competence' by late adolescence, feels very dated, uncomfortably like a jargon presentation of commonsense. On the other hand one notices that parenting is evaluated by present-day standards rather than by those of the period. And the historical differences are particular obvious when we read the conclusions which Clausen has drawn on gender. They clearly reflect the experience of a cohort whose women had to choose between motherhood and a career.

Overall it is clear that inheritance and childhood shape most lives decisively. The most powerful influences in recovery and success for both boys and girls are parental social class, followed by intelligence (but more for boys) and physical attractiveness (but more for girls). These could be undermined by inadequate parenting, and especially by conflict in the family, both in childhood and in marriage.

These gender differences are striking in many ways. Thus we find that the 'competent' men are reported to have fewer rather than more friends. This can be explained by the almost universal habit of American men of this generation, even when unhappily married, to confide in their wives. Women by contrast have more friends, perhaps because fewer than half of them confide in their husbands.

It is particularly interesting that 'competence' proves more useful for the men than for the women. The success of women, in contrast to men, depended much more on their physical attractiveness than their intelligence, and the crucial factors in their adult lives were their choice of spouse and the fate – in terms of career and marriage – of their offspring. Yet at the same time women are more powerfully affected by their childhood memories. Over half the 'incompetent' women came from conflictual or pathological childhood families. And all the women, but only half the men, took their parents' marriage as the model for their own. It is this which shaped their adult lives most decisively.

Clausen's book, I suspect, only touches the surface of what may still be learnt from this extraordinary lifelong documentation. It is particularly important that the documentation is not just one-sided. Along with the original summarized interviews and observations with the parents and the cohort child, there are the perspectives of brothers and sisters, husbands and wives. There is both the contemporary documentation, and the reflective life-story interviews which were carried out in 1982. The personal and social dynamics in the interviews are often clearly revealed by the plentiful and uninhibited comments of the researchers. One can almost hear the bristling in the caustic description of one middle-class thrice-married 'semiprofessional' man: 'a very tense, anxious individual who seemed to need control in the interview at all times . . . He remains distanced by excessive rambling . . . He is extremely immature in relation to his wife.'

Very rarely, however, one feels that the subject did manage to get the upper hand over the interviewer. One case was a downwardly-mobile man called Reb, who had a petty criminal record, and in 1982 was on his deathbed. When the interviewer asked him, 'How would you like most to be remembered?' Reb replied:

> The only kind of immortality that anyone ever gets is to [have] left an unforgettable memory somewhere. . . . So I hope people will remember some very good things I have pulled off, some beautiful capers.
> *What comes to mind?*
> The blowing up of the munitions train.

After he had given some more examples of capers, she asked him, 'Do you have a theory of how your life was shaped?' After a long pause he smiled, and recited:

'There once was a girl, quite mild
Who kept herself all undefiled
By thinking of Jesus, infectious diseases
And the dangers of having a child.'

Something like that, sure.

The now utterly baffled interviewer struggled to offer him an interpretation. He finally shut her up with: 'If a man asks for bread, don't give him a stone'.

If your taste is more for 'qualitative' retrospective interpretation of this kind, there is of course no need to spend millions of dollars in building up a vast archive. It is relatively cheap to launch an autobiographical collection. The technique was first systematically developed by Polish sociologists and Scandinavian ethnologists from the late 1920s, and has a British parallel in the work of Mass Observation at the University of Sussex. It makes it possible to collect hundreds of in-depth reflective accounts, either of full lives, or on a selected theme. At the Nordic Museum in Stockholm, for example, thematic autobiographical essay competitions are held every year, and the indexes of the material have been entered into a database available to researchers throughout Sweden.

Marianne Gullestad's *Everyday Philosophers* (1996) is a particularly welcome book, because it is a rare recent discussion of the practice and significance of this method of research. She is herself an anthropologist who clearly also has talents as an artist, for the cover picture is a self-portrait of herself as a housewife, conveying a Munch-like agony.

Gullestad's book is certainly an important contribution to understanding the value of autobiography for researchers, which she clearly situates both within literature and the social sciences. She describes the Norwegian competition on which the book is based, which attracted six hundred entries, and analyses the diverse types of story which were sent in.

The body of the book consists of lengthy presentations and interpretations of just four selected stories, two by women and two by men. The authors of these written stories were also interviewed orally. They range from a man who had been a child in a remote fishing settlement to a working class woman from Oslo. The detailed discussion gives a very good sense of the key issues raised by twentieth century social change in Norway, and the different searches for identity which they express.

By now it has become clear what Gullestad means by 'everyday philosophers'. She goes on to argue that most ordinary people are philosophers, for 'social life is theorized by those who live it', and 'their reflections – crude or sophisticated – contribute to social understanding'. Gullestad also suggests that because of the complexity with which each individual identity is created, only 'thick' descriptions are adequate, and that they can 'provide a necessary corrective to modernist thinking'.

While this argument for 'everyday philosophers' is certainly attractive, it is somewhat undermined by the way in which it is delivered. The presentations remain firmly in the hands of the anthropologist: we are given extracts between comments rather than the full texts. More seriously for our purpose here, the abundance of 'thick' description has squeezed out the sustained cross-analysis of the material which would be needed to convert unconvinced social scientists to Gullestad's method.

In particular, we are left with little sense of how typical this ability to philosophize may be of the general population, and especially of whether writing an autobiography might not be an activity characteristic of precisely those who have most successfully come to terms with their life problems.

Gullestad does show that the autobiographies represent a wide range of experience, and she picks out various sub-genres among them. Interestingly, one type was a direct reflection of an earlier academic fashion, the ethnographic village stories sent in by some older rural men, conveying collective rather than personal memories. At the other extreme, a few men wrote long accounts revealing their intimate sexual lives, most often in the Don Juan mode. However, only a small minority of authors wrote about problematic relationships. In these the reader is typically addressed 'as a compassionate stranger, a confessor, or even a therapist'. The style of these more confessional narratives seems to be influenced by the agony columns in women's magazines and the popular press. It was women who most often wrote about feelings and relationships, and also about illness. The younger authors tended to be more open than the older.

There was, however, not only a marked absence of descriptions of severely traumatic experiences, but even a very pervasive reluctance to write much about couple relationships in married life. Gullestad attributes this to the conflicting loyalties which authors feel when writing about those nearest to them. One is forced to conclude that while open autobiographical competitions may give useful indications of how many – perhaps most – people deal with the ordinary setbacks of life, because these life stories are essentially public rather than (like a good interview) confidential in context, such competitions cannot provide a reliable method for understanding how people remember or survive traumatic experiences.

Of the four authors examined in detail there is however one who certainly does write of traumatic experience. She is Kari, a woman born into a working class Oslo family in 1924. Brought up with a father and grandmother who were both drunks, she describes her life as difficult from infancy onwards, and eventually in her fifties she suffered serious mental illness. Her most 'brutal' experience was when at the age of 13 'the foundation of my life disappeared'. This was through the death of her grandmother, who had mainly brought her up, and by Kari's subsequent sudden eviction by an aunt who thought that her husband was trying to seduce her. Kari explains how she survived because she 'encapsulated grandmother in her memory' as a positive moral exemplar.

However this interpretation, which overlays Kari's memories, seems to owe a good deal to a 'doctor at the hospital' who she met forty years later, after being admitted for depression. Equally strikingly, she seems to have developed a special role there as a *'skrivoman'*, a 'graphomaniac', writing incessantly, and using this as a therapy to express the emotional conflicts which had been previously 'locked in'. She describes how she felt 'a tremendous need to write. It diverted all kinds of thoughts that bothered me'. Even at the hospital she became well-known for her exceptional facility in self-expression on paper. She recalls how as an inmate 'I learned about many difficult life stories'. The paradox of her situation was brought home to her one day when she found herself talking with two professional writers:

> I was sitting, as usual, on a chair in the corridor with the writing pad in my lap. Then two men stopped right where I was sitting. One was a well-known author, the other a journalist. The author . . . said to the journalist, as they were standing there: 'Isn't this life strange? The two of us live by our writing, but we cannot write, and here sits an ordinary housewife, and she cannot stop writing.'

Kari stood out equally when she was in her home setting. Her torrent of letter-writing was so immense that 'at the local post office I am famous because of that', and she herself worried that she was putting too much pressure on her less fluent correspondents: it could 'almost be a problem, because other people are always owing me a letter'.

It would clearly be rash for us to take Kari's 'everyday philosophy' in coming to terms with her traumatic past as typical of others who have suffered similar experiences. Nor is atypicality, especially in the use of writing as a kind of internal confidante, unique to Kari. In a similar way Cecilia, a lower-middle-class teenager born in 1974 in a small town by the sea, also has a special love of writing which emerged remarkably early: she won a prize as an author as early as the age of twelve, and she says, 'The words have always been my best friends'.

Of course responding to a personal interview is also an unevenly spread skill, and encouraging hesitant oral self-reflection is a basic therapeutic technique. We know too from recent research that the ability to present a 'coherent' life narrative may in itself be an indication of a psychic wellbeing rooted in secure emotional attachments. *Any* form of effective communication thus privileges the emotionally secure and successful. But the resulting bias becomes much stronger when we move from the sample-based in-depth interview, in which the researcher acts as a catalyst for the transmission of experience, towards the autonomous self-directed writer who enters an autobiography competition.

The autobiographical competition nevertheless does have two great strengths. The first is the obverse of its weakness: while the testimonies undoubtedly reflect the wider social contexts in which they are produced, they need not be shaped by the research team (although the more advice and guidance and thematic suggestions are given in order to encourage entries from the less confident, the greater that likelihood becomes). But at the very least, competition writers are not boxed in as 'respondents' to the detailed preformulated hypotheses of over-determined researchers. Good interviewers, of course, avoid this anyway, but any interview must be a two-sided encounter and the agenda of the interviewer is bound to help shape the outcome. The written authors are self-propelling. While this quality sets them apart, it also gives their testimony much more independence.

A second advantage is practical: the autobiographical competition is cheap. It need entail no fieldwork costs. The only essential expense is in analysing the material. At the opposite extreme, the Berkeley cohort studies must have been incredibly expensive, initially involving a whole team of social workers continually visiting and observing each study family. This is a luxury which few social scientists can hope to enjoy. Nevertheless I am unconvinced that the cheapest mode of research can offer us a sufficient window on the problem: the informants are too special a group. The retrospective life story grounded in a longitudinal study also has its problems, but they can be mitigated by quantitative social scientists who felt a genuine willingness to interact practically with in-depth qualitative researchers. It is in such co-operation, I believe, that the best hope lies for understanding how ordinary men and women most often succeed in overcoming setbacks and traumatic experiences in their lives.

References

Clausen, J. (1993) *American Lives: Looking Back at the Children of the Great Depression*, New York: Free Press.

Barnes, G. C., Thompson, P., Daniel, G. and Burchardt, N. (1997) *Growing Up in Stepfamilies*, Oxford: Oxford University Press.

Gullestad, M. (1996) *Everyday Philosophers: Modernity, Morality, and Autobiography in Norway*, Oslo: Scandinavian University Press.

13

REVIEW ARTICLE

Tina Papoulias

Paul Antze and Michael Lambek (eds), *Tense Past: Cultural Essays in Trauma and Memory* (London and New York: Routledge, 1996)

The fruit of the close collaboration of a group of (mainly Canadian) scholars, this collection of essays testifies to the development of an exciting interdisciplinary approach to the study of memory as a cultural object. Moving in the main within an anthropological framework, the essays in this volume represent an attempt to flesh out and problematize the discursive contexts within which a focus on memories of trauma becomes the sanctioned way of thinking about the relation between past and present.

The contributors are for the most part informed by and responding to the work of Ian Hacking, whose recent book, *Rewriting the Soul,* is an imaginative attempt to historicize current debates about the therapeutic and political significance of memory and trauma. He argues that our present conception of memory – which includes the clinical writing on disorders of memory – can be understood in the context of what he calls 'the sciences of memory': a discursive nexus which took shape in the 1870s with the foundation of the new discipline of psychology. This nexus not only allows for the emergence of memory as an object of study which can lead to knowledge about the self, but is crucially premised upon the paradoxical notion that 'what has been forgotten is what forms our character, our personality, our soul' (Antze and Lambek 1995: 70).

In an elegant and incisive introduction, the editors establish the parameters through which Hacking's framework will be inflected in the essays that follow. While acknowledging an emphasis on a social production of 'memory', they propose a move away from a macro-historical approach, towards a location of 'memory' in discrete practices of remembrance. Such practices are seen to arise in the intersection of individual and collective narratives and are further mediated by political, juridical, and institutional formations. This emphasis on the plurality of discourses shaping the experience of memory is signalled in the book's structure: the essays in *Tense Past* are divided into three sections, starting with the invocation of memory in narratives of sexual victimization, moving on to the historicization of medical and therapeutic discourses around trauma, and concluding with an attempt to theorize the production of models of memory and trauma within a variety of cultural contexts.

In the case studies constituting the first part of the book, the popularity of narratives of sexual abuse is seen to intersect with a process of 'political disengagement' (ibid.: xxiv) in which the focus on specific acts of violence suffered by an individual may serve to disavow 'the really difficult questions of social etiology and the real, if diffuse, loci of responsibility' (ibid.: xxvii).

In a compelling and incisive analysis, Donna J. Young discusses the uses of memory in the production of life stories of three generations of women in an impoverished rural area of New Brunswick, Canada. In the two older women's narration, subjective experience offers insights into the social and economic transformations shaping their community. By contrast, the youngest woman's filtering of childhood pain through the idioms of abuse, trauma and memory recovery produces a series of snapshots of atrocity removed both from historicity and from a complex understanding of social marginalization. In other words, as Young suggests, the tropes of recovered memory therapy assist in rupturing the link between individual and collective realities, thereby transforming 'historical trauma' into 'individual drama' (ibid.: xxiv).

If Young's case study demonstrates how therapeutic discourses of memory recovery may serve to reify the past, other contributors are concerned to show how practices of remembrance exceed the frameworks of memory which mediate them . In looking at the kinds of self-narration available to people diagnosed with multiple personality disorder (now re-named dissociative disorder), Paul Antze argues that such people do not simply reproduce the received psychiatric narratives of dissociation, in which multiplicity is seen as a result of repeated childhood trauma. Rather than subscribing to the vocabulary of victimization and surrendering responsibility to a body of memory experts, individual sufferers may use the trope of dissociation to negotiate psychic conflicts and develop a sense of accountability and relation to others.

In the same vein, Jack Kugelmass takes up practices of commemoration undertaken by American Jews through the 'secular ritual' of visits to Poland and the camps, and argues that these practices cannot simply be understood as empty gestures, compulsive returns to what Pierre Nora (1989) has memorably called *'lieux de mémoire'* – desiccated commemorative objects which attest to the loss of a living community of memory. Refusing what he sees as the reductionism of Nora's definitions, Kugelmass situates these practices as an active engagement with the relics of a past that can no longer be grasped otherwise, but which can nevertheless be reconstructed through public performance. This restaging, Kugelmass argues, cannot be simply equated with the loss of historical consciousness: rather it is to be understood as the only way to keep history alive in a way that is directly relevant to the present generation's concerns.

The question of how the Holocaust can be remembered is reopened in Laurence Kirmayer's contribution, this time through a fascinating foray into the clinical literature of trauma. In the light of current debates over the possibility of repression and recovery of memories of childhood abuse, Kirmayer's article sets up a bold comparison between Holocaust and child abuse survivors and suggests that amnesia of the traumatic event is only seen to occur in the latter case. The camp survivor's intrusive nightmares and flashbacks, in contrast, testify to an inability to forget, an inability which is at least partially linked to a 'public space of solidarity' around the reality of the camps (ibid.: 189). Kirmayer sets up these two distinct clinical pictures of traumatic memory (dissociative amnesia and compulsive recall), in order to suggest that the after-effects of trauma are composite structures: their origin at once psychic and social. His paper, like a number of other contributions, explicitly directs itself against the popular psycho-biological approaches to trauma, in which traumatic memory is seen purely in terms of brain functions and is thereby universalized. Equally, however, this paper could be said to wage an oblique battle against the use of 'trauma' in recent literary theory – and in the work of Shoshana Felman and Cathy Caruth in particular – in which holocaust testimonies and literature are used as exemplary texts through which the so-called fundamental unrepresentability of trauma may be grasped.

Generally, *Tense Past* offers an impressive range of material and originality of research, a combination which is rather uncommon in edited collections. However, some of the essays resort to rather problematic counter-strategies in their attempt to contest the alleged universality of psychological frameworks of memory function. In Kirmayer's case, the distinctions between 'private space of shame' and 'public space of solidarity', between amnesia and involuntary recall, circumvent the way in which questions of trauma serve to destabilize these very categories. His positing of a space of solidarity around the Holocaust is in itself questionable, particularly in the light of phenomena such as survivors' guilt, the painful transmission of parents' secrets to the second generation and, on a collective level, the popularity of Holocaust revisionism since the mid-1980s.

In a different context, some of the more conventional anthropological essays operate through a rather uncritical typology of 'western' versus 'non-western' societies. This resort to classical anthropological tools is out of synch with the book's overall project of defining memory as a variable practice at the intersection of numerous discursive arrangements, and such essays testify to an uneasy cohabitation of Foucauldian methodologies with an understanding of 'non-western' cultures as spaces of tradition rather than sites of discursive struggle.

Finally, of all the essays assembled here, it is only the contribution of Ruth Leys that problematizes the definition of 'memory' as an act of representation which is foundational to the subject. Leys' fascinating excursion to the clinical literature on the traumatic neuroses of war examines the history of the legitimation of contemporary definitions of psychic trauma. According to Leys, this history highlights a crisis in the post-Enlightenment definition of the subject and it is precisely this crisis that current clinical work around trauma may serve to disavow. In short, the use of hypnosis in the treatment of traumatic neuroses opens the question of whether patients get better because they are able to represent their past to themselves, or because of a process of suggestion to which they are susceptible.

In this essay as in her other work on trauma, Leys offers a historical reconstruction of the relationship between concepts of suggestion and memory. Her insights therefore problematize the basic understanding of practices of remembrance as practices of self-representation, opening a set of questions which workers in cultural as well as clinical studies on trauma and memory would do well to consider. For if it is a fallacy to suggest that the past can be apprehended 'as it really was', it may be equally fallacious to suppose that an imaginative reconstruction of the past to serve one's ends is a satisfactory, or indeed a feasible alternative.

References

Antze, P. and Lambek, M. (eds) (1996) *Tense Past: Cultural Essays in Trauma and Memory*, London and New York: Routledge.

Caruth, C. (1991) 'Unclaimed experience: trauma and the possibility of history', *Yale French Studies* 79, pp. 181-192.

Hacking, I. (1995) *Rewriting the Soul: Multiple Personality and the Sciences of Memory*, Princeton: Princeton University Press.

Leys, R. (1996) 'Death masks: Kardiner and Ferenczi on psychic trauma', *Representations*, no. 53: 44–73.

Nora, P. (1989) 'Between memory and history: Les lieux de mémoire', *Representations* no. 26: 7–25.

14

REVIEW ARTICLE

Epidemics of our time: trauma or fantasy?

Susannah Radstone

Elaine Showalter, *Hystories: Hysterical Epidemics and Modern Media* (New York: Columbia University Press, 1997)

British Publication: *Hystories: Hysterical Epidemics and Modern Culture* (London: Picador, 1997)

The ground broken by Freud and Breuer's pronouncement, in the 'Preliminary Communication' concerning the psychogenesis of hysteria, that '[h]ysterics suffer mainly from reminiscences' (Freud and Breuer 1991: 58) brought to view the tangled roots linking the developing concept of a hidden and powerful unconscious with nineteenth century anxieties concerning memory's absence and excess. Freud's later emphasis upon fantasy, rather than memory, in his revised writings on hysteria's aetiology can be regarded, in part, as the vanquishing of memory's unbiddability by fantasy's origins in unconscious wishes and anxieties. The latter are formations, whose origins analysis roots firmly in the subject, rather than in memory's complex relation to external events.

Two qualifying currents ran through this new emphasis upon fantasy and desire rather than upon involuntary memory. First, the issue of personal responsibility raised by this new emphasis on unconscious sexual and violent fantasies was mitigated by Freud's consolation to his earliest hysterical patients that 'we are not responsible for our feelings' (ibid.: 227). Second, the possible association *only* of fantasy with the determining force of unconscious inner processes was undercut by Freud's continuing stress on the part played by unconscious revision or associative modification in the construction of *memory*. Nevertheless, the shift from memory to fantasy arguably reveals psychoanalysis's strivings to bring hysterical (and other neurotic) symptoms under the sway of the subject's (albeit unconscious) determinations, and, with analytic aid, modifications, rather than to consign them to the paradoxical intractability and volatility of memory's relation to events.

The 'discovery' of the unconscious arguably undercut notions of self-determination and placed limits on 'agency'. However this must be set beside the part played by Freud's adoption of fantasy in the development of a therapy in which the analysand is encouraged to recognise – and to take some responsibility for – the part played by the unconscious in shaping 'reality' and determining 'destiny'. For Freud, it was this recognition that promised to extend the ego's capacity to shape a life, rather than to be steered by unrecognised unconscious fantasies and desires.

The relative 'empowerment' effected by the turn to fantasy was arguably accompanied, moreover, by a 'democratizing' and 'universalizing' tendency in the revised understanding of psychical life that it produced. The 'discovery' of fantasy's centrality to all psychical processes – that fantasy shaped the internal worlds of the 'mad' and the 'sane' – replaced that binary with a more nuanced appreciation of gradations of psychical stability and 'disease'.

Yet if the turn to fantasy can be narrativized in psycho-politically progressivist terms, the infamous and much-documented Freud/Masson debates (Masson 1984) represent only the fiercest and most bitter edge of an opposing position that interprets its politics more darkly. In Masson's terms, the move to fantasy is construed in relation not to Enlightenment principles of democracy and universality, but to the silencing of patriarchy's abused victims. The 'retreat' from memory is understood to be accompanied here not by a potential expansion of the capacity to grasp and to act in and upon 'reality', but by the striking out of the historical reality of abuse, as testified to by memory and its pathological excesses and absences. In place of a testimonial therapy that could read symptoms as signs of unspeakable abuse, Masson and his followers see, in Freud's turn to fantasy, the development of an approach to hysteria whose imputations implicate, rather than exonerate, the subject.

Masson's polemical 'retrieval' of memory formed part of – some might say spearheaded – a movement in which trauma has taken centre-stage. Whether in the pages of psychiatric journals or on the 'self-help' or 'personal growth' shelves of community bookstores, this movement emphasizes the pathological effects of trauma (especially trauma resulting from sexual abuse) upon future mental and emotional life. Within this frame, trauma is linked with particular pathologies of memory which typically produce dissociative states, memory gaps, and so on.

Freud's shifting account of hysteria's aetiology, and the memory/fantasy debate that it continues to provoke, touches upon complexly inter-woven and over-determined histories: the historical production and re-production of memory as a site of cultural anxiety; contested histories of the Enlightenment project, most specifically, in their feminist variants; and most complexly, the wider feminist debates concerning hysteria's relation to psychoanalysis' sexual politics. Does (Freudian) psychoanalysis, that is to say, contribute to the social oppression of women, as Masson and his feminist fellow travellers would have it? Or do its post-seduction theory insights concerning fantasy and identification reveal the sheer difficulty, if not impossibility, of success-fully negotiating the developmental stages enjoined upon woman by the patriarchal construction of sexual difference?

Hystories, which continues its author's earlier study of hysteria in *The Female Malady* (1985), is both formed and informed by these interweaving histories and debates, at times consciously and, at other points, perhaps less so. Showalter's intervention constitutes a critique of the 'return to memory' established by Masson and his followers, exemplified in 'trauma survival movements', such as that of 'recovered memory'.

Hystories associates this return with the development of a divisive 'sur-vivor' culture characterised by blame and vengeful litigation. Showalter's fundamentally Enlightenment critique of this culture suggests that only a renewed emphasis upon fantasy can rescue contemporary western culture from the distortions that threaten its stability and limit its capacity for healthy and democratically organized public life. In short, Showalter calls for the nurturing of a psychically enlightened culture within which collective or individual *responsibility* can be acknowledged for violent, fearful, or sexual fantasies. These will otherwise overrun our culture in the form of the 'hysto-ries' which her thesis names and interprets.

The thesis propounded in this polemical and accessible work is that hys-teria, despite the views of the psychological establishment, is 'alive and well' in the late twentieth century western world, though in transformed guise. Hysteria's domain has shifted, argues Showalter, from the clinic to the popular narrative, or 'hystory', in which various arguably 'traumatic experi-ences' take centre-stage. TV, the popular press, and e-mail spread hystories with which growing numbers of troubled individuals are coming to identify. These hystories of ME, Gulf War Syndrome, recovered memory, multiple personality disorder, satanic abuse and alien abduction each provide explanatory narratives that allow somatic or psychical symptoms, which Showalter inter-prets in relation to anxiety and repression – in relation, that is, to unac-knowledged unconscious fears and desires – to be understood in relation, rather, to various trauma-inducing external causes linked to conspiracies (often, of silence).

In ME, physical symptoms as well as feelings of anxiety are understood to be caused by a virus, or contaminant element(s) surrounded by conspiratorial cover-ups or silences. In Gulf War Syndrome, symptoms are attributed not to the contemporary equivalent of 'shell shock' – not, that is, in relation to unacknowledgeable terror – but rather to the effects of toxic contaminants such as organo-phosphates, surrounded by a military and governmental wall of silence. In 'recovered memory', diffuse and diverse symptoms ranging from physical illness, to depression or low self-esteem are linked to the forgotten occurrence of childhood sexual abuse surrounded by familial cover-ups. In multiple personality disorder, a similar range of symptoms accompanied by 'unacceptable' types of behaviour are attributed to 'alters' or split-off personalities formed as a result of physical or sexual abuse, whose actions cannot be attributed to their 'host' since their presence is unknown to the host, prior to therapy. In satanic abuse, an individual's current shortcomings and symptoms are linked to their having been compelled to take part, as children, in unspeakably terrible rituals by their Satanist families, evidence of whose activities and histories remain totally hidden behind brilliantly maintained screens. Finally, in alien abduction, unacknowledgeable (usually sexual) desires are attributed to the forced seductions and investigations performed by aliens whose presence on our planet is known to but unacknowledged by those in authority.

To her credit, Showalter readily acknowledges that those who succumb to these 'hystories' are suffering and experiencing difficulties that must not be dismissed. Her quarrel is not with the sufferers for whom hystories provide consolatory narratives, notwithstanding the caustic tone of several of her case-histories. Neither is her dispute specifically with academics who lend their credentials to those narratives, though her descriptions of their contributions to the development of particular hystories can be acerbic to say the least. Neither is she mounting an attack on psychotherapy, *tout court:* for Showalter, only good psychotherapy and psychoanalytically informed cultural criticism can save us from the bad psychotherapies which are contributing to hystory's current escalation.

The sub-title of the US version of *Hystories* and aspects of its argument foreground the part played by the speed and spread of contemporary electronic communications in the escalation of hystories. However, *Hystories'* argument, in keeping perhaps with the book's critique of hystories themselves, eschews direct accusation. Nevertheless, the sharpest edge of Showalter's cultural critique of hystories is directed against their crossing of the line from private narratives that enable therapeutic (though not necessarily 'truthful') sense to be made of a life, to media-spurred, public, political and judicial 'rituals of testimony' (Showalter 1997: 204) that involve accusation and persecution. In a final chapter that warns – a little hysterically perhaps – of the coming hysterical plague, Showalter likens the emergence and proliferation of these public discourses to the witch-hunts of the seventeenth century. She concludes that this development, like Arthur Miller's *The Crucible* which dramatized those witch-hunts, demonstrates the 'human propensity to paranoia' (ibid.: 206).

At base, *Hystories* calls for a return to those insights and values arguably delivered by Freud's turn towards fantasy. For Showalter, hystories appear to represent a withdrawal from the hard task enjoined by those insights: that of grasping as our own unconscious fantasies the violent, destructive, or sexual forces that hystories locate and persecute elsewhere and in others. Showalter's impassioned plea is both a *cri du coeur* and an unashamed appeal for a return to enlightenment values. 'The hysterical epidemics of the 1990s continue to do damage', she concludes 'in distracting us from the real problems and crises of modern society, in undermining respect for evidence and truth, and in helping support an atmosphere of conspiracy and suspicion. They prevent us from claiming our full humanity as free and responsible beings' (ibid.: 206). Thus if the Freudian turn can be narrativized as a politically progressive one, then Showalter's thesis follows that Enlightenment tradition. For it is the recognition of *universal* human propensities and, in particular, the grasping of responsibility for our own projections that promises to move us beyond a culture of blame inhabited by perpetrators and victims, and towards a freer and a more equal society.

Though *Hystories'* construction of hystory as genre is a convincing and gripping one, the book's Freudian cultural critique of the genre's emergence and proliferation begs as many questions as it answers: questions that circle around memory, history, and psychoanalysis and its complex relation to feminism. Showalter's historiography is shaped both by notions of cyclical return and by a psychoanalytically-informed *legerdemain* of the *plus ça change* variety concerning humanity's eternal propensities to paranoia, anxiety and disavowal. She suggests that the current hysterical epidemics are prompted, in part, by *fin-de-siècle* anxieties similar to those which gave rise to seventeenth century witch-hunts and 'apocalyptic anxieties that always accompany the end of a century' (ibid.: 6).

The former tendency is most evident, perhaps, in *Hystories'* partial association of contemporary cultural hysteria with women. Here, Showalter's feminist analysis suggests that women's arguably greater susceptibility to hystories stems from society's continuing refusal to acknowledge the full force of female sexuality as well as women's capacities for violent or hostile feelings. Thus, she calls for a change in social attitudes while enjoining women to take individual responsibility – perhaps with the aid of good psychotherapy – for feelings that might otherwise become displaced through hystories.

Here, Showalter's accent on the social construction of *gender* difference sidesteps the issue of hysteria's arguable imbrication with those psychical processes that accompany the production of *sexual* difference itself. This is a surprising and diminishing sidestep given Showalter's commitment to both feminism and psychoanalysis. Here, then, it would appear that Showalter's emphasis upon the unchanging relation between hysteria and woman might have been pushed further, beyond the confines of the social construction of gender and towards the realm of the psychical origins of sexual difference. Yet *Hystories'* somewhat ahistorical arguments concerning hysteria's relation to the social construction of femininity also appear rather tired, if not inaccurate, for surely women's arguably continuing difficulties in acknowledging sexual desire need to be set against a whole raft of changes wrought, over the last century, in the sexualised constructions of 'man' and 'woman'?

If *Hystories'* *plus ça change* approach to historiography produces its own problems, so too does the 'cyclical return' approach which is evident, though not fully spelt out, in Showalter's description of hystories' cyclical emergence. Showalter suggests that contemporary hystories constitute, in part, a response to *fin-de-siècle* anxieties which return to haunt Western society at the end of each century – a postulation which appears to return us to Freud's initial theory of hysteria's aetiological association with traumatic memory. Unfortunately, the return of memory to the hysterical centre-stage is not analysed further, leaving a number of intriguing avenues unexplored.

Most puzzlingly, perhaps, given the centrality of the memory/fantasy opposition to Showalter's initial thesis, the book lacks any analysis whatsoever of what appears to be a central aspect of hystorical discourses: their central preoccupation with – or better put, their production of – memory itself. This omission seems to arise from the book's somewhat uneven historicization of the phenomena it describes – its mixing, that is of an ahistorical and universalistic deployment of psychoanalytic concepts with an historiographical approach that oscillates between the cyclical and the apocalyptic. While the book implies that some things change, some stay the same, and some come round again and again, it is not clear why it distributes these qualities as it does.

Showalter's thesis would seem to have it that anxieties about the future, together with the psychical problems that continue to accompany patriarchal constructions of masculinity and femininity, prompt hystories which transform unacknowledgeable unconscious ideas, or fantasies, into 'memories': that the wheel that brings memory round again is turned by cultural anxiety. Here, the 'wheel' of history appears to turn according to Freudian notions of unconscious repetition, while the forces determining changes in cultural forms and genres remain somewhat obscure but appear to be largely technologically driven. Showalter's stress on the fantasies screened by hystories needs to be accompanied by an examination of what hystories needs to be accompanied by an examination of what hystories reveal about contemporary constructions of *memory*. These constructions – as the 'postmodernism debates' reveal – may differ in significant ways from the late nineteenth century constructions to which Showalter's thesis suggests contemporary culture is returning.

Similarly, *Hystories'* case rests both on the arguable contemporary return of hysteria and upon humanity's eternal propensity to paranoia. Here Showalter's eschewal of memory in favour of fantasy appears also to have produced an eschewal of history. To be more accurate, it eschews the possibility that the relation between the inner and the external worlds – between the psychical and the historical – may be more two-way than her thesis would seem to allow. *Hystories'* understanding of, say, Gulf War Syndrome maps a complex relation between traumatic memory, disavowal and conspiratorial fantasies concerning the external world. Yet Showalter's model of cyclical return cannot accommodate the possibility that new geopolitical relations, together with new types of warfare, *might* play some part in transforming the landscape of our inner worlds. Perhaps, that is, social-historical forces may play some part not just in determining the abeyance or return of particular neuroses, but in producing new versions and varieties of psychical ease and disturbance, sidelining older forms of psychical disease and producing new ones.

In the case of Gulf War Syndrome, Showalter's psychoanalytically 'correct' concentration on the inner world's capacity to shape the sense made of the outer world tips over into what looks like a refusal to acknowledge that the external world can have *any* determining force whatsoever. Within this scenario, any questioning of the part played by chemical warfare, insecticides and the like in the production of mental or physical disease risks being labelled 'hysterical'. Here, perhaps, the book enters the terrain of 'wild' psychoanalysis, rather than good cultural criticism. It positions itself on one side of a reductive binary opposition between traumatic memories related to actual experiences and fantasies emerging from unconscious process.

But perhaps such scholarly caveats are out of keeping with *Hystories'* purpose and intent. This anxious and no doubt speedily written book clearly seeks to counter the 'hysterical plague' that is arguably sweeping the US and Great Britain, rather than to constitute the authoritative history of the contemporary psycho-social phenomena with which it is concerned. In so doing, it makes convincing claims about the hysterical identifications and paranoia shared by apparently disparate social movements and the popular narratives around which they develop.

Not surprisingly, Showalter's remedy is very much in keeping with her diagnosis. In place of the 'actings-out' she identifies in the vengeful excesses of survivor-culture's court-room dramas, Showalter calls for a culture within which 'unacceptable' desires and fantasies can more readily be acknowledged: a culture in which citizens can take responsibility for fantasy, rather than displace it elsewhere. But fantasies cannot be generated in a vacuum. Whether individual or cultural, fantasies are inextricably intertwined with, rather than formed in opposition to, memory. Moreover historical constructions of memory have not remained constant. Showalter's study of the fantasies screened by hystories' 'memories' urgently calls for the study of constructions of memory in contemporary social movements and popular narratives.

Perhaps the most valuable contribution made by *Hystories* is its attempts to recover an ethic of responsibility from the heart of a 'trauma survivor' culture within which, as Showalter so amply illustrates, collective and individual responsibility is constantly and repeatedly disavowed through the construction of 'other' who act upon the individual or collective 'survivor'. Yet Showalter's exclusive focus on fantasy leaves me uneasy, for history has its responsibility and burden too: to bear witness to traces of 'happenings' which leave their traumatic and enigmatic marks upon the memories of peoples and individuals. *Hystories'* theoretical substitution of fantasy for memory splits fantasy too violently from history and memory, thus (paradoxically) risking repeating trauma's violent cut.

The task that remains, therefore, is to conceptualise culture and history itself not in terms of the false dichotomy of memory or fantasy, but as the enigmatic interweaving of the traces deposited by both.

References

Freud, S. and Breuer, J. (1991) *Studies on Hysteria,* Penguin Freud Library vol. 3, London.

Masson, J. (1984) *The Assault on Truth,* New York.

Showalter, E. (1997) *Hystories: Hysterical Epidemics and Modern Media,* New York: Columbia University Press; London also published as *Hystories: Hysterical Epidemics and Modern Culture,* London: Picador.

INDEX